I hated going to the beach—no bathing suits for me!—and with arthritis in my hands and knees, it was tough to do any physical activities. That was until I met Dr. Gerry Mullin and learned about the Gut Balance Revolution.

I lost 40 pounds following the Gut Balance Revolution program, and I look and feel 15 years younger! I went from a size 10 dress down to a 0! The weight loss makes me feel terrific.

Before the program, I was plagued by debilitating irritable bowel syndrome symptoms, fatigue, joint pain, and brain fog. I also had allergies and skin problems. Every one of these symptoms has been resolved. I feel like a new person!

So many people ask me what I've done to look and feel so great. I can't believe that this simple program—it really is a simple way of eating—can transform your life. The Gut Balance Revolution is an easy way to lose weight, eat healthy, and curb carb cravings. I strongly recommend this program to everyone!

—Terri

Before the Gut Balance Revolution, I wasn't able to climb a flight of stairs without being short of breath. On this program, I've lost 19 pounds, I am down a couple sizes in my clothes, I feel great about myself, and I look fantastic! Now I can handle the stairs with no problem and breathe normally when I reach the top.

I have tried many programs before, and some worked for the time I was on them. But this one not only worked for me while doing it but it made me feel so good afterward that I am compelled to continue on it for a life change so that I not only lose weight but remain healthy. It's a mind-set thing. I am now determined to be healthy and beautiful at the same time and am loving life! I would recommend anyone to just try it. The results speak for themselves.

Dr. Gerry, thank you so much! I appreciate people like you taking the time to care for others and to help us be what God intended us to be in the first place: healthy! I have learned that to be healthy, it doesn't mean you have to stress about it or be sad. Be happy in what you are doing, which is bettering your body, mind, and well-being. Thank you for helping me get on the right track. Now I am able to help others. For you have to partake first and be an example to show that it really works.

From my heart, I thank you so much! My body is grateful for your program.

—Bernadette

I lost 20 pounds on the Gut Balance Revolution! I can't tell you how much better I feel. I'm not tired all the time like I used to be. I sleep better. My clothes fit better and aren't as tight. I feel great!

This program is different because it teaches you which foods will help you feel better and lose weight.

I am still going through the program now and probably will continue it for the rest of my life. It's so easy to follow. And I know if I go back to eating like I was eating before, I will not feel like I do now.

—Stephanie

On the Gut Balance Revolution, I lost 10 pounds. I don't get sick or have a bulging stomach after I eat anymore (which is the best part!). My clothes fit again. I feel energized, healthy, and clean. My cholesterol levels even went down. I changed my mood, my bowels are working regularly, and I am no longer fatigued. Now if I even try to cheat, I get sick. My body has changed. It doesn't recognize processed unhealthy foods anymore. I don't have cravings or get the 3:00 p.m. hunger headache anymore. It's great!

It's a real learning experience to see all of the "bad" in the food you used to eat, and it makes you ask, "How am I not 300 pounds?"

–Jennifer

Originally, I went on the Gut Balance Revolution program, because I was plagued with digestive issues. I struggled to find a solution to the constant gut distress. It really limited my life. I was exhausted all the time and constantly worried about what I could eat–and where the bathroom was. But all that changed when I went on the Gut Balance Revolution.

Within 6 weeks, my symptoms were nearly gone. And there was an unexpected bonus. My husband, Scott, who'd been trying to lose weight for years, went on the diet with me and dropped 19 pounds. Both of us began feeling so much better just by eating healthy foods and getting rid of all that processed stuff.

Now when I travel to conferences, the business lunches are no longer a nightmare. And Scott and I can enjoy having dinner with friends, take in a movie, and even go to football parties.

Our world has opened up again.

–Cindy

I've gone on lots of diets over the years. I tried everything from Weight Watchers to Jenny Craig. But nothing really worked until this program. In 8 weeks, I lost 12 pounds–and I felt so much better.

–Monique

THE

GUT BALANCE REVOLUTION

THE

Gut Balance Revolution

Boost Your Metabolism,
Restore Your Inner Ecology, and
Lose the Weight for Good!

GERARD E. MULLIN, MD

Associate Professor of Medicine at The Johns Hopkins University School of Medicine

RODALE.

Copyright © 2019 by Gerard E. Mullin, MD

All rights reserved.

Published in the United States by Rodale Books, an imprint of Random House, a division of Penguin Random House LLC, New York. Published by Rodale Inc. as *The Good Gut Diet,* a direct mail hardcover, in 2014. First published in trade hardcover by Rodale Inc. in June 2015.

rodalebooks.com

RODALE and the Plant colophon are registered trademarks of Penguin Random House LLC.

Exercise illustrations on pages 223–233 © 2014 Rodale Inc.

The content on pages 200 and 202 to 209 is reprinted by permission from SAGE Publications: Bernstein A BJ, Ehrman JP, Goulbic M, Roizen MF, *American Journal of Lifestyle Medicine* (vol. 8, issue 1), pp. 33–41, Copyright © 2014 by SAGE Publications.

The following recipes are reprinted courtesy of Stone Mill Bakery: Greek Village Salad, page 280; Wild Rice and Turkey Soup, page 314; and Dr. Gerry's Super Salmon Salad, page 317.

Originally published in hardcover in the United States by Rodale, an imprint of the Crown Publishing Group, a division of Penguin Random House LLC, New York, in 2015.

Library of Congress Cataloging-in-Publication Data available upon request.

ISBN 978-1-62336-778-7 trade paperback
Ebook ISBN 978-1-62336-402-1

Printed in Mexico

Book design by Christina Gaugler
Illustrations by Karen Kuchar

6 8 10 9 7 5

First Paperback Edition

To the loving memory of my parents,
Frances R. Magnanti Mullin and Gerard V. Mullin Jr.

To my family and loved ones for their unwavering support

To those who struggle with weight-related problems, the
clinicians who care for them, the researchers looking for a cure,
and the organizations and individuals who promote awareness
and research

To Drs. Anthony Kalloo, Myron Weisfeldt, Linda Lee, my
colleagues and friends, administrators, and staff who support
my work at Johns Hopkins

CONTENTS

INTRODUCTION: IT'S NOT YOUR FAULT!

The year was 1977. A 17-year-old high school student and his mother walked into a new doctor's office for the first time looking for answers to a recent and inexplicable sore throat, loss of appetite, fatigue, and fever. The esteemed doctor was referred by a leading physician in their small community of Wayne, New Jersey. The physician was fresh out of training in endocrinology and metabolism and was beginning his practice in the region's top multispecialty group.

When the doctor walked into the room wearing his white coat, he gazed up and down at the boy, shot him a dismissive frown, then looked over at the boy's mother with disapproval in his eyes.

In the few minutes allocated for the visit, the doctor stated he was certain that this young man had mononucleosis and ordered confirmatory blood tests. As he was leaving the room, the boy's mother asked, "Doctor, he has a difficult time eating. Do you have any suggestions?"

The physician turned around with an angry scowl and sharply rebutted, "Ma'am, if he didn't eat for a week, it wouldn't hurt him. Given his size, it may make a healthy dent!" With that, he stormed out of the room. The chill that followed was like a blast of arctic air. The boy and his mother were momentarily frozen by the doctor's painful words.

This young man was 293 pounds the day he visited that doctor, and his shame about his weight was immense. If you haven't guessed by now, the young man in that doctor's office was me.

Unfortunately, that doctor was more interested in assigning blame than he was in offering solutions. We now know that this type of stigmatizing and shaming approach toward overweight people is counterproductive and can actually cause weight gain.[1] In fact, blame, shame, and lack of support are feeding directly into the obesity epidemic.[2] But after all these years, I now realize that doctor did me a favor. He gave me an example of what *not* to aspire to as a physician. Doctors are healers who are bound by the Hippocratic oath to provide empathetic care to those in need.[3] That man broke the spirit of his oath.

Though disappointed and hurt by my first encounter with this physician, I went back for another visit to be cleared for return to school following my bout of mononucleosis. The illness had been more severe than usual, and I had lost 12 pounds in only a few weeks. When I walked into the office, the doctor remarked, "I'm glad that the illness was therapeutic," and smiled.

As he looked over my chart, he noted that my high school football team was ranked as number one in the state and asked me what I was studying at DePaul High School. "I'd like to be a doctor," I replied. That's when he dealt the final blow. He chuckled, looked me up and down once again, and said, "Not looking like this, you won't." Our relationship ended.

Despite the doctor's rudeness, he communicated an important and sobering message to me: "Physician, heal thyself." If I wanted to be a doctor, I should first look at my own body and take care of it. Back then, the prevalence of obesity was low and most doctors were thin. So a morbidly obese person aspiring to be a doctor was being unrealistic. I needed to lose the weight if I wanted to be a physician.

That's when my own weight-loss journey began.

HOW I ALMOST DIDN'T BECOME A DOCTOR

Shortly after my visit to that physician, I graduated from high school and entered college. I was morbidly obese, and it quickly became plain that I wasn't living up to my potential academically. I was strongly advised by the head of the university's preprofessional committee to consider another profession–such as podiatrist or physician assistant–since I wouldn't be recommended for medical school. That's when I hit rock bottom. My life's dream had been to become a doctor, and it looked like I wouldn't achieve it.

That Christmas, I spent some time at my brother Tim's house. The movie *Rocky* was on television. That's when I had my aha moment. All I had to do was figure out what steps I needed to take to make it happen, as Rocky did in the movie.

I had a vision of myself as an empathetic doctor who would help others who struggled to lose weight, but I knew that first I had to find my own path to health. I found my inspiration and my focus. I spent hours in the library researching diet programs and the effects of different foods on human metabolism. I tested several "diets" and failed at many, but I was committed to succeeding. I knew that if I searched hard enough, I could find an answer to my weight problem.

At the checkout counter of my local grocery store, I came across a book about the health benefits of fiber. I purchased it and read it over winter break. The author explained why fiber was important for maintaining a healthy weight–and it dawned on me that my own diet had always been fiber poor. I realized that the diets I'd attempted–like the "grapefruit diet," popular in the late 1970s–were futile because they contained little or none of this critical substance.

So I decided to create my own diet plan, one that was rich with fiber. One of my staples was oat bran (to bolster my fiber intake) with plain low-fat yogurt, sweetened with a pinch of molasses, pure maple syrup, or raw honey. I also began to switch my protein sources to mainly seafood and away from red meat. I used olive oil and nuts as my principal sources of fat.

I went for long walks across campus or rode a bicycle during study breaks for exercise. In no time, I was dropping weight and feeling fantastic. My energy skyrocketed, and so did my mental clarity.

After losing my first 50 pounds, I began running and lifting weights and engaging in a number of athletic activities with my brothers Patrick and Tim, along with my friend Chris Houlihan. It was like *Rocky* come to life.

By the end of 1979, I got down to 175 pounds—a result that rivals gastric bypass surgery. My aptitude and scholastic performance dramatically improved. A year later I was accepted into medical school. Today, I am an academic gastroenterologist among an elite group of doctors at one of the leading hospitals in the nation. I'm not sure I could have achieved all this had I not been able to drop the weight and *persevere*.

But how did I make the change when so many others can't? Why did the diet plan I developed on my own actually work?

20/20 HINDSIGHT

I now realize that I'd developed a way of eating that restricted foods that promote inflammation and spike blood sugar and fat-forming insulin. I was also supporting the growth of friendly bacteria in my gut with prebiotic fiber-rich foods and live yogurt cultures. As you'll learn in this book, this may be the key reason the diet worked. We know today that the trillions of bacteria housed in our digestive tract have a significant influence on our ability to gain or lose weight. I'll explain more about this in a moment.

First, I want to share another key discovery I made during this time.

I realized that it wasn't my fault that I was so large. I hadn't been eating lots of junk food. I was just unknowingly eating the wrong foods that were promoting inflammation, reducing the diversity of microbes in my gut, and leading to fat accumulation.

If you're overweight, it's likely not your fault either. Nobody wants to be overweight, but it happens to many despite their best intentions.

We live in a world where obesity is a global epidemic, and it didn't come about because people are lazy or stupid. Something else is at work. At one time, just getting enough to eat was the most basic problem of survival. Now we face the opposite problem.

Seventy percent of Americans are overweight and 36 percent are obese.[4] Globally, 1.5 billion people are overweight and half a billion are obese. Today, one-third of all women and one-quarter of all men in America are on a diet. In the United States alone, more than $60 billion is spent on weight-loss products per year.

Studies estimate that up to two-thirds of those dieting will gain back more weight than they lost when they stop their diet programs. You've probably seen popular celebrities and even former contestants from *The Biggest Loser* regain weight months after successful dieting. In fact, most Americans can only sustain a behavioral-modification-diet lifestyle program for 3 to 6 months before falling off and rebounding. And amazingly, one-third of those who undergo gastric bypass obesity surgery regain the weight because the underlying problem was not fixed.

Obesity has crippling effects on health and well-being, shortens life expectancy, hinders quality of life, and adversely impacts the economy. Treating obesity and obesity-related conditions costs billions of dollars a year. By one estimate, the United States spent $190 billion on obesity-related health-care expenses in 2005–double previous estimates.[5] Looking ahead, researchers have estimated that by 2030, if obesity trends continue unchecked, 50 percent of America will be obese, and obesity-related medical costs alone could rise to $66 billion a year. Obesity is a major driver of Medicare costs and contributes to our growing federal debt.

HOW DID THIS HAPPEN?

I blame the food industry's promotion of processed foodlike substances that I call "ingestibles" and rich proinflammatory and disease-promoting crops that become affordable junk food. We rely on a "food industry" to promote our health, while our health-care industry fails to promote the role of sound nutrition in healthy living and disease prevention. The "food industry" does an excellent job of designing and selling tasty and addictive products that make consumers continuously buy and eat more than what they need. Big Food knows all too well how to make its products appealing, tasty, irresistible, and cheap, so that people keep coming back for more–despite the consequences. Americans now consume 150 pounds of sugar sweeteners (cane and beet sugar and corn sweeteners)[6] a year–about 22 teaspoons daily–and the food industry is partially to blame. Historically, our sustenance came from foods high in nutrition and low in calories, but the products designed by food conglomerates today are low in nutrition and high in calories. Most Americans are overfed yet nutritionally starving. As government continues to subsidize the food industry's mass production of fast-food staples such as wheat, dairy, and soy over real food, we're likely to see these trends continue.

But we cannot put all the blame on the food industry and the government subsidies it receives. The behavior, mind-set, and lifestyle of the present generation are a vital part of the dynamics of obesity and weight-related illness. We need to look at the greater ecosystem of biological, microbiological, sociological, and psychological influences that lead to weight gain to find a solution to this problem.

They teach us in medical school–in the few hours devoted to the subject–that weight gain and weight loss are merely a reflection of total caloric consumption, metabolism, *and nothing else.* But this concept doesn't explain why people can't drop weight despite eating less food. Why are so many people gaining weight, and what can we do to help them lose it?

That's what this book is about.

THE REAL REASON FOR THE OBESITY EPIDEMIC

The truth is that you gain or lose weight for multiple reasons. We now know that glycemic control, insulin spikes, inflammation, and even hormones that regulate metabolism are all factors that determine your weight. Obesity is a complex disorder resulting from a combination of genetic, behavioral, lifestyle, and psychological factors that influence food choices and activity.

Sure, overconsumption of calories may be part of the reason people gain weight. But why are these folks overconsuming food in the first place? There are many reasons. If you trace only one possible biochemical chain of causality, you get something like this: Overeating stems from imbalances in the network of brain biochemicals called neurotransmitters (like dopamine), along with gut-derived hormones that regulate satiety and short-term appetite (like ghrelin) and control our urge to eat. As we overconsume calories and become inactive, our fat cells continue to grow and become insensitive to insulin. This results in diabetes, atherosclerosis, cardiovascular disease, and a number of other complications.

But there are *many* other ways to gain weight. Science is now showing us that obesity can result from a number of imbalances in the body, from inflammation to endocrine and metabolic dysregulation. The story of weight loss is much more nuanced than most of modern medicine would have us believe.

Fascinating new research points to yet another contributing factor I've long known played a role in the weight-loss drama–the gut microbiome, the ecosystem of flora in your intestines. Research is showing that it's the balance and diversity of these microbiota in your gut that may ultimately determine the fate of your weight.

In retrospect, this is the precise reason I was able to drop the weight that had plagued me for so many years–I rebalanced the flora in my gut. In 1979, I was ahead of my time in forming my own blueprint for weight-loss success. Impressed with my results, friends and family started asking for dietary advice. Although only a junior in college, I was counseling people about diet and weight loss, and I've done so ever since. Even then, I found that my approach allowed people to eat more, weigh less, and feel more vibrant. Over the years, I've refined this plan based on my education and experience as a doctor. But you'd be surprised how much of my approach is the same as it was in the '70s.

Why? Because the diet I developed happened to focus on improving gut microbial balance and diversity. My original vision of becoming a doctor was to help others lose weight once I found a system that worked. What I didn't know was that my mission to help people would come to fruition through serendipity.

My accidental discovery has now been borne out by two new major areas of research that have revolutionized our understanding of why people gain weight. Both point to a disordered digestive tract as playing a central role.

First, the human gut microbiota have been found to play a pivotal role in weight maintenance because of their influence on food metabolism, appetite regulation, energy expenditure, endocrine regulation, gut barrier integrity, inflammation, and insulin resistance. Distortions in the composition of normal, healthy intestinal flora have been found to contribute to obesity.

Second, weight gain has recently been linked to chronic low-grade systemic inflammation in the gut that results from the seepage of gut-derived bacterial toxins through a porous intestinal lining into the bloodstream. This further drives problems with insulin resistance and fat accumulation.

When people address these two core systemic processes by focusing on rebalancing the flora in their gut, the results are often miraculous. I've witnessed the turnaround of patients who have followed the same program you'll learn in this book. I've observed many patients in my clinic lose as much as 10 to 15 pounds every 4 weeks. They were able to burn fat and keep it off for the long term. They were succeeding on my plan even though other diet programs had previously failed them. With my plan, their weight loss has been seamless and sustained. And miraculously, many of their chronic digestive symptoms disappeared as well.

ONE UNFORGETTABLE CASE

A woman named Rose came to see me after being treated by several other doctors for troubling gas and bloating. Despite her search, Rose couldn't find relief and was eventually diagnosed with irritable bowel syndrome (IBS). Although she "starved herself," Rose gained weight, and no doctor could find a metabolic cause.

I suspected that Rose's gas, bloating, and abdominal discomfort after meals were due to the rapid fermentation of foods by an overgrowth of bacteria in her small bowel. This condition is called small intestinal bacterial overgrowth (SIBO). My suspicion was confirmed by lactulose hydrogen breath testing. I placed Rose on the Gut Balance Revolution and treated her with antimicrobial herbs to help kill off the overgrowth of gut bugs in her small bowel.

Six weeks after her initial visit, Rose came in for her follow-up. Repeat lactulose hydrogen breath testing showed the SIBO was gone, and Rose no longer had gas, bloating, or abdominal discomfort. Plus, she was proud of her new figure–she'd lost 20 pounds in 6 weeks, though she'd never dropped a single pound on one of her many previous diets.

Why did Rose lose weight on this program when so many others had failed?

Gut bugs. That's right. Gut bugs.

Around the same time I treated Rose, the science behind the role of gut microbes in weight gain, obesity, and diabetes had begun to explode. Research showed that lean mice can be made overweight by simply transferring gut microbes from obese mice. Likewise, the transfer of gut microbes from lean mice into obese mice improves diabetes.

In this book, I'll tell you more about exactly how a healthy balance of gut flora holds the key to maintaining a healthy weight. I'll also outline a complete program that will allow you to overcome your struggle with sustained weight loss. When you follow the plan, you'll likely find that you not only lose weight but also feel energized and vibrant, and many of your chronic health complaints may simply disappear.

Diet plays a special role in fostering the growth of microbes that favor obesity or feed bacteria that promote a lean metabolism. By tilling the soil of your gut microbiome, reseeding your gut with good fat-burning bacteria, fertilizing these friendly flora with special foods like prebiotics, and enhancing the overall biodiversity of your inner eco-system, you can easily reboot, rebalance, and renew your health. I'll give you all the steps to do that. Along the way, I'll provide step-by-step meal plans, shopping lists, restaurant guides, recipes, recommendations on dietary supplements, stress-reduction techniques, exercise programs, and more.

The gut microbiome appears to be the mysterious factor that may drive weight gain despite our best efforts. Yet no other program has approached weight loss by rebalancing the gut flora. After seeing the success stories in my clinic, I felt it was time for me to share with the public the program I've been developing for decades.

If we take an integrative, whole-systems approach to health, healing, and weight management—when we learn to balance our body ecology and think about the species that live within us—we have greater hope for long-term success with weight loss and health outcomes.

By remapping your gut ecology, you can shed weight, rejuvenate your health, and feel vibrant. That's what the Gut Balance Revolution and this book are all about.

THE
GUT BALANCE
REVOLUTION

CHAPTER 1

The Hidden Secret to Weight Loss

WEED, SEED, AND FEED YOUR INNER GARDEN

Eat less and exercise more.

We've all heard it—from our doctors, on TV, on the Internet, in magazines, from friends and family. At one time or another, most of us have even tried it. But let me ask you: How has this recipe for weight loss worked for you?

It seems like such a simple formula—it matches our understanding of the physical principles of the universe. Energy in, energy out. What we don't spend, we store. It's common sense. It *must* be right.

There's just one small problem. It doesn't tell the whole story of why people gain weight. And it doesn't tell us how to lose it.

The calories in/calories out theory of weight loss is outdated. Modern science has proven beyond any shadow of doubt that your weight and your health are dependent on much more than how many calories you consume. You'll learn about some of this evolving science in this book. However, common sense and personal experience tell us that if weight and health were all about the amount of calories you consume each day, you could eat 1,800 calories of Oreos and Diet Coke and stay fit and healthy. But, of course, we all know that doesn't work. The food you eat has a far greater influence on your body than solely the amount of energy it provides. It has wide-ranging effects on numerous biochemical and physiological processes. While it's true that most of us could afford to eat a little less, and reducing total caloric intake is necessary to a certain point to incur weight loss, the quality of the calories you consume is far more important in the long run.

That's especially true if you want to burn fat and keep it off for good. Anyone can go on a starvation diet, burn out the treadmill, and drop a few pounds. You might even lose a couple of pants sizes or notice that you look a little better in your bathing suit. But the sad reality is that most of the pounds you drop will be water weight, and some fat-burning muscle to boot. Without altering your lifestyle and eating habits, revisiting your relationship to food, and systematically enhancing the overall quality of the calories you consume, your diet is doomed to fail in the long run.

In fact, research has shown that the vast majority of calorie-restricted diets fail long term. A study conducted at the University of California in Los Angeles showed that people who go on calorie-restricted diets typically lose 5 to 10 percent of their body weight within 6 months–but regain everything they've lost within 4 to 5 years.[1]

And this yo-yo effect causes downstream biological complications that make it even more difficult to lose weight in the long run. Your body is a complex ecosystem (actually, an ecosystem *within* an ecosystem, as we'll see shortly), and all complex biological systems have mechanisms in place to maintain homeostasis. The dictionary defines homeostasis as "the maintenance of relatively stable internal physiological conditions (as body temperature or the pH of blood) in higher animals under fluctuating environmental conditions." It's easy to see why this is important. If you didn't have a built-in biological mechanism for maintaining basic physiological processes such as body heat, survival would be far more complicated.

What does this have to do with weight? Well, the rate of your metabolism and the amount of fat you carry are tightly regulated by a complex array of homeostatic internal processes. Some doctors call this internal thermostat your "body weight set point," and it's influenced by a number of factors such as hormones, neurotransmitters, intestinal peptides, your gut microbiome, and more.[2, 3]

Several studies have shown that your body weight set point remains fairly constant, maintaining your body weight in a stable range despite minor changes in energy intake (calories in) and expenditure (calories out). It's also been shown that your body is very efficient at holding on to weight during periods of caloric deprivation. That's because your body set point has shifted downward and is telling your body that your metabolism needs to be slowed to minimize weight loss during periods of caloric deprivation. This provides a clear survival advantage but demonstrates how low-calorie diets that are based solely upon energy deprivation have short-term efficacy as the new set point limits ones weight loss. Your body weight set point will also try to keep you from gaining weight when you eat too much by burning more calories, but this effect is short lived. Overall, it's harder to lose weight than it is to gain weight–an experience many of us are all too familiar with. Yo-yo dieting is a very common result of weight-loss programs and causes one to ultimately weigh more. Yo-yo dieting has been shown to raise the body's set point, which is your brain telling your body "Hey, we ought to now weigh more to reach this new equilibrium" and sending control signals throughout your body to slow metabolism so you gain body weight and fat mass–the new normal. Thus, you weigh more than before with each failed energy-deficit diet program and it becomes harder and harder to lose weight as the set point is raised each time a weight-loss regimen fails.[4]

To effectively lose weight and keep it off, you need to strategically alter your body weight set point. Emerging evidence suggests that bariatric surgery, particularly gastric bypass, may work in part by helping the body establish a new set point by altering the physiology governing body weight.[5] And that's the real problem with yo-yo dieting—every time your weight rebounds, your set point gets pushed higher, so your body acclimates to the new body weight set point as "the new normal." Hormonal and metabolic adaptations now make it more and more difficult to lose weight.[6]

Calories in/calories out doesn't work for the masses, because it *can't* work. It can't work, because simply reducing the amount of food you consume and spending more energy exercising doesn't necessarily influence your body weight set point. Sure, there are some people out there who can lose weight by eating less and jogging 100 miles a week, but they're the exception. We may admire (or even be a little jealous of) them, but they don't point the way for the majority of us to lose weight and stay healthy.

So if eating less and exercising more isn't a realistic, sustainable way to lose weight, what is?

This is where things get interesting. When you talk behind closed doors to doctors or scientists who specialize in metabolism, they'll reveal that we aren't 100 percent certain *why* there is an obesity epidemic in this country in light of the fact that we are consuming fewer calories as a nation.

Yep, you read that right. We are getting fatter, even though we are taking in fewer calories than we did a decade ago. A new study published in the *American Journal of Clinical Nutrition* shows that the average daily caloric consumption of Americans fell by 74 calories between 2003 and 2010. Despite this shift, obesity rates among women have stayed at a whopping 35 percent, and for men they continue to increase.[7]

This finding confused the authors of the study. "It's hard to reconcile what these data show, and what is happening with the prevalence of obesity," said coauthor Dr. William Dietz, former director of the division of Nutrition, Physical Activity, and Obesity at the Centers for Disease Control and Prevention.[8] The data simply don't bear out the whole calories in/calories out concept.

But there's no question we're in trouble. The constellation of obesity, metabolic syndrome, and type 2 diabetes is arguably the greatest single health-care challenge in the industrialized world, and it's rapidly spreading to less-developed nations. Until a few decades ago, obesity was rare. Now the people who are obese or overweight outnumber those suffering from malnutrition. This is an unprecedented state for our species.

And it's spawned an industry of celebrity "experts," each of whom claims to have found "the single most important reason America is overweight." These people will try to convince you their special method can help every person drop many pounds overnight. Many will hype an exotic food-based supplement that no one has heard about except on celebrity talk shows, while others talk about detoxing, juicing, and bizarre rituals that grab our attention based on pure sensationalism. More evidence-based health experts deliver the message that stabilizing insulin resistance and blood sugar is key, while others focus on reducing inflammation. Other authorities tell us about the importance of balancing our hormones. Then there's the "Paleo" prophets and the vegan aficionados, and a million others.

So which of them is right? None of them and all of them.

There are *many* factors that lead to weight gain and weight loss. There's no question insulin resistance and blood sugar balance play a vital role, and they may indeed be one of the core reasons so many of us are overweight, exhausted, and unwell. They are the key factors in metabolic syndrome and type 2 diabetes. We also know that low-grade systemic inflammation and creeping weight gain, especially around the belly, are intimately linked. In fact, the adipose tissue that collects around the belly is inflammatory and leads to a cycle of hormonal imbalance and further weight gain. Do hormones play a role? Absolutely. Insulin, leptin, ghrelin, thyroid, and other hormones are all pieces of the weight-loss puzzle.

Recent research has even linked certain environmental toxins, such as persistent organic pollutants (POPs), to weight gain. These chemical substances—often referred to as obesogens—persist in the environment, bioaccumulate through the food web, and pose a risk of causing adverse effects to human health and the environment. POPs mimic hormones like estrogen that encourage your body to put on weight, and they block cellular docking stations that trigger weight loss.

Genetics plays a role, too, and so does your community—people who have good social support networks tend to weigh less and live healthier, longer lives. Yes, calories play a role and how much you eat does seem to matter, but it's not the whole picture.

And there is one, until now largely unrecognized factor that connects many of these pieces. . . .

New research is showing us that this factor has a far more profound impact on long-term weight-loss results and overall health than anybody expected. Medical scientists are beginning to find that when you balance this area of your health, weight tends to drop off more easily and your results last longer. My extensive experience as a leading digestive health specialist and medical nutritionist at The Johns Hopkins University School of Medicine bears out what this cutting-edge science is now revealing. Your gut microflora—the vast ecosystem that lives in your intestines—is a crucial factor in weight gain and illness and holds the key to permanent weight loss and vibrant health.

THE HUMAN GUT MICROBIOME: THE GARDEN OF LIFE AND KEY TO HEALTH

As human beings, we do not live in isolation. We are part of a complex social network of people who collectively interdepend on one another for just about everything. Whether it's food, mail delivery, energy to run our homes, or whatever else we want or need, we're reliant on tens of thousands of people to optimally live our lives. Modern industrialized society has evolved to a highly sophisticated synchrony of symbiosis.

The human body is not so different. It's not a sterile island but a complex network of trillions of microorganisms. These tiny beings surround us and lie deep within us, and we are utterly dependent on them for our health and well-being.

This may be difficult to fathom, since we're taught that we need to get rid of germs and maximize our hygiene to optimize our health. In fact, at the first sign of any apparent illness in childhood, we're doused with antibiotics, though medical science has little idea and virtually no research regarding the long-term consequences of these treatments.

We didn't evolve in a glass bubble, and we don't live in a germ-free world today. Nor would we want to. As you'll learn in this chapter, these microorganisms are crucial for the development of a healthy immune system and play a role in many other vital functions.

Living deep in your lower intestines is a complex ecosystem of microorganisms—a veritable garden of life. This magnificent orchard is composed of viruses, bacteria, and fungi, all of which collectively constitute what's called the human gut microbiome. When we care for this garden and nourish our flora, our health flourishes. But when we feed these microorganisms poorly and treat them poorly, the biodiversity of this ecosystem plummets and our health is compromised.

The modern movement of "going green" has taught us a lot about the importance of developing practices that support environmental sustainability. Each of us participates in a larger ecosystem, and our actions influence the health of that ecosystem. If we want our world to be healthy, we have to act in ways that help make it healthy.

But what about the ecosystem inside of you? It's something few of us think about. Just as our actions influence the ecosystem around us, they influence our ecosystem within. Balance and biodiversity in this ecosystem create health—imbalance and reduced diversity in the ecosystem create illness. There are many mechanisms by which microbes can protect us from disease or make us sick, help us lose weight or pack on the pounds, and we'll discuss many of them throughout this book. Indeed, the most important lesson is that the solution to your weight problem as well as many of the diseases we face today may never be found if research remains focused on you, the host. We must pay due attention to the host-environment interface—the complex set of relationships that constitute the human–gut microbiome connection.

The average human being has about 100 trillion of these organisms at any given time. Although most are located in your lower intestines, you're literally bathed and surrounded by microbes. Despite the best hygiene, we carry billions of microbes that hide under fingernails, lounge between teeth, stick to our skin, coat our eyes, hang out in our hair. There are more than 600,000 bacteria living on just 1 square inch of skin. The same holds true at internal passages: your respiratory system, genitourinary system, eustachian (ear) tubes, and much more. Just like in the 1999 sci-fi movie *The Matrix*, the naked human eye sees only an altered reality. It's incapable of seeing the trillions of microbes that constantly surround us. How would you feel if you could see every one-celled organism?

The microflora in your gut alone weigh about 3 to 5 pounds. These microbial cells outnumber your own human cells by a factor of 10 to 1, and microbial DNA outnumbers your human DNA by 100 to 1. Take a moment to think about what that means. Inside your body, there are more bacterial cells and DNA than human cells and DNA. Do you think this might have an impact on your health?

While we haven't yet identified all the strains of human gut microflora, the Human Microbiome Project, a collaboration led by Dr. Jeffrey Gordon of Washington University School of Medicine in St. Louis, made substantial advances in accomplishing this incredible feat. With $173 million in funding from the National Institutes of Health, this project's mission was to comprehensively characterize and analyze their role in health.[9, 10]

So far, they've isolated 1,000 species across dozens of different phyla–an astounding variety of microbes. There are few ecosystems on the planet that are as complex as the one inside of you. The species density and biodiversity of the human large intestine is nearly equal to that of the Amazon rain forest.

Our relationship with this ecosystem is symbiotic. We house our flora and provide them with food. In turn, these organisms serve us in a number of ways. They:

- **Break down complex carbohydrates.** Humans lack the enzymes to do this. You wouldn't be able to properly digest a single fruit or vegetable without your gut microflora.

- **Produce vitamins and nutrients.** You'd otherwise be unable to manufacture these on your own, including vitamin K, vitamin B_{12}, niacin, pyridoxine, and others.[11]

- **Produce short-chain fatty acids (SCFAs).** We'll spend a good deal of time in the next chapter on what these are and why they're important, but for now, be aware that they're involved in regulating immunity, healing, and combatting inflammation, and they may protect you against cancer and other diseases.[12]

- **Protect against pathogens.** Your gut microflora are your first line of defense against foreign invaders.

- **Help train the immune system.** Bacterial genes send signals to your gut's immune system that control local and systemic inflammation and play a role in determining whether you develop allergies and autoimmune diseases.[13]

- **Support detoxification.** When you metabolize your food, toxic metabolites (including carcinogens) are formed in your liver and carried by your bile into your digestive tract for elimination. Your gut flora degrade these potentially harmful biochemicals so they can be safely eliminated.

- **Modulate the nervous system.** Emerging research shows a connection between your gut microbiota, your digestive system, your nervous system, and your brain that may affect everything from appetite regulation to behavior to mood.[14]

For all these reasons—and many more—your gut microbiome has a profound impact on your weight, your health, and the quality of your life. Balance in this ecosystem leads to health and optimal weight. Imbalance contributes to weight gain and a plethora of diseases including type 2 diabetes,[15] irritable bowel syndrome,[16, 17] inflammatory bowel disease,[18-23] cardiovascular disease,[24] allergies,[25, 26] mood disorders,[27] and many others.

How Does the Gut Microbiome Get out of Balance?

There are lots of ways.

Consider, for instance, where your founding populations of intestinal bacteria came from—their origin impacts your weight and health. When you're in the womb, your intestines are relatively sterile. Babies acquire their gut microbiota from their mothers while passing through the birth canal and via breastfeeding.

When babies are born by Caesarean section (C-section) or bottle-fed, their gut flora aren't as fully developed. Several studies have shown that babies who were breastfed appear to be protected against the development of childhood obesity,[28] and that being born via a C-section puts young people at higher risk for developing this condition.[29] In Chapter 2, you'll learn more about these studies. I'll go into greater detail about the importance of early exposure to flora and explain how our hygiene-obsessed culture may be setting the stage for illness and weight gain by killing off our friendly gut microbes.

Obviously, you have no control over how you were born or whether you were breast-fed. But the good news is that there are plenty of other factors you do have control over that influence the balance of your gut microbiome. For example, your diet.

As Dr. Stig Bengmark explained in his article "Nutrition of the Critically Ill—A 21st-Century Perspective": "Diet has the most powerful influence on gut microbial activity."[30] Everyone knows the saying "You are what you eat." Dr. Sanjay Gupta went a step further when he wrote: "If we are what we eat, then Americans are corn and soy."[31] His sobering report shows how ubiquitous these disease-promoting, proinflammatory food commodities are in our bodies. Dr. Gupta actually had a strand of hair analyzed by Dr. Todd Dawson from the University of California, Berkeley, revealing that 69 percent of the carbon in that sample was derived from dietary corn. Our bodies are reflections of our dietary choices–all food is ultimately digested then metabolized by our gut flora, so it's actually more accurate to say "You are what *they* ate!"

Increasing evidence shows that how you feed your gut microbiome is a critical factor in your health and weight. Eating a diet rich in high-fat, sugary, processed foods reduces the overall biodiversity of your gut microbiome. These changes can happen in as little as 24 hours, and growing evidence shows that when the diversity of your gut microbiome is altered, you pack on pounds. A review paper published in the journal *Future Microbiology* that looked at the role of the gut microbiome in weight gain and obesity stated, "The gut microbiome's influence on obesity is likely to involve a microbial-dietary interaction."[32]

Diet isn't the only factor that affects the health and biodiversity of the gut microbiome. The unnecessary use of antibiotics also plays a role in the balance of the gut microbiome, as highlighted by Dr. Martin Blaser's new book, *Missing Microbes*.[33] We give antibiotics to children at record rates. In the United States, the average child now receives one course of antibiotics per year and has received 10 to 20 courses of antibiotics by the age of 18.[34] While antibiotics can be useful medications, they're overprescribed, and they have a detrimental long-term impact on the human intestinal microbiome. This may be one reason for the skyrocketing of childhood obesity rates. Indeed, a recent report showed that infants given broad-spectrum antibiotics before the age of 2 have a higher chance of becoming obese while children.[35]

That's to say nothing of the hidden antibiotics we're exposed to every day. Our meats are loaded with detectable levels of antibiotics, which adversely impact the balance and biodiversity of our gut microbiome.

Is this overuse of antibiotics and its impact on our gut microbiome responsible for the boom in obesity rates? It's obviously not the sole factor, but growing evidence is showing that it may be an important–and until now underrecognized–contributor to the obesity epidemic in this country. I'll explain more about why and how in the next chapter.

Other factors contribute to an out-of-balance gut microbiome, including stress, physical inactivity, and personal relationships. Each has an important influence on your health that can positively or negatively impact the symbiotic helpers in your gut.

So how do you keep the friendly flora happy and healthy? You become a good gut bug gardener.

Becoming a Good Gut Bug Gardener: Weeding and Seeding Your Inner Flora

By now you may be thinking, "Okay, I've heard some of this before. I know there are bugs in my gut. Don't I just need to eat some yogurt or kefir or take probiotics to keep them healthy?"

It's a lot more complicated than that. Yogurt, kefir, and probiotics can be very helpful, and each is an important part of this program, but these alone aren't enough. Just as you can't support a rain forest by dropping a few pine seeds or spreading some nitrogen fertilizer, a couple cups of store-bought yogurt a day won't provide your gut microflora the complete nourishment they need to thrive.

You have trillions of tiny beings living inside of you—an ecosystem so complex human science has yet to understand it fully. As you live and eat, so does your gut microflora live and eat. When you're healthy, the ecosystem is healthy. Perhaps the most important mark of a healthy ecosystem is biodiversity—the more types of species present, the healthier the overall ecosystem is likely to be.

As with all ecosystems, different species constantly vie for power and superiority. When one gets a strong enough foothold and starts to outcompete the others to the point of extinction, the health of the overall ecosystem plummets. Imagine what happens if a species of predators hunts its prey to extinction. This can create obvious problems: The predators, for example, now have nothing to eat. But these changes in species can have effects that reverberate throughout the ecosystem in ways we may not expect, because all the species in an ecosystem are dependent on one another in numerous ways.

The same is true of your inner ecosystem. When certain strains of gut bugs get too strong a foothold, they can outcompete their counterparts, with broad effects throughout your gut microbiome and your body. Some bugs are flat-out bad actors. Salmonella, shigella, and others will make you sick even if they are found at low levels in your gut. Other strains can cause problems only if they predominate. You may gain weight, develop chronic illness, and experience other difficulties. As we'll see in Chapter 2, there are at least seven pathways that lead from gut microbiome imbalance to weight and health problems—and science is discovering more connections every day.

On the other hand, there are trillions of gut microbiota that are commensals (friendly microbes typically found in healthy humans), which we know play a role in supporting proper weight regulation and are important for optimal health and well-being. These include bifidobacteria, some strains of lactobacillus, and many others.

The number and type of bugs throughout your gut are also important. The vast majority of your gut microbiome is located in your large intestine, and that's where the vast majority should be. However, there are relatively smaller quantities of bacteria throughout your small intestine and the other parts of your gut as well. This is normal. Problems can arise if too many bacteria begin to inhabit your small intestine, leading to a condition called small intestinal bacterial overgrowth (SIBO), which we'll discuss later.

Of course, you want to have plenty of the commensal flora or good bugs in your large intestine, but you *always* have strains of potentially helpful and noxious bacteria in your inner ecosystem. Indeed, some species seem to have positive effects under some circumstances and negative effects in others. The name of the game isn't "eliminating bad bugs"–you couldn't do that even if you wanted to without extensive and counter-productive collateral damage (though it's imperative in the event of a gastrointestinal infectious illness). Instead, medical science is showing us that the basic biological laws governing the ecosystem around us also apply to the one within. It's the overall balance and biodiversity of your inner ecosystem that's important, and the Gut Balance Revolution program is designed to help you enhance your gut's biodiversity and regain balance.

To achieve this, I've created a three-phase diet and lifestyle change system based on the best research current science has to offer. It's supported by my personal experience as well as my experience as a clinician. I have treated hundreds of patients (some of whom you'll meet along the way) using the methods in this book with positive results. Here's how it works.

- **Phase 1: Reboot.** In this phase, you'll till the soil of your gut microbiome, setting the stage for a lush garden to flourish. It's a 30-day higher-protein, ketogenic, low-glycemic-load, low-FODMAP diet (if you don't know what those terms mean, don't worry–you'll learn along the way). It's designed to enhance your digestive health, speed up your metabolism, reduce inflammation, improve insulin sensitivity and blood glucose balance, burn fat and help you lose weight and keep it off for good, enhance your mood, and set the stage for the resolution of many chronic illnesses.

- **Phase 2: Rebalance.** Once you've tilled the soil of your gut, you're ready to plant seeds and fertilize them so your inner garden will flourish. In this phase, I'll teach you how to strengthen and diversify your inner ecosystem by fertilizing it with special foods and supplements that are like Miracle-Gro (or compost, if you prefer an organic gardening analogy) to your good gut bugs. These include prebiotics, probiotics, and other foods that help them thrive.

- **Phase 3: Renew.** Once you've completed Phase 2, your gut microflora will be properly balanced, biodiversity will have returned to your inner ecosystem, and you'll naturally lose weight and feel more energetic. You may find feelings like depression and anxiety evaporate and make tremendous strides in overcoming chronic illness. Now your job will be to integrate a long-term, flexible, sustainable eating plan that will help you keep the weight off. This is where the vast majority of diets fail and why so many studies show that diets don't work. Many programs can help you lose weight for a little while–6 months to a year–then your body weight set point slows metabolism and gradually induces weight gain, as we've already learned. But I want you to have the tools to achieve and maintain optimal weight, health, and gut microbiome balance *for life*. That's what you'll learn to do in Phase 3.

As you walk down this path toward a healthy, thriving personal ecosystem, I will provide you with the tools and information that you need to rebalance your gut microbiome, optimize your nutrition, exercise more effectively in less time, live a less stressful and more fulfilling life, achieve optimal health and weight, vitality, and more. You will discover:

- Superfoods that will support your gut microflora, help you lose weight more effectively, and may protect you from a wide variety of chronic illnesses (eat these and you will see your health bloom as your waistline shrinks)

- Foods to avoid to keep your gut microbiome balanced for life

- A complete eating program—including delicious menus and recipes—that will keep your gut bugs happy and healthy

- When you should include fermented foods in your diet and when to avoid them (eat them at the wrong time and you send your gut microbiome further out of balance)

- How stress adversely impacts your gut microbiome and how one special relaxation technique may help nourish the friendly flora within

- Why getting the right amount of sleep is critical if you want your inner garden to thrive

- Simple, effective, quick exercise routines you can do at home that will amp up your metabolism

- The truth about supplements for weight loss: which ones work, and which are absolute bunk (I will also teach you what to look for in a high-quality probiotic)

- And more . . .

I'm eager to get started and share more about the surprising ways your gut microbiome impacts weight and health. But before I get to that, I want to address one critical question you may be asking yourself right about now.

IS THIS PROGRAM FOR ME?

You may be a little skeptical about this program, and I want to be honest and let you know it's not for everyone. There's no one-size-fits-all diet that works for every person. Despite what many experts might tell you, humanity has thrived on a wide variety of diets. From the Maasai, whose diet largely consisted of blood and yak milk, to the Pima, who ate acorns and cactus, one thing is clear: Homo sapiens is an adaptable species.

As we learn more about human biology, we move ever closer to a truly personalized model of medicine where specific interventions are developed for specific individuals. I believe that at some point in the future, we may be able to develop diet and lifestyle recommendations tailored to every person's specific requirements.

But we're still a long way from that, so for now we have to take what we know of the science today and apply it in a way that makes the most sense for the general population. That's what I've attempted to do with this program.

It's highly likely your gut microflora are not optimally balanced. If you've struggled to lose weight or keep it off; if you had several courses of antibiotics in your youth or have undertaken a course of them in the last year; if you suffer with digestive discord; if you struggle with a chronic illness (one-third of Americans do); if you have allergies or asthma; or if you're coping with depression, anxiety, or other mood disorders, it's highly likely that your gut microbiome is not in optimal condition—and it may be *way* out of balance.

You have nothing to lose in learning more about your gut microflora and trying this program. The good news is that the same things that support your inner ecosystem optimize your entire biology. So the worst-case scenario is that you'll learn to eat and live in a way that supports your body, reduces inflammation, rebalances your hormones, enhances insulin sensitivity, and reestablishes a lush garden in your digestive system. Plus, you'll likely learn a few things you didn't know about your digestive health along the way.

But honestly, I think you'll get a whole lot more than that out of this program. Most of my patients who have tried this diet have lost at least 10 to 12 pounds in a matter of weeks, felt more energized than they had in years, and watched many chronic symptoms simply fade away.

THE GUT BALANCE REVOLUTION SUCCESS STORIES
Ted, 79

Ted, a 79-year-old gentleman from Iran, came to see me accompanied by his daughter. He presented with metabolic syndrome, severe cardiovascular disease with two cardiac stents and subsequent angioplasty, type 2 diabetes, and hypertension, and he was morbidly obese. He came in to my office because he had started suffering from bloating, abdominal swelling, excess gas, and he was exhausted. He began to wonder if something in his gut may be the core of many of his health problems.

Ted ate a standard American diet (SAD)—high in inflammatory fats and processed carbohydrates and low in omega-3 fatty acids, fruits and vegetables, and fiber. I realized immediately that Ted's gas, bloating, and sudden abdominal distention after meals is typical of small intestinal bacterial overgrowth (SIBO), which could easily be the outcome of how he was eating and living. SIBO occurs when gut bacteria overpopulates the small intestine. In SIBO, the bacterial counts in the small intestine are markedly elevated and are imbalanced with the enrichment of anaerobes. This leads to a host of metabolic complications that you will learn about in the next chapter.

To confirm my suspicion of SIBO, I ran a lactulose hydrogen breath test, the standard test for the condition, in which the patient drinks a sugary solution. The bacteria present in the gut ferment the sugar, producing gases that are diffused into the bloodstream and exhaled into a tubelike breath analyzer.

Teds test was off the charts for SIBO. I placed him on a diet low in a category of fermentable foods called FODMAPs (fermentable oligo-, di-, monosaccharides and polyols) to starve out the heavy burden of bacterial overgrowth in the small intestine. To further weed out these bugs, I advised Ted to take some antimicrobial herbs for an additional month while he continued on the diet.

After 60 days, Ted felt like a new person. He lost 27 pounds and felt more energetic than he had in years. His gas and bloating after meals disappeared, and his metabolic syndrome improved.

Ted then returned to Iran. I advised him to begin fertilizing his flora with pre-biotic and probiotic foods like kimchi, miso soup, pickled foods, asparagus, and homemade yogurt. After another 30 days of fertilizing his inner garden, he lost another 10 pounds, and every symptom he entered my clinic with disappeared. Ted was a new man.

Ted, like many of my patients, lost weight while healing his gut and rebalancing his intestinal flora. I invite you to join me on the same journey that he took: to go where no weight-loss book has gone before. We'll travel deep inside your gastrointestinal system, where an array of flora lives that rivals even the most fecund rain forest. Along the way, you'll learn how these bacteria support your health and how you can support them. You'll learn to live in balance and harmony with your gut microflora. And by doing so, you will lose weight, feel better, and be happier than you have in a long time.

To begin the journey, let's take a more careful look at the ways your gut microbiome influences your health. I want you to understand some of the basic biochemical pathways that connect the flora in your gut to the rest of your body. This will help you realize just how powerful these microscopic organisms are and give you the knowledge you need to better care for them so that they can better care for you.

CHAPTER 2

Dysbiosis— Gut Microbe Imbalance

SEVEN PATHWAYS TO WEIGHT GAIN AND ILLNESS

S trange but true: Growing research suggests that the bugs in your gut send messages to your brain causing the release of hormones that make you feel full and satisfied and help you lose weight. Your gut flora also influence the chemical pathways that help regulate blood sugar and insulin balance. And your gut microbiome teaches your immune system how to function correctly and even helps regulate how fast–and how well–your metabolism works.

Your gut flora represent a highly diverse ecosystem whose composition is as unique as your fingerprint. The more diverse it is, the healthier you are. Your gut ecosystem is also delicately balanced between many friendly symbiotes and a limited number of potentially harmful pathogens that are prevented from gaining a foothold and triggering an aggressive immune response.

There are times, however, when your gut's garden gets out of balance, resulting in an overabundance of pathogens and/or a deficiency of beneficial bacteria. This is called dysbiosis–a state of microbial imbalance related to your gut ecosystem, your skin, your inner ear, or any of the other communities of microbes in your body. The scientific literature is quite robust in connecting dysbiosis of human ecosystems to adverse health outcomes.

But the key news is this: We're beginning to understand that your gut microbiome has a far broader impact on your health and weight than scientists originally knew. The influence appears to be so strong that some researchers refer to the gut microbiome as a "hidden organ" whose health is a strong indicator of your long-term weight and well-being.

In this chapter, I'll review seven ways your gut microbiota influence your health and weight. We'll take a journey into the fascinating relationship between your brain and your gut bugs, and we'll look at how your gut flora influence your metabolism. We'll

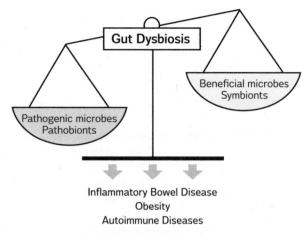

Inflammatory Bowel Disease
Obesity
Autoimmune Diseases

GUT DYSBIOSIS—CONSEQUENCES

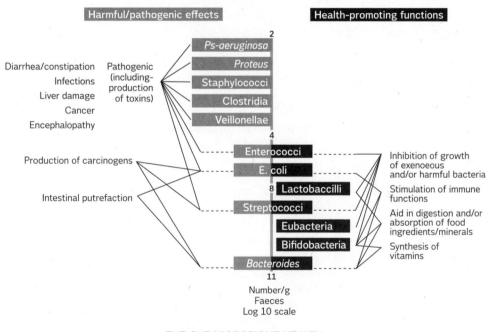

THE GUT MICROBIOME HEALTH

even talk about how these commensals (friendly microbes) communicate with your genes to influence your health. Along the way, we'll review some of the most recent, cutting-edge research in the fields of gastroenterological well-being and metabolism that demonstrates just how powerful these tiny symbiotic microbes are.

The take-home message: *The type of flora in your gut profoundly influences your weight.* But how? What do these bugs do in your body to tell it to store fat or drop it?

Could a Poo Transplant Help You Lose Weight?

Scientists at the Center for Genome Science and Systems Biology at Washington University in St. Louis asked themselves a simple question: Does gut flora influence weight gain? To find the answer, they designed an interesting experiment.[1] They took two groups of mice whose digestive tracts had been sterilized. In the first group, they colonized the mice's intestines with the fecal flora from an obese cage mate. In the second group, they colonized the intestines with gut flora from a lean mouse. They then fed these two groups of mice the same diet for 2 weeks. At the end of 2 weeks, the mice that were inoculated with feces containing gut bugs from the obese mice had gained more weight than the mice exposed to the lean mouse's gut microbiome, despite equivalent food intake and activity.

This experiment shows that there are specific types of gut flora that cause you to gain fat—and other types that lead to weight loss. The type that's dominant will dictate how much fat you accumulate.

There are more recent and compelling fecal transplant experiments that further illustrate the importance of the gut flora in determining body weight. For instance, there is a study that examines the gut flora of pregnant women. In pregnancy, maternal gut microbes shift to a mix that favors fetal growth in the 3rd trimester of pregnancy which is associated with accelerated growth of the unborn and metabolic alterations in the mother such as insulin resistance and inflammation. The study found that fecal transfer from 3rd trimester pregnant women into germ-free mice causes obesity whereas 1st trimester donors remain lean.[2]

Another series of fecal transplant experiments provide further insights into the therapeutic potential of fecal transplants to treat obesity. Again, investigators from Washington University led by Dr. Jeffrey Gordon transplanted the feces from human twins that were discordant for body weight into the colon of germ-free mice. Mice receiving feces from the obese twin became obese while mice who were fecal recipients from the lean mice stayed lean. In the second part of this experiment these mice (lean and obese) were co-housed resulting in the exchange of fecal material. The scientists knowing how diet influences the gut microbiome then fed these co-housed mice either a high fat, low fiber or a low fat, high fiber diet. The obese mice receiving the low fat, high fiber diet lost weight and had the thin twins gut bacteria take over their flora while those fed the high fat, low fiber diet remained fat. These experiments are the first in humans to show that leanness is transferrable but only in the presence of a diet that promotes the growth of healthy flora.[3]

There have been interesting preliminary human trials using fecal bacteriotherapy (FBT)—the transfer of intestinal flora from one individual to another to establish a healthy gut microbiome in the recipient. In other words, these "poo transplants" take the feces of someone with a healthy microbiome and introduce it into someone who lacks one.

Most of the FBT studies so far have been conducted to determine whether this intervention would be an effective way to fight recurrent *Clostridium difficile* infection (CDI), which is usually seen after the use of antibiotics. Once successfully treated with antibiotics, CDI has a high recurrence (greater than 25 percent), since these antimicrobials generate dysbiosis that is characterized by a reduced diversity of the microbiota and the favoring of the growth of pathogenic species. CDI is a highly contagious diarrheal illness that is increasingly common in hospitals and can be lethal. Of the more than 400 cases of recurrent CDI that have been treated with FBT so far, the cure rate is over 90 percent for those with a potentially life-threatening infection that is resistant to all other aggressive medical therapy protocols. This is a powerful model for showing how dangerous dysbiosis can be and how rebalancing the gut ecosystem by infusing a healthy mix of gut microbes can produce dramatic results. There is even new research showing that swallowing a capsule of strained feces from a donor (poop pill) also works for recurrent *C. difficile*.[4] While other scientists are working on a synthetic stool solution.[5]

The million-dollar question: Are poo transplants an effective intervention for weight problems? Though they're not a cure for obesity, they appear to be capable of shifting one toward a lean metabolism.

In 2010, a randomized, double-blind, controlled trial on the use of FBT for diabetes and obesity was conducted in 18 male subjects.[6] Half received fecal material from lean male donors; half were implanted with their own feces. After 6 weeks, those who received fecal transplants from lean donors saw a marked reduction in fasting triglyceride levels and significant improvement in insulin sensitivity. This is a small test group, but the results were replicated in a similar follow-up study by the same researchers, so the science is promising.

Does that mean you'll be able to walk into your doctor's office in the near future and ask for a poo transplant to improve diabetes or lose weight? Not likely. The safety of fecal transplantation has never been formally investigated long term, and clinicians have expressed concerns about FBT "opening up a can of worms after 4 of 77 patients developed a de novo autoimmune disease after FBT."[7] Furthermore, the FDA limited the practice of FBT to those with CDI-associated diarrhea that failed to respond to conventional medical therapy, provided donors are properly screened and patients are informed that fecal transplants are still experimental.[8]

This is an exciting area of research. The Johns Hopkins University School of Medicine and its dean, Dr. Paul Rothman, have formed a microbiome interest group led by Drs. Cynthia Sears and Glenn Treisman to set priorities and to collaborate and pool resources. I'm fortunate to be working with this distinguished team of investigators. Dr. Linda A. Lee* leads the Johns Hopkins FBT program. Research on FBT may pave the way for more targeted, safer interventions for obesity, irritable bowel syndrome, inflammatory bowel problems, metabolic syndrome, and more.

---

* Dr. Lee is a pioneer and leader in the field of integrative gastroenterology and director of the Johns Hopkins Integrative Medicine and Digestive Center and is clinical director for the division of gastroenterology at The Johns Hopkins Hospital.

What implications does this have for your health? And most important, what can you do about it?

This book will guide you in shedding inches and pounds and gaining health and vitality by rebalancing your gut flora using an inside-out approach. But I've found that people have the most success in programs like this when they know *why* the interventions work.

So let's look at some of the ways imbalanced gut microbiota set the stage for weight gain. Then, in the remainder of this book, I'll explain precisely what you can do to rebalance your gut microbiome. What you're about to read is by no means a comprehensive review of the scientific literature on this subject. Instead, I've focused on key discoveries to give you a sense for how important your gut microbiome is for your weight and health.

First, let's look at how the bugs got in your gut in the first place and how this early inoculation may set the stage for your lifelong health.

PATHWAY 1: ORIGIN—WHERE YOUR GUT BUGS CAME FROM IS IMPORTANT

In your lower intestines is an ecosystem as complex as a rain forest. How did those bugs get there? Remember that the intestines are sterile *in utero*—there were no bugs in your gut when you were in the womb. You got them from the environment. So the first place most people acquire flora is via the birth canal. The female vagina is one of the few places besides the gut that harbors a significant population of microflora. Some vaginal fluid is almost always swallowed at birth, so the flora in it contain the first bugs that colonize the infant's gut.

The next significant influence on your gut microflora is breast milk, which contains bifidobacteria, a powerful probiotic we'll look at later in this book. It also appears that breast milk enhances the growth of biofilms—layers of friendly flora that adhere to and line our gastrointestinal tract, protecting against pathogens and infection.[9]

Growing data show that these early influencers on the gut microbiota may have long-term health impacts. A new study has found that C-sections and formula-feeding disrupt the development of intestinal microbial communities in infants. Researchers evaluated the composition of gut microbes of 24-month-old infants. When compared to vaginally delivered children, infants delivered by C-section were deficient in a specific genus of gut bacteria called *Bacteroides*, which helps break down complex molecules in the intestine, and in some studies appears to protect against obesity.[10]

In addition, researchers found significant differences between the gut microbes of infants who were strictly formula fed and those who were breastfed. For example, formula-fed infants had higher levels of the pathogenic organism *Clostridium difficile*, which can potentially cause an aggressive course of diarrhea.

Researchers have also proven that children born via C-section start life with fewer

THE GUT BALANCE REVOLUTION SUCCESS STORIES

Brenda Davis Gandy, 52

Back in the day, Brenda was a skinny kid and a slender, active teenager. But soon after college, that effortlessly slim girl became a stress eater and began to pack on the pounds. "For some reason," she says, "I'd go for the rice and pasta and bread whenever I was anxious—the stress would just make me want to eat everything in sight." Diets? Brenda tried them all. She'd drop a few pounds, then go off the program and gain the weight back.

But by February 2014, she'd gone up to a size 18 and was having trouble walking up a flight of stairs without getting short of breath. "I decided that I needed to do a complete life change," she recalls. "I didn't want to die young because of health problems—I wanted to change my lifestyle. Even if there were stressful situations that I had no control over, I realized that I could control what I put into my mouth." That's when she decided to try the Gut Balance Revolution.

For Brenda, the program was simple. "I liked that there were foods to favor, foods to have a few of, and foods to just forget about," she says. "Before, my diet consisted mostly of carbs—bread was really my weakness— but now I can go through a whole meal without having a slice of bread. My cravings haven't gone away completely, but I've tamed them quite a lot. And I've also found better ways to deal with stress." A surgical technician who works in the operating room, assisting the nurses and doctors, Brenda would often come out of a lengthy session filled with anxiety and grab a candy bar to calm her down. Now? "I just have a cup of yogurt and some fruit," she says. "It makes me feel better than a Snickers bar ever did, and it's way better for my health."

And now that she's lost 20 pounds—in just 6 weeks—a lot of things are better for Brenda. She's gone from a size 18 to a size 12, and she's had fun shopping for new clothes. Reluctant to exercise when she was heavier, she's now taken up Zumba and she's not afraid to rock a bathing suit. She sleeps better, too, and her acid reflux is pretty much a thing of the past. And, best of all, she has a brand-new sense of confidence. "I love all the compliments," she says. "I feel good, I look good, and it feels great to have my self-confidence built up."

healthy microbes in the gut, resulting in a higher risk for developing serious disease,[11] that these microbial imbalances may last up to 7 years after delivery,[12] and that Caesarean birth is a risk factor for allergies, asthma,[13] inflammatory bowel disease, celiac disease, type 1 diabetes, and autoimmunity.[14] It even predicts which babies will develop colic.[15] Additional studies show that babies born by Caesarean delivery are at higher risk for developing obesity, while those who are breastfed are more likely to be lean during childhood.[16, 17]

The rate of Caesarean births has steadily increased in recent decades. In 1965, the national Caesarean birth rate was 4.5 percent.[18] Today, nearly 32.8 percent of babies are born via C-section.[19] During this same time, the rate of childhood obesity has steadily increased. Correlation doesn't equal causation—that these two trends took place at the same time doesn't necessarily mean that an increase in C-sections is leading to increased rates of childhood obesity. But the coincidence invites the question: Are the two connected?

That's *not* to say that C-sections and formula-feeding are wrong. In many cases, Caesarean birth is the safest delivery method for mother and baby, and some women have difficulty breastfeeding. The point here is to illustrate how important our gastrointestinal flora are to our long-term health. One of the outcomes of studies like these is that medical researchers are now looking for ways to provide babies born by Caesarean, as well as formula-fed babies, the critical food for the gut microbiota.

But even if a baby is born by C-section or isn't breastfed, its gut microbiome can be rebalanced over time. That's because as we age, our environment, our lifestyle, and our diet continue to influence what kinds of bugs are in our guts and where they live.

In Chapter 10, we'll examine lifestyle factors like diet, exercise, and stress, but for now, let's take a moment to look at the ways we continue to acquire bugs through our childhood and learn about some of the specific challenges our children face in a world riddled with agents that kill these friendly flora.

Some of My Best Friends Are Germs: The Hygiene Hypothesis

Remember when your grandma told you that playing in the dirt would give you bugs? Well, she was right, but the bugs you collected were probably not the kind she referred to.

After vaginal birth and breastfeeding, the next place your gut bugs come from is the environment around you. Playing in the dirt, being around other children, even snuggling with the family pet provide important species of flora that help fill out our inner ecosystem. There's accumulating evidence that the intestinal bacteria acquired in postnatal development play an important role in "training" our immune system to function properly.

The prevalence of allergic disease sufferers has increased from 15 million in 1998 to 25.7 million in 2010.[20] The highest proportion is among children ages 5 to 14. Gut microbiome balance may hold one of the keys to unlocking the mystery of why we see this sudden increase in immune system imbalance.

Research has shown that children raised in rural environments, where playing in the dirt and being around farm animals are more common, have lower incidences of allergies and other autoimmune conditions.[21] Why? Well, these kids have a different relationship to the bugs in their environment.

In her fascinating book *Farmacology,* family doctor Daphne Miller investigates this relationship between rural environments—specifically small family-owned sustainable farms—and health. The book is a beautiful view of how the soil truly feeds us. One of the recurring themes in the book is that the microbial biodiversity of the soil breeds the diversity of our gut microbiome and impacts our health in a variety of ways. First, there is the simple fact that people who live on farms have more exposure to a broad array of microbes—from the soil, from the dung of farm animals, from the milk products of ruminants, and more. This exposure to a diverse microbial environment offers health benefits.[22] The amount of exposure children have to other kids also makes a difference, because they're exposed to more microbes. Scientists at the University of Arizona examined the incidence of asthma in 1,035 children and the prevalence of frequent wheezing related to the number of siblings or whether the children attended daycare.[23] They found that having older siblings protected against the development of asthma, as did attendance at daycare during the first 6 months of life. That's because increased germ exposure early in life confers protection against the future development of asthma. Since people who live and eat on farms are exposed to even more bugs, it's reasonable to assume that they receive further health benefits. Indeed, a study recently published in the *New England Journal of Medicine* showed that children raised on farms had lower incidences of asthma than those raised in urban environments; exposure to a broader array of microorganisms is the probable cause.[24]

But the relationship between microbes, farms, and health goes deeper. As Dr. Miller explained, the soil in sustainable organic farms has a broader biodiversity of microbes, which assimilate nutrients from the earth. The plants grown in this soil are more nutrient rich than their conventionally grown counterparts. Animals that eat these plants or humans who eat this nutrient-rich food acquire health benefits. One study revealed that organically farmed soils have higher biodiversity and that fruits grown in this rich microbial environment have higher levels of antioxidants, phenolics, and ascorbic acid.[25] Organic gardening has been shown to improve soil biodiversity and protect plants against harmful soilborne pathogens.[26] (This is a core principle of the organic movement, for which my publisher, Rodale, has long been an advocate.) In contrast, soil "treated" with antibiotics and pesticides results in reduced soil microbiome diversity and the selection of antibiotic-resistant microbes whose genes eventually are conferred to the gut microbiome of consumers. Farm animals add yet another link in the chain. As they eat and digest the nutritionally enriched food on sustainable farms, they fertilize the soil with manure that's chock-full of a diverse array of microbes, which in turn feed the soil, which feeds the plants we eat, and so the cycle continues.

These connections between microbial diversity of the soil, the nutrient profile of foods that results, and the microbial diversity of humans are profound, and we're only beginning to understand them.

"The impact of the gut microbiome on our health is very much like the influence of the soil microbiome on plant nutritive composition and its health," said Dr. Miller. In a sustainable model whereby human stool compost is used as plant fertilizer, our fecal microbiome enriches the soil microbiome biodiversity, establishing a symbiotic cycle between the soil and human microbiome and leading to improved health outcomes.

Concepts like these and the studies highlighted here have led to growing support for a theory known as the hygiene hypothesis,[27] which suggests that living in an oversterilized environment where early vaccination is commonplace and antibiotic use is prevalent may set the stage for the epidemic of allergies, asthma, autoimmunity, type 1 diabetes, and obesity and the growing problem of inflammatory bowel conditions in children.[28, 29]

Originally proposed by Dr. David P. Strachan in 1989, when he noticed an inverse correlation between family size and incidence of hay fever,[30] this theory has gained traction in medical circles over the last 2 decades and was updated by Professor Graham Rook as the "Old Friends" theory.[31] The premise: Our "old friends"–the microorganisms that we are exposed to in early life and that eventually inhabit our gut–coevolved with us, and over time they've come to play an essential role in helping us establish healthy immune function. Our immune systems, through exposure to these friendly organisms, learn how to properly recognize ally or intruder and are trained to attack the right invaders. According to Dr. Rook, "the rise in allergies and inflammatory diseases seems at least partly due to gradually losing contact with the range of microbes our immune systems evolved with, way back in the Stone Age. Only now are we seeing the consequences of this, doubtless also driven by genetic predisposition and a range of factors in our modern lifestyle–from different diets and pollution to stress and inactivity."

According to the "old friends" theory, children who aren't exposed to the diverse array of these immune-educating microorganisms early in life have a reduced biodiversity of commensals in their gut. The result is that the underdeveloped gut immune system is overreactive to foreign invaders, resulting in harmful inflammatory responses that become sustained and lead to chronic allergic and inflammatory disease.

Today, children receive antibiotics at record rates. The average child in the United

States and other developed countries receives 10 to 20 courses of antibiotics by the time he or she is 18 years old, antibacterial soaps adorn many bathroom sinks, and there's a bottle of sanitizing gel in every home—if not every room.[32] How do all these sterilizing agents affect our body's microbiome, and what are the long-term consequences on our health? What happens when we are consciously killing off our "old friends"?

Researchers have begun looking for answers to that question, and what they're finding isn't pretty. Even a short 5-day course of a common antibiotic like ciprofloxacin has been shown to kill up to one-third of the gut microbiome, resulting in an unbalanced and reduced biodiversity of the gut microflora. While some of these bugs recover once the patient goes off the antibiotic, scientists have found that many species remain dormant for up to 2 years after treatment.[33] What's more concerning is recent evidence suggesting every course of antibiotics may produce *permanent* and unfavorable alterations in the composition of our gut microbiome.[34]

So is avoiding overuse of prescription and over-the-counter antibiotics enough to reverse this trend toward a permanently altered gut microbiome? Unfortunately, the answer is no.

Our meat supply is loaded with detectable levels of antibiotics that adversely impact the balance and diversity of the flora in our gut. The FDA has estimated that the livestock industry now uses 20 million pounds of these antibiotics annually.

These drugs were originally dispensed to keep infection down in the horrific conditions that used to be called feedlots and are now known as CAFOs (concentrated animal feeding operations), where animals are kept for more than 45 days in extremely confined areas that produce no vegetation. But farmers noticed something interesting—antibiotics not only kept infection at bay, they also seemed to fatten up the livestock. That's why, since the 1950s, antibiotics have been used in low *nontherapeutic doses* to increase the body weight of cows, sheep, pigs, and chickens.[35]

Are the antibiotics used to "beef up" our meat actually fattening up America? A study at New York University Medical Center sought to answer that question. Dr. Ilseung Cho and his colleagues administered antibiotics commonly used in livestock to weaning mice at doses similar to those used in agriculture, and the conclusion was that these drugs may well be a contributing factor to the obesity epidemic in this country.[36]

The team found that antibiotics led to significant changes in the composition of the gut microbiome, resulting in modifications and copies of key genes involved in the metabolism of carbohydrates to short-chain fatty acids. This is a key finding, because short-chain fatty acids govern how much energy we harvest from carbohydrates. Increases in colonic short-chain fatty acids meant more energy was extracted from the foods these mice ate, which led to increased weight gain. After about 6 weeks, the study mice had gained approximately 10 to 15 percent more than their untreated counterparts, despite being fed the same diet. Other important metabolic changes included alterations in the metabolism of lipids and cholesterol by the liver. Disrupting the finely balanced ecosystem of the gut microbiome through the use of antibiotics clearly has consequences. It disrupts metabolism and leads to weight gain.

Does this mean that overuse of antibiotics and the resulting disruption in *your* gut ecosystem lead to weight gain? The evidence seems to point in this direction. Does it mean that the antibiotics used to fatten up livestock are also fattening up many of us who consume significant quantities of these livestock? Probably. There's no question antibiotics kill off our gut microflora and that this has an effect on our health.

Could altering our gut microbiome and changing our relationship to our "old friends" be part of a cycle of ill health that leads to increased inflammation, which leads to even more weight gain and poorer health in a spiral that spins ever further out of control? To answer that question, we need to discuss the next pathway and look more carefully at the relationships between gut microflora, inflammation, and weight.

PATHWAY 2: INFLAMMATION—YOUR SYSTEM ON FIRE

One of the keystone discoveries of modern medicine is the relationship between systemic inflammation and a host of chronic illnesses, including cardiovascular disease, dementia, gastrointestinal disorders, type 2 diabetes, weight gain, and more. Virtually all specialties in the medical sciences recognize inflammation as a major player in the development of chronic disease states.

Inflammation is important, but in some ways it's gotten a bad rap. It's not inherently good or bad. It's about balance—yin and yang; acute versus chronic; controlled versus uncontrolled. You hear a lot about how important it is to "cool down" or "turn off" the inflammatory response, and for most Americans, that's essential. But to properly moderate inflammation, you need to know what it is, how it works, and how you got so inflamed in the first place. And, as we'll see, the gut microflora are important actors.

When Your Immune System's Sprinkler System Fails

Our immune systems are cellular forces that have evolved to protect us from infectious elements. When you get a splinter and the area turns red, swells, and becomes warm— that's your immune system at work. When you have a fever and you feel like you're about to burn up as you try to fight off a cold, it's a sign your immune system is mounting a healthy response to clear the infection.

Your immune system involves a lot of inflammation because immune and inflammatory reactions are basically the same thing. Virtually every aspect of your health operates on a spectrum from optimally balanced to completely out of control. Weight is like this—you could be a few pounds too big to look supersexy in this summer's bikini, you could be morbidly obese, or you could be somewhere in between. The numbers on the scale (and your lab tests) creep in one direction or the other, depending on where you fall on this spectrum. And your gut controls your body curves. If you want to look sexy outside, start fixing the inside.

Your immune system exists on the same kind of spectrum. When it's optimally balanced, the immune system releases cells that attack foreign invaders when needed, but otherwise it rests. When it's out of balance, it's constantly sending cellular messengers that say "attack," and in the worst cases, these cellular protectors turn on your body and start to beat up your own cells. This is called systemic inflammation.

The condition may sound familiar. We talked about how the incidence of allergies, asthma, and other autoimmune (*auto* means "self," so the term means "self-immune") conditions is on the rise. Inflammation is at the very core of this process. Inflammation also leads to weight gain. Here are a few highlights illustrating the connection between runaway systemic inflammation and fat accumulation.

- **Insulin resistance.** Inflammatory cytokines block insulin receptors, reducing your sensitivity to the hormone. As you become more resistant to insulin, your body has a more difficult time converting the calories you consume into energy. Instead, you pack on fat. That's why metabolic syndrome, type 2 diabetes, and obesity are intimately interwoven conditions.

- **VAT.** Visceral adipose tissue, also known as belly fat, is metabolically active and encourages further inflammation in the body. So fat makes you inflamed, which causes you to gain more fat in a vicious cycle.

- **Leptin resistance.** Inflammation of the hypothalamus leads to resistance to leptin, the chief hormone that makes you feel full. When you've eaten enough, your body senses this and sends this hormone to your hypothalamus to tell you to stop. When you become resistant to leptin, you feel hungry more often and it's difficult to satiate that hunger, so you eat more and you gain weight.

Remember, the flora you're exposed to when you're young train your immune system to differentiate friend from foe. If you don't have the right bugs in your gut at an early age, the stage is set for immune imbalance, inflammation, and thus weight gain. But what if your immune system *was* properly trained when you were young? Is it still possible for your immune system to swing out of balance?

Absolutely. There are many dietary, lifestyle, and environmental factors that can lead to inflammation. Too much sugar in your diet (Americans eat about 150 pounds per person yearly–way too much), too little or too much exercise, stress, environmental toxins, food sensitivities, and more can all lead to chronic systemic inflammation.

However, one overlooked player in this cycle of inflammation, weight gain, and disease is your gut microflora. In Chapter 1, we talked about the consequences of failing to support the healthy bugs in your gut. Under normal circumstances, the gut flora

Can Bad Bugs Make Your Liver Fat?

The production of endotoxins by bugs in your gut doesn't only set off systemic inflammation, it also makes your liver fat. Nonalcoholic fatty liver disease (NAFLD) is a condition characterized by fatty infiltration of the liver in people who don't drink excessive alcohol. In NAFLD, 5 to 10 percent of your liver turns to fat, impacting its function in a number of ways. Lipid and glucose metabolism are affected, and you have a more difficult time detoxifying your blood. It's estimated that from one in three to one in four people have a fatty liver, and it's clear that the condition is linked to overweight/obesity, metabolic syndrome, and diabetes.[37]

While many physiological processes drive the condition—including inflammation, insulin resistance, and oxidative damage—new evidence suggests that endotoxins from gut bacteria are involved in the development of NAFLD.[38, 39]

Dysbiosis may weaken the tight junctions that are the glue holding together the cells of your intestinal lining, allowing bacterial toxins to enter the liver. These endotoxins then foster an increase in free fatty acid uptake and production by the liver, ignite inflammation, and promote insulin resistance—a harmful trifecta that injures the liver.

People with NAFLD also have a higher prevalence of small intestinal bacterial overgrowth[40] (SIBO—a condition we'll discuss later in the chapter). Ironic though it may be, the organ meant to detoxify your body may be dramatically impacted by gut-derived bacterial toxins that result from dysbiosis. Probiotics have been shown in laboratory animals to prevent and treat NAFLD by rebalancing the gut flora and restoring gut barrier integrity.[41]

represent a tremendous variety of species (500 to 1,000). The biodiversity in your intestines is a marker of health. This is actually a primary law of all biology: The greater the diversity of an ecosystem, the greater its health.

A sudden shift away from a healthy mixture of bugs reduces the biodiversity of our microbial friends and diminishes our ability to adapt. In the case of your gut microbiome, as biodiversity diminishes, the preponderance of pathogenic species of bugs tends to increase.

This can be problematic, because certain strains of bacteria produce endotoxins (toxins generated inside your body) that, if absorbed into the bloodstream, can be harmful to human health. Among the many endotoxins microbes can produce, lipopolysaccharide (LPS)–an essential component of their cells–is among the worst, because it triggers a powerful immune response that when left unchecked can develop into chronic systemic inflammation.

Your body doesn't like LPS, so it primes your immune system to go after LPS with all its might. It sends cytokines into action–powerful immune messengers that stimulate several classes of cells, including macrophages, monocytes, dendritic cells, and others. This begins the inflammatory process. And that's the issue with having an underdeveloped immune system with a faulty braking mechanism that permits inflammation to go unimpeded like a runaway train.

Intestinal inflammation loosens the adherence of your gut lining cells at critical junctions, creating breaches in this lining—which allows LPS and other bacteria-derived toxins to enter your bloodstream.[42] Some label this situation the *leaky gut syndrome*. When your immune system senses that these toxins are leaking into the bloodstream, it cranks up the inflammatory response even more in a vain attempt to beat back the LPS.

Systemic inflammation from gut bacteria–derived LPS has been implicated as an early driver of obesity and insulin resistance, and this process is probably the reason.[43] Plasma levels of LPS are higher in people with obesity and type 2 diabetes, and increased levels of a powerful inflammatory molecule induced by LPS called serum amyloid A proteins are found in obese people.[44, 45] Associations between serum levels of LPS and serum levels of insulin and triglycerides were reported in patients with type 2 diabetes and obesity.[46] And researchers have shown that subcutaneous infusions of LPS can cause weight gain and insulin resistance in mice.[47] Short-term antibiotic administration that kills off the intestinal bacteria that produce LPS in obese mice has been shown to decrease weight and body fat.

How does your gut become overrun with bugs that set off this inflammatory chain reaction? Well, many factors are involved, but your diet—specifically the amount and type of fat you eat—is probably the most important. Eating too many inflammatory fats induces changes in the gut microbiota that lead to endotoxemia and the resultant inflammation.[48] Investigators have demonstrated that a high-fat diet leads to detrimental changes in flora that set off the exact kind of LPS-driven inflammation we just reviewed. We also know that when you get this inflammation under control, the weight naturally drops away.

Fats aren't necessarily evil. The *type* of fat you eat is what's critical. In Chapter 4, I'll explain exactly what kinds of fats you should focus on and which you should avoid to reverse and avoid the intestinal inflammation that can lead to weight gain.

Supplements may help protect you from this process, too. Augmenting levels of bifidobacteria in the gut, either with probiotics or prebiotics, has been shown to reduce inflammation and improve glucose tolerance.[49] Replenishing bifidobacteria has also been shown to reduce gut leakiness, allowing less inflammatory LPS to pour into your bloodstream.[50] We'll review how to use supplementation to support your weight-loss efforts in Chapters 4 and 11.

However, before we get to all that, we need to complete our exploration of the ways in which imbalance in your gut microbiome can lead to weight gain. So let's talk about how the overall profile of your flora may be the best indicator for how likely you are to gain or lose weight.

PATHWAY 3: TYPE—HOW YOUR GUT BUG "FINGERPRINT" AFFECTS YOUR WEIGHT

Could you have a "gut microflora type" like you have a blood type? Emerging science is showing that different people have gut microbial combinations that are as specific to them as their fingerprints. And we're beginning to learn that the type of bacteria that is dominant in your gut–your personal floral fingerprint–may have a dramatic impact on your weight and health.

The overall consensus is that obesity and weight gain are characterized by an over-abundance of a class of bacteria belonging to the phylum Firmicutes, which many doctors now call "fat-forming bugs." While there's some variation in the findings, most of the studies show that a preponderance of bacteria from the phylum Bacteroidetes correlates with leanness.[51]

Scientists at the Washington University School of Medicine are leaders in this field of research. To begin determining whether or not a gut floral fingerprint could have an impact on weight, they analyzed the gut microbiota of genetically altered mice (the genes that control the appetite-regulating hormone leptin production were rendered inactive or were "knocked out"). You may remember from earlier in the chapter that leptin governs satiety–the feeling of fullness. Mice without these genes are constantly hungry, so they eat all the time and get fat. When the scientists looked at the gut microbiome of these obese mice, they found that they had more bacteria from the Firmicutes phyla of bacteria and less from Bacteroidetes.[52] Their lean mice counter-parts showed exactly the opposite floral fingerprint.

Excited by these findings, these scientists conducted follow-up research in humans that demonstrated similar microbial patterns. In one study, 12 obese participants were ran-domly assigned to either carbohydrate-restricted or fat-restricted diets. Both groups lost weight and both groups had a reduction in Firmicutes and an increase in Bacteroidetes.[53]

To confirm these findings, these investigators, looking for patterns between micro-bial clustering and leanness or obesity, compared the fecal microbial communities between adult female twin pairs and their mother. The twins who were obese showed reduced bacterial diversity, fewer Bacteroidetes, and more Firmicutes, just as predicted. Similar to the results found in mice, lean twins showed the opposite pattern–enhanced biodiversity, a greater number of Bacteroidetes, and fewer Firmicutes.

Why are Firmicutes associated with overweight and obesity? It appears these bugs have an impact on carbohydrate and lipid metabolism. They may actually be *too* efficient at extracting energy from the food you eat, which may explain the reason a Firmicutes fingerprint is associated with weight gain.[54] We'll discuss this further in Pathway 5 (page 32).

Studies have also shown that the burden of Firmicutes in obese people decreases after weight loss, even after gastric bypass surgery.[55] The improvement in gut microbial balance appears to occur soon after gastric bypass surgery and may contribute toward the rapid improvements in insulin sensitivity after the procedure prior to any substantive changes in weight. In fact, some researchers are now suggesting that the weight-loss results of this surgery may result to a certain extent from a change in gut microflora.[56, 57]

Understand that the aforementioned Bacteriodetes-Firmucutes story is more consistently observed in mice than in humans and that there are other organisms that may influence obesity. For instance, methane-producing bacteria, such as Methanobacter smithii,[58] is felt to increase the risk of obesity by speeding up the breakdown of food, boosting the production of fatty acids, and leading to the formation of fat, which over time, results in obesity.[59] In contrast, others such as A muciniphilia, and H. pylori and Christensenellaceae minuta[60] appear to be protective and favor being lean. Ultimately, the combination of genetics and diet determine which bacteria are more predominate in our gut. Overall, a balanced, robust, and diverse community of gut flora are the key to good health and a lean metabolism.

Again, we see the powerful influence that gut bugs have on your ability to create a lean metabolism. Now you may be asking yourself, "Hmm, how can I get a fat-burning floral fingerprint that will help me lose weight?" The answer brings us to Pathway 4 and diet.

PATHWAY 4: DIET—THEY ARE WHAT *YOU* EAT

You know the old saying "You are what you eat." But when we eat, we're feeding more than ourselves—we're feeding an entire ecosystem. What you feed your gut bugs determines a great deal about what species of bugs predominate at any one time. And as you now know, the balance of bugs in your gut has a tremendous impact on your health and weight. What you feed your gut microbiome—how you fertilize your inner garden—may be the key determinant in whether you are able to lose weight.

It's repeatedly been shown that the standard American diet (SAD)—high in inflammatory fats, high in processed carbohydrates, and low in fiber—negatively impacts gut flora in several ways.

First, animals and humans experience unhealthy shifts in both bacterial and metabolic profiles when fed a high-fat, high-sugar, low-fiber diet. The SAD diet shifts the relative balance of bugs in your gut toward the Firmicutes phylum—the fat-forming bugs.[61] It appears that a dramatic shift to these fat-forming bugs can occur in as few as 24 hours[62] after consuming a high-fat meal. That an alteration in gut microbiota can happen this quickly is an astounding finding, revealing what a powerful influence diet has on health.

If you want to have a fat floral fingerprint, just keep eating in a SAD way. But if you want to fertilize bugs in your gut that will help you lose weight, then you should cut back on inflammatory fats, dramatically reduce your sugar intake, and increase your levels of fiber. But you need to do this in a specific order or you may inadvertently encourage the wrong bugs to grow in the wrong places in your gut. (Learn details about the steps you need to take in the chapters that follow.)

Then there's the diet-inflammation-gut microbiome link we began discussing earlier in this chapter. Foods you eat have a dramatic impact on how much systemic inflammation you experience–there's no longer any question about that. Inflammatory saturated fats and high-glycemic-index carbs spark the fires of inflammation. When this conflagration creeps into your intestines, like a forest fire within, it devitalizes the gut's terrain so that bad bugs can proliferate.

As you learned when we talked about Pathway 2, these bad gut bugs may produce harmful metabolic by-products that further increase inflammation, promote fat accumulation, and increase insulin resistance. Left unchecked, this process can punch holes in your gut, causing it to become porous–which only serves to exacerbate this cycle of inflammation, poor health, and weight gain.

The answer is deceptively simple. You just need to stop eating foods that set your system on fire and start eating the foods that cool it down. I'll give you all the details in the next chapter.

Finally, the foods you eat impact your genetic expression, and your gut microflora may be one of the primary means by which this occurs. Let's take a step back and discuss the difference between your genotype, your phenotype, and how your gut microbiome "talks" to your genes.

Genotype, Phenotype, and Genetic Cross Talk

It was once thought (and many people, including some doctors, still believe) that your genes are unchangeable. In some respects, this is true. Unless we learn how to genetically modify humans, the color of your eyes, your height, the shape of your face, and many other fundamental aspects of who you are won't change no matter how powerful the environmental influence. Similarly, we have genetic predispositions toward the amount we weigh, what diseases we're prone to, and more. These "hard-coded" aspects of your physiology are known as your genotype.

However, your genotype tells only part of the story about who you are and who you will become. Environmental influences *do* impact the expression of certain parts of your genetic code. Diet, exercise, stress levels, toxins, and more can trigger receptors in your genes that will alter the messages they send your body. That means what you do, what you eat, how you exercise, how much stress you have, and how you behave every day actually affects you at the deepest possible biological and physiological levels. These environmental influences can reprogram the translation and/or expression of the genes that control your body systems. The ability of environmental influences like these to alter your genes is called epigenetic modification. While we don't have control over our genotype, we can influence the expression of our genes to alter health outcomes.

One of the key influencers of epigenetic modification is diet. The foods you eat send messages to your genes. A new branch of science called nutrigenomics has been developed to uncover how the foods you eat modify genetic expression of body physiology. As it turns out, the gut microflora play an important role.

The bugs in your gut have a special superpower—they can communicate genetically. This is called "quorum sensing,"[63] and your gut flora use this power to communicate with one another and with you, their human host. Bacteria can actually "swap" DNA with one another by sending signals that alter the genetic pattern of their neighbors. A fascinating study conducted at the University of Victoria in Canada provides an example of how this occurs.[64, 65] Scientists sought to discover why Japanese people extract more nutritional value out of nori* (the seaweed in sushi) than other folks do. As it turns out, genetic cross talk between microbes is at the very center of the story.

Zobellia galactanivorans is a bacterium that lives on several species of seaweed, including those used to make nori. When people eat seaweed, they unwittingly consume this microorganism that has hitchhiked onto the plant and then takes up residence in the gut microbiome of the host. Once there, *Z. galactanivorans* sidles up to its bacterial counterparts and says, "Hey, check this out. I can digest seaweed better than you. Want a piece of this action?" The surrounding bacteria engage in "horizontal gene transfer," stealing the genes that allow *Z. galactanivorans* to get more nutrients out of the seaweed. Once that happens, they can digest seaweed just as well as the ocean-based bacterium can. It's almost like a magic trick.

Overall, gut bugs communicate with your DNA by emitting proteins that impact receptors on the gene. These alterations in genetic expression may drive fat accumulation and change the way you process sugar. So the foods you eat impact the kind of flora in your gut, which then send messages to your DNA telling it to pack on fat.

The key takeaway is pretty straightforward: What you eat affects your gut flora, which in turn send messages to your body to either pile on fat or burn it off. To have a lean metabolism, you need to rebalance your gut microbiome to help you lose weight.

In the next chapter, we'll discuss how to make the needed changes in your diet to shift your microbiome back to a balanced state. For now, let's look at a few more ways that disruptions in the gut ecosystem and a reduction in the diversity of the gut microbiota can cause you to pile on the pounds.

---

* Nori is the Japanese name given to various types of edible seaweed and algae. Nori's origin dates back to ancient China and Japan, around the 8th century. It is usually used as a wrap for sushi, in miso soup, or just eaten plain. Nori has a high content of minerals, fiber, and many different types of vitamins.

PATHWAY 5: METABOLISM—THE IMPORTANCE OF SHORT-CHAIN FATTY ACIDS

The role of the gut microflora in metabolic function is now well recognized. The amount of energy you harvest from the foods you eat is largely determined by the type of bugs you have in your gut. Let's look at what this means and why it's important.

Eating is an interesting process. As you chew your food, salivary enzymes are added to it, turning it into a substance called chyme. This is then swallowed, and the chyme moves down to your esophagus and drops into your stomach, where it's exposed to hydrochloric acid and additional enzymes that pull it apart into its chemical constituents. These are delivered to your small intestine, where most of the nutrient absorption in your body occurs. What's left over drops into your large intestine, where the vast majority of your gut microflora live. Then your bugs have a feast.

One of their favorite foods is fiber. Human beings can't digest fiber without the help of our flora. That's why a certain amount of fiber simply passes through us—what our bugs don't eat comes out in our poo. This is one among many reasons fiber is such an important dietary substance. Without enough fiber in your diet, your flora starve, biodiversity plummets, and dysbiosis can set it.

As your gut flora eat fiber, they break it down into short-chain fatty acids (SCFAs), which are extremely important to human health. SCFAs increase the gut's absorption of water, regrow gut cells, and may provide defenses against colon cancer, inflammatory bowel disease, and more.[66]

The amount of SCFAs your gut bugs produce is incredibly important—as usual, balance is the key. Too few SCFAs and you don't get their protective benefits. Too many and weight gain, glucose imbalance, and increased triglyceride production may result.

As their name indicates, SCFAs are fatty acids that are energy dense and calorie rich. The more short-chain fatty acids you produce, the more calories in your diet. In normal humans, SCFAs provide from 80 to 200 calories per day, depending upon the amount of daily dietary fiber intake.[67] However, certain species of your gut microflora overproduce SCFAs from carbohydrates, so there is interspecies variation in the efficiency of the fermentation of fiber to SCFAs. Remember the Firmicutes bacteria from our discussion about gut bug fingerprints? They're thought to be fat-forming gut microflora by most scientists today, and the SCFA connection tells us why.

A shift of either 20 percent more Firmicutes or 20 percent fewer Bacteriodetes results in more SCFAs extracted from fiber and absorbed to provide a gain in caloric energy. Why do the Firmicutes bacteria produce more SCFAs? They overdigest the fiber you eat. That means less is left undigested as fiber that comes out in your poo and more SCFAs are absorbed and turned into energy in your body. What happens with the additional energy you can't use? It gets stored as fat by a complex mechanism that we discuss later on in this chapter, but this is likely the reason SCFAs trigger increased triglyceride production in your liver.

But this isn't the only way that Firmicutes influence your metabolism. A new study[68] shows that this class of bacteria encourages your body to also *absorb* more of the fat you consume in your diet, creating a double whammy of increased SCFA production and increased dietary fat absorption that has been concretely associated with weight gain.

These facts alone show that the calories in/calories out diet approach is hopelessly out of date—there's no way for you to accurately track how many calories your gut bugs are harvesting for you. It also shows that the type of food you eat is probably much more important than the amount.

Does this mean you should eat less fiber, so your food won't be converted into SCFAs? No! As we've already learned, when you eat a high-fat, low-fiber diet, your gut bug profile swings toward Firmicutes and ultimately turns into fat. Once these fat-forming bugs take over, what little fiber you do eat is overdigested and turns into more fat—all of which is another step in the wicked cycle of weight gain. Fiber is not your enemy. In fact, it's one of your dearest dietary friends. You just need to balance it with proper amounts of healthy fats, high-quality protein, and low-glycemic carbs so that it can do its job correctly.

As if runaway Firmicutes and the problems associated with it weren't enough cause for concern, studies have now shown that your gut microbiota govern another important regulator of lipid metabolism called angiopoietin-like protein 4 (ANGPTL4), also known as FIAF (fasting-induced adipose factor).[69] ANGPTL4 helps regulate the proportion of triglycerides deposited in your adipose tissue (your fat). When too little of it is floating around in your body, more triglycerides are sequestered as fat. Research on ANGPTL4 is in its early days, but studies show that the type of bugs in your gut seems to influence how much of the protein is in your blood.[70, 71] This may be another mechanism by which your flora impact your metabolism and your ability to gain or lose fat.

This is all more evidence that your gut flora have a significant impact on your ability to lose weight. As you'll learn in Chapter 3, you can create a lean metabolism by feeding your gut bugs right and changing your lifestyle to support theirs.

But for now, let's look at two more pathways leading to weight gain. You see, it's not only the type of bugs in your gut that's important, but where they live.

PATHWAY 6: PLACEMENT OF GUT BUGS—THE SIBO EPIDEMIC

Under normal circumstances, most of your gut microbiota live in your large intestine, closer to the end of your digestive tract, an oxygen-poor environment inhabited predominantly by anaerobic bacteria. The small intestine, where most of the nutrients from your food are absorbed, is a relatively sterile and better oxygenated environment that favors the growth of aerobic bacteria under controlled circumstances. The growth of gut bugs in your upper digestive tract is limited by the suppressive actions of stomach acid, digestive enzymes, bile, the sweeping movement of peristaltic waves, and more.[72]

In some cases, however, gut bugs either crawl up into your small intestine from the large intestine or aren't cleared from it properly. When this happens, these gut bugs disrupt the way the small intestine functions. This is called small intestinal bacterial overgrowth (SIBO), and it can be a serious problem. SIBO is defined as having more than 100,000 bacterial organisms per milliliter of fluid in the small intestine. Compare this to the small intestine's normal low levels of a mix of aerobes and anaerobic bacteria at a concentration of 1,000 to 10,000 organisms per milliliter of fluid, and you can see the problem.

SIBO symptoms typically include gas, bloating, and flatulence after meals but can include loose stools, constipation, abdominal distention, and abdominal pain. SIBO has also been associated with chronic fatigue syndrome, fibromyalgia, rosacea, restless leg syndrome, and more. Many patients say that when their SIBO is finally resolved, chronic symptoms disappear and they feel more vibrant and energetic than they have in years. Irritable bowel syndrome (IBS) has been shown in many studies to be associated with gut dysbiosis,[73] including SIBO. Systematic reviews of the research have revealed that the majority of patients with IBS suffer from this condition.[74, 75] Furthermore, individuals with obesity have been reported to have a higher prevalence of functional gastrointestinal disorders such as IBS.[76] This connection of obesity, SIBO, IBS, and dysbiosis further supports the foundation for the Gut Balance Revolution approach for Ted, whose story you read in Chapter 1.

I have felt that SIBO was a factor in weight gain for a long time. I've observed that when patients are treated for SIBO, they seem to naturally lose weight while gaining energy (weight down = energy up). Ted's story is a perfect example. When we resolved his dysbiosis and treated him for SIBO, he lost weight and his energy skyrocketed. Recall that Ted was originally referred to me for assistance managing his IBS, not his obesity. Observations like this are part of what drove me to write this book. The weight gain/weight loss story is more complicated than most people think, and my gut instincts convinced me that the intestinal microbiota play a role. My clinical observations (and my gut instincts) are finally being borne out by research.

A provocative study was recently conducted that shows SIBO leads to increased intestinal permeability—an issue we discussed earlier in this chapter—which allows more gut bacteria–derived endotoxins into your bloodstream, setting off the cascade of events highlighted in Pathway 2. Researchers analyzed 137 morbidly obese individuals who had been referred for bariatric surgery and 40 healthy controls for SIBO by glucose hydrogen breath testing (the standard test for the condition) and liver biopsy (to assess liver injury). These investigators reported that SIBO was more common in obese than lean participants. The obese subjects testing positive for SIBO also had more severe liver problems, suggesting that the condition contributed to fat accumulation in the liver.[77] There are many other scientific studies in laboratory animals that demonstrate how

SIBO weakens the integrity of the intestinal lining, permitting bacterial toxins to escape into the liver and cause injury.[78]

These findings have been confirmed by a recent study showing the results of hydrogen breath tests can accurately predict whether you have too much body fat and whether or not you're at risk for weight gain and obesity. Dr. Ruchi Mathur and colleagues showed that participants with higher concentrations of methane and hydrogen in their breath—sure signs that the small intestine has been overgrown with *Methanobrevibacter smithii*—had a higher body mass index (BMI).[79] Dr. Mathur, director of the outpatient diabetes treatment center at Cedars-Sinai Medical Center, stated, "It's possible that when this type of bacteria takes over, people may be more likely to gain weight and accumulate fat. . . . Obesity is not a one-size-fits-all disease."[80] More proof that calories in/calories out is far from the whole story.

Does this mean if you're overweight you definitely have SIBO? Not necessarily. However, if you've tried many diets but the fat is still stubbornly on your body and you suffer from the typical symptoms of SIBO, there may be bugs in the wrong part of your digestive system.

Antibiotics that kill these bugs are presently the gold standard of medical practice to treat this condition, but they can be problematic. For one thing, they don't selectively kill the misplaced anaerobic colonic flora that have found their way into your small bowel. They simply wreak havoc on your entire gut microbiome, as all antibiotics do. There is extensive collateral damage that can last for years. In my experience, and that of many of my colleagues, SIBO tends to reappear quickly if the root causes (such as poor diet, poor digestive function gut movement, and structural abnormalities in the gastrointestinal tract) are not addressed, which leads to recurrent courses of antibiotics. Seems like a catch-22, doesn't it?

Fortunately, diet has been found to play a prominent role in treating this condition. Less severe cases of SIBO can often be improved by "starving out" the overpopulation of microbes in the small bowel with a change in diet. In mild to moderate cases, I've been able to combine herbal preparations designed to suppress the growth of these bugs with diet to eliminate SIBO.[81] In persistent cases, antibiotics may be the only option. If this is the case for you, it's still best to take a careful look at the underlying causes driving the condition and optimize your diet and lifestyle to reduce the risk of SIBO recurring. So the Gut Balance Revolution is most certainly for you.

Now let's turn our attention to the last pathway leading from an imbalanced microbiome to weight gain and disease: the ways bugs talk to your brain and the rest of your body.

PATHWAY 7: COMMUNICATION—HOW YOUR GUT TALKS TO YOUR BRAIN

It's long been known that your gut communicates with your brain. In fact, the connection is so profound that it inspired author Dr. Michael Gershon to call the human digestive tract "the second brain."[82] Your gut tells your brain when you've had enough to eat and when to send messages to the pancreas to release insulin. It has a dramatic impact on your mood and so much more.

One of the most rapidly expanding areas of research is around gut-brain-microbe communication. We now know that hormones and neurotransmitters in your gut aren't alone in talking to your brain but that your intestinal flora have a conversation with your head, too.

A number of biochemical pathways lead from your gut to your brain, and several are affected by flora. But let's focus on the most important of these: your hypothalamic-pituitary-adrenal (HPA) axis, because as far as gut-brain communication is concerned, your HPA axis is an interstate freeway.

The HPA Axis: A Freeway of Information

The hypothalamic-pituitary-adrenal axis is a complex set of interactions between the hypothalamus in your brain; your pituitary gland, which controls several hormones in your body; and your adrenal system, which governs your stress response. It's the major freeway of information in your neuroendocrine system responsible for a wide variety of physiological processes including stress, digestion, immune function, energy storage, appetite and expenditure, mood, and sexuality.

Gut bugs may play a role in the development of your HPA axis. It's been shown that a healthy microbiota early in life is critical for the proper development of the HPA axis in rats.[83] If this turns out to be true of humans as well, we'll know that your microbiota have a far wider influence over your health than we originally thought. Improper development or dysregulation of your HPA axis can lead to an exaggerated stress response, impaired cardiac function, alterations in neurotransmitters and brain hormones, and increased caloric intake. This may be one of the reasons why mood disorders such as depression and anxiety and even autism have been tied to dysbiosis and why administering probiotics helps improve these conditions.[84, 85]

The gut uses the HPA axis to communicate with your brain through enteroendocrine cells. These cells are regulated by your gut microbiota and thus influence them in important ways.[86] They impact the secretion of incretin hormones, including glucagon-like peptides 1 and 2 (GLP-1 and GLP-2). A series of studies has shown a close connection between gut microbes and levels of both GLP-1 and GLP-2.[87]

These two hormones are important because they stimulate the release of insulin from the pancreas, slow gastric emptying, promote satiety (the feeling of fullness), promote insulin sensitivity, and reduce gut permeability—all of which counter obesity.[88, 89] For example, if there's too much GLP-1 in your blood, your pancreas will release more insulin that can, over time, lead to insulin resistance and weight gain. But if you don't have enough GLP-1, your stomach will empty more quickly, dumping sugar into your blood, causing insulin resistance and weight gain.

GLP-1 and GLP-2 also decrease your appetite. So if you have too little of them, you will be hungrier and likely to eat more. The way your gut talks to your HPA is critical. When that communication goes haywire, you're much more likely to pile on the fat.

As always, balance is key. How is optimal hormonal balance obtained? With diet—by eating plenty of nondigestible carbohydrates, specifically oligofructose, found in fruits and vegetables like bananas, onions, Jerusalem artichokes, asparagus, leeks, and others. This class of fiber is so important because your gut bugs *love* to eat these fiber-rich and fermentable carbs, and when they get them, they send out "happy" messages encouraging your body to produce these chemicals in the right amounts. That's why this class of fiber has been found to help people lose weight, reduce hunger, moderate caloric intake, and balance insulin and glucose.[90] But as I mentioned earlier in this chapter, we will take a systematic approach toward rebalancing your gut microflora and weight loss by recommending food groups in discrete phases.

LOOKING AHEAD

All this science is showing us that the human body is an ecosystem. And ecosystems are complex entities requiring attention and care to remain healthy. Most of the one-dimensional formulas for weight loss on the market today fail to take this fact into account. We've been led to believe that the number of calories you consume is the decisive factor in weight loss. I hope this chapter has illustrated that this idea is simply false.

So what's the solution? You can change your diet in ways that will help your gut bugs tell your body to burn fat. You can weed, seed, and feed your inner garden and help a lush orchard to grow within. You just need to know which foods to eat, which to avoid, and how to design your meals for each phase of this program so you can create a lean metabolism. In the chapters that follow, I'll show you how.

CHAPTER 3

The Gut Balance Revolution Overview

You are about to embark on a journey—one that will take you deep into the Amazon rain forest that lives inside your gut. On this journey, you'll have some unexpected adventures and be confronted by strange, counterintuitive facts—for example, that you can eat more (not less) and still lose weight, and that you can burn fat and rebalance your gut microbiome by simply relaxing.

You'll also meet a host of odd creatures that cause you to gain fat and others that help you burn it off. You'll be introduced to bugs like bifidobacteria[1] and lactic acid bacteria.[2] Some of these creatures will be your friends on your weight-loss journey. Others will be your foes.

During your trip, something profound is going to happen. You will revolutionize your understanding of weight loss, health, and the nature of the human body. You will restore your metabolism so you can experience a lifetime of great health and vitality. You will create a new relationship with the complex ecosystem that lives inside you.

Welcome to the Gut Balance Revolution.

At this point, I hope I've convinced you that the reason why you pack on fat or burn it away is far more complex than the old calories in/calories out story you've been told for decades. As I described in Chapter 1, weight loss is about much more than simply eating less and exercising more. The factors that lead to weight gain and weight loss are far reaching and include genetic predisposition, phenotypical influences (like diet, lifestyle, and stress), blood sugar and insulin balance, hormone regulation, inflammation, energy metabolism, and more.

And as you've learned, your gut microbiome—your inner garden, the rain forest you're about to journey into—is a key player in the story of weight loss and health that has been largely ignored.

Until now.

You see, despite all of the complexities of the science of why people gain weight, there's a wonderfully simple approach you can take to shedding pounds and rebalancing your health. All you have to do is eat and live in a way that makes your gut bugs happy. You need to become a good gut bug gardener.

By focusing on rebalancing your gut microbiome and taking a community-based ecosystems approach to the whole puzzle of weight loss, you cut through the junk science, the late-night infomercial claims of "automatic weight loss," and instead go right to the heart of weight gain and the obesity epidemic that haunts this country.

Eating in a way that supports your gut microbiome means you're also eating in a way that avoids the primary drivers of unwanted weight. When you feed your flora the foods they love, when you till the soil of your inner garden and then seed your gut with friendly

Can Gut Bugs Regulate Hunger?

Leptin and ghrelin are the two primary appetite-regulating hormones in your body. Leptin, made by your fat cells, sends signals of fullness and satiation. Its counterpart, ghrelin, made predominantly in your stomach, sends signals of hunger to your brain. When either one is out of balance, or when your cells become resistant to their messages (as happens in cases of leptin resistance), your appetite (and your weight-loss attempts) can go haywire.

But the bugs in your gut affect your appetite. Ghrelin is suppressed by *Helicobacter pylori*.[3] More ghrelin in your blood means you feel hungrier more often.

Nobel Laureate Barry Marshall, MD, has shown that *H. pylori* is connected to heartburn, acid reflux, and ulcers, and he developed an antibiotic regimen to treat these conditions by killing off *H. pylori*. But what if this sends the gut microbiome out of balance? Could treating patients with antibiotics that eliminate *H. pylori* make them hungrier and cause them to gain weight?

Maybe. One study has shown that 92 veterans treated with antibiotics for *H. pylori* gained significant weight compared to their untreated counterparts. That's because when the *H. pylori* was killed off, levels of the appetite-regulating hormone ghrelin increased sixfold—a profound change. The physiological expectation is that the resultant increase in appetite would lead to significant weight gain.

It's been noted that *H. pylori* has virtually disappeared in our children due to multiple courses of antibiotics, with only 6 percent of kids showing evidence of this strain of flora in their guts. Could our escalating obesity rates be connected to the reduction in *H. pylori* due to these treatments? Could *H. pylori* be at times a commensal (friendly microbe) in disguise while at other times a pathogen? It's too early to say for sure whether *H. pylori* is a "Dr. Jekyll and Mr. Hyde" bug, but some scientists are suggesting that treating *H. pylori* infections may have opened up a Pandora's box.[4]

flora, you not only rebalance your gut microbiome and optimize all the pathways high-lighted in Chapter 2, you also:

- Rebalance blood sugar and insulin levels, in many cases reducing or reversing insulin resistance.
- Cool off chronic systemic inflammation—one of the major contributors to all chronic illness.
- Reestablish optimal levels of appetite-regulating hormones like leptin and ghrelin.
- Reverse damage done to your body by a high-sugar diet.
- Rev up your overall metabolism so you can keep fat off long term.

This all happens automatically when you shift your focus to eating and living in a way that's good for your friendly flora of gut bugs. Remember, the commensal microbes in your gut thrive on the same things you thrive on, and vice versa. Eating in a way that makes sense for your gut bugs means eating in a way that makes sense for you.

That's why, starting right now, I invite you to think of yourself as more than an individual person. Instead, think of yourself as an entire ecosystem. The digestive tract is the inner core of your body's ecosystem, and these microbial communities have a powerful influence on your fat-burning machinery—your metabolism—as well as your overall health and well-being. Your job is to keep your gut microbial ecosystem balanced and strong in order to obtain optimum health.

Here's how you do it.

WEEDING , SEEDING, AND FEEDING YOUR INNER GARDEN: AN ECOSYSTEMS APPROACH TO WEIGHT LOSS

The Gut Balance Revolution is a three-phase program designed to reduce dysbiosis, reseed your gut microbiome with friendly flora, and then fertilize that inner garden so it stays healthy for a lifetime.

This isn't some gimmicky crash diet that leads to yo-yo dieting, poor long-term results, and a harmfully raised metabolic body weight set point, as we discussed in Chapter 1. Instead, it's a science-based program designed to help you restore a healthy metabolism and enhance the vigor of your life by reestablishing a robust inner ecology.

To achieve this, you have to address what I call the Three Rs:

- **Reboot** your inner ecology. This is a time of renewal when you "till the earth" to set the stage for a healthy garden in your gut while priming your fat-burning metabolism.
- **Rebalance** your flora. After you've weeded your inner garden, you rebalance your gut microbiome by seeding your gut with healthy bacteria and fertilizing those bugs with the right foods.

■ **Renew** your health for life. This is the ongoing, long-term, lifestyle change part of the plan, where you integrate the healthy habits you've learned into a manageable program that fits your personal needs.

By following these Three Rs, you'll burn off fat and rebalance your gut microbiome. And you'll feel more energetic and happier than you have in a long time.

The program is simple–though that doesn't always mean it will be easy! Here's how it works.

Phase I: Reboot—Weed Your Inner Garden and Rev Up Your Metabolism

The first 30 days of the program will help you reestablish a healthy relationship with food. For most of you, this will naturally lead to accelerated weight loss. Many of you will lose 10 to 15 pounds (or more!) during the first month of the program, and you'll do this by making a few dietary and lifestyle modifications that starve out the bad bugs in your gut, reduce systemic inflammation, and rebalance your blood sugar.

The key to this phase is a low-carbohydrate, moderate-fat, higher-protein ketogenic diet that specifically reduces a class of highly fermentable carbohydrate-rich foods called FODMAPs.

FODMAPs is an acronym for "fermentable oligo-, di-, and monosaccharides and polyols." I know that's a mouthful, but don't worry–you don't have to remember all of those terms. What it really refers to is a class of carbohydrates that contain short-chain sugars that gut bugs can readily ferment, which promotes their growth and leads to a host of digestive symptoms including gas, pain, bloating, and more.

By limiting these foods and dramatically reducing your intake of starchy and highly processed carbs, you'll remove from your diet the primary food sources that sustain the imbalance in the microbial communities in your digestive tract.

Reducing these carbs and focusing on lower-glycemic-load meals also has the happy benefit of rebalancing your blood sugar, reversing insulin resistance and fat accumulation, and reducing overall systemic inflammation (a process that's further enhanced in this phase by eliminating inflammatory oils from your diet).

Instead of eating inflammatory, sugary foods that lead to imbalance in your gut microbiome, you'll focus on fat-burning superfoods (like blueberries, green tea, and chile peppers) that will rev up your metabolism while supporting the community of your gut's beneficial bacteria. In fact, I'll provide you with a list of my top 10 fat-burning superfoods to include in your diet–all of which are also featured in the delicious, gut-bug-balancing meal plans and recipes you'll find in Chapter 11.

By the end of Phase 1, you will:

■ Lose up to 15 pounds (or more)

■ Set the stage for a rebalanced gut microbiome

- Improve your blood sugar balance and reduce systemic inflammation
- Reduce any digestive complaints[5, 6]
- Enhance your energy levels
- Improve your mood and cognition

You may notice that, barring a few exceptions like the reduction of FODMAPs, this reboot phase of the program parallels a few highly successful low-carb healthy eating plans that are proven to be effective[7-14]—at least in the short term. That's intentional. I wanted to leverage the best of all the weight-loss science that exists for this program.

Unfortunately, though, other weight-loss programs do poorly long term[15] because they're difficult to stick to—and because they also kill off some good gut bugs that sustain our health (like bifidobacteria) and are important for a lean metabolism.[16, 17] That's why, with this system, I want to take things a step further. I want to provide you with all the tools you need to rebalance your metabolism, burn fat, and reestablish a healthy gut microbiome. I'll do that by teaching you how to seed and fertilize your inner garden and achieve inner ecological harmony for life. That way, this program will be the last, best diet you'll ever need!

That is what Phase 2 is all about.

Phase 2: Rebalance—Seed and Fertilize Your Inner Garden to Restore Ecological Harmony

After 30 days of rebooting your gut microbiome and revving up your metabolism, it'll be time to shift your focus toward rebalancing your inner flora by fertilizing the friendly helpers that support your health. Now that you've weeded your inner garden, it's time to seed and feed it.

In Phase 2, you will be increasing your carb intake. Our focus will be on healthy, whole-foods carbohydrates that are packed with fiber and healthy prebiotic fibrous foods that feed your fat-burning friendly flora, instead of the junk carbs that got you into trouble with your weight in the first place. Specifically, we'll do that by reintroducing into your diet some key fibrous, complex carbohydrates—fruits and vegetables that are high in insoluble fiber that your human digestive tract can't break down but that are the perfect fuel for fat-burning bugs. Burn, baby, burn! I'll add plenty of fermented foods that are filled with the healthy bacteria your gut microbiome needs to flourish.

Low-carb diets have their place, particularly when you're starting out in the reboot part of this program. Many popular diets have proven—and the research has shown—that reducing your overall carbohydrate intake is important for rebalancing blood sugar, reducing inflammation, losing weight, and generally improving your health. I'm with them on that.

However, maintaining these programs doesn't usually work. In the long run, low-carb diets have a high "recidivism rate," which just means people tend to fall off the wagon and regain everything they've lost—and then some.

One of the reasons these diets may not work in the long run is that they tend to kill off certain species of friendly bacteria in your gut. For example, recent studies have shown that a gluten-free diet can cause a reduction in key species of healthy beneficial gut microbes such as lactobacillus and bifidobacteria.[18, 19] Long-term energy-restricted diets, which form the foundation for the vast majority of weight-reduction programs, are also associated with a decrease in bifidobacteria.[20] Why is this important?

Remember the bifidobacteria from Chapter 2? That little bug appears to support a lean metabolism.[21] Children who maintain a normal weight have been reported to have higher stool bifidobacteria counts than those who become obese.[22] Studies have linked low levels of bifidobacteria to obesity in adults.[23, 24] And it's not just your waistline that suffers when these species of friendly flora are killed off. Bifidobacteria, one of the primary probiotics found in places like mother's milk, has a broad range of health effects. Low levels of bifidobacteria in the digestive tracts of infants have been linked to an increased risk for allergy, asthma, autoimmune disorders, and, yes, obesity.[25] This may be one reason why feeding infants breast milk, which is loaded with prebiotics and even bifidobacteria, prevents the future development of childhood obesity.[26, 27]

Your metabolism doesn't like long-term low-carb eating. Your inner garden doesn't like it. And your waistline doesn't like it. The results of low-carb diets are, unfortunately, very predictable: People fall off the wagon, they regain weight, and, often, they pack on even more pounds than they had before. As you know, the more yo-yo dieting you do, the higher your body weight set point is raised and the more weight you're liable to gain—it's a horrible rebound effect.

We're going to take a different approach on this program. One that will rejuvenate your inner garden *and* provide you with long-term weight loss. And it all comes from taking that ecosystems approach to eating I mentioned earlier.

Phase 1 has been designed to "reboot" your metabolism by basically hitting the proverbial reset button. You will be eliminating foods that are high in sugar, promote inflammation, and sustain an unhealthy and imbalanced gut ecosystem. These bacterial communities are interacting to slow down your metabolism, accumulate fat, and hold on to weight. In Phase 1, the fat-burning machinery is turned on by cutting out the unhealthy refined carbs that got you into trouble while shifting the gut microbial communities to a more healthy mix that favors a lean metabolism. In a sense, you are tilling the garden in preparation for the planting of new life. In Phase 2, you fertilize your inner garden with healthy foods to support the growth of commensal flora that shift the microbial communities in your gut ecosystem back to health and promote a lean metabolism. So in this phase, I ask you to increase your intake of fermented foods such as sauerkraut, kimchi, yogurt, kefir, and miso. These foods help seed your gut with good bugs that will rebalance your gut microbiome. Then we'll feed these good bugs with prebiotics—a special class of fiber-rich, very filling carbohydrates such as oat bran, artichokes, Jerusalem artichokes, and others that the good bugs in your gut love to feast on.

By doing this, you'll increase your high-quality carb and fiber intake over the course of Phase 2. This will not only set the stage for a rebalanced gut microbiome—one that will help you kick your metabolism into high gear—but will also curb your appetite and help avoid the kinds of hormonal and metabolic adaptations that can lead to trouble.

As long as you're on Phase 2, you can expect a sustained weight loss of about 5 to 10 pounds of excess body weight per month. I want you to stay on this phase until you achieve your goal weight. You'll find that it's a healthy plan for long-term eating, and you can certainly remain on it as long as you like.

In the rebalance phase, you can expect:

- Enhanced energy as your mind and body become accustomed to this new way of eating and living
- A renewed sense of well-being
- If your doctor checks your blood chemistries, an ongoing reduction of inflammation and continued rebalancing of your blood sugar and insulin levels

You may want to make this way of living and eating your lifelong path. If you do, that's fine. Or perhaps you'd like to reintegrate a few more foods and even allow yourself a treat every once in a while (I know I do!). That's where the last phase of the program comes in.

Phase 3: Renew—Keep Your Friendly Flora—and You—Healthy for Life

Once you achieve your goal weight, you'll feel renewed, your gut microbiome will be rebalanced, and you'll have set the stage for long-term health and optimal weight.

When you reach this point, you'll have the metabolic flexibility to integrate more foods into your diet and even eat off the plan once in a while. Here's a key point to remember: The dose makes the poison. As long as your gut microbiome is healthy, your metabolism is balanced, and you focus on real foods, small amounts of comfort food—even a little pasta or dessert from time to time—will not pack on the pounds. The human body is designed to eat a wide variety of foods, and when it's operating optimally, it still has resilience.

You'll find that some foods have a larger impact on your weight and health than others. Everybody is different, every metabolism is different, and every gut microbiome is different. Remember that the flora in your gut are as specific to you as your fingerprint. No one else has quite the same mix of gut bugs as you do. Little wonder that we all respond to dietary and lifestyle influences so differently.

That's why I designed this phase to provide you the flexibility to create your own ideal, personalized eating plan for life. I'll teach you how to identify foods that support you and your gut microbiota and eliminate foods that don't. This will give you the secret key to unlock the door of lifelong health and optimal weight.

I created this part of the program with real people in mind, people who live busy, hectic lives—just like you do. You see, another problem I have with most of the diet programs out there is that they set up an impossible standard and then get judgmental when you can't meet it. For example, I've met precious few people who eliminate all processed sugar for life. Sure, reducing it is a great idea. But are you really *never* going to have a scoop of ice cream or fresh homemade cookies again? When the holidays hit, are you really going to skip the pumpkin pie or the cookies? I doubt it. Even if you could, who would want to? There's no point in being healthy and thin if you can't have fun so relax and enjoy life! Why set impossible goals like these as the standard? It just doesn't make sense.

More to the point, unless you have very specific health problems, you don't have to stick with a severely regimented eating program for the rest of your life to maintain a healthy weight.

That's why during the renew phase you're going to take holidays off (you deserve it!) and rest from your diet on the 7th day (if you want to). Once you achieve your goal weight, as long as you stick to healthy real foods most of the time, limit sugars and processed substances, and remain mindful of the foods you know don't nourish your body or your gut microbiome, you'll be able to maintain your weight effortlessly for life.

During the renew phase, I'll teach you how to do that. I'll also explain what to do when the program is over (it's actually never really "over"; you just keep eating healthy for life).

LOOKING AHEAD

Okay, that covers the basics. Now it's time to roll up your sleeves. We will begin like any good gardener does by tilling the soil and preparing your inner garden for all the goodness to come. In the next chapter, you'll discover how to mitigate the dysbiosis that is sending your inner ecosystem out of balance by improving the biodiversity of the microbial communities in your gut.

I will also explain how to limit foods in your diet that could be disrupting your gut microbial balance and causing a wide range of uncomfortable symptoms (i.e., bloating and flatulence). I will teach you how to replace these foods with healthy, satiating, anti-inflammatory alternatives that will support your health inside and out.

Finally, you'll learn about my top 10 superfoods for Phase 1. If you don't believe food can be used as medicine, I have a feeling I will change your mind once you read about these amazing nutritional superstars.

That's all coming up in Phase 1. Ready to dive in?

CHAPTER 4

Phase I: Reboot

WEED YOUR INNER GARDEN
AND REV UP YOUR METABOLISM

Imagine a patch of ground overgrown with weeds. The soil is hard, dry clay. The only plants that grow are invasive species of weeds–hardy and durable, but hardly the type of plants you'd want in a lovely, healthy garden.

Now let's pretend you want to start a garden on this piece of untended land. What's the first thing you'll do? Clear out the weeds and prepare the soil, right?

Well, the steps are not so different when it comes to preparing the "soil" of your gut for the healthy ecosystem of gut microbiota you wish to plant in it. You want to increase the overall biodiversity of this inner ecosystem, shifting it toward a robust set of microbial communities that work together in a symbiotic way to support your health and help you achieve an optimal weight.

That's precisely what Phase 1 is designed to do. During the first 30 days of this program, you'll focus on weeding your inner garden and tilling the soil of your gut. You'll do this by:

1. Rebooting your gut ecosystem

2. Reestablishing good eating patterns

3. Revving up your metabolism

Here's how it works.

REBOOTING YOUR GUT ECOSYSTEM: TILLING THE SOIL IN YOUR INNER GARDEN

Living deep in your lower intestines is a complex ecosystem of microorganisms that constitutes a garden of life. This magnificent orchard is composed of trillions of highly diverse organisms that have evolved to a sophisticated synchrony of symbiosis. When we care for this garden and nourish our flora, our health flourishes. But when we feed our friendly gut bugs poorly and treat them poorly, the diversity of gut microbes is diminished and our health is compromised. Just as your stockbroker advises you to diversify your portfolio, my goal is to teach you to biodiversify your gut microbiome to improve your overall health and promote a lean metabolism. As with our own communities, reduced diversity results in stagnation and decay. We all need a diverse and balanced community of microbes whose functions complement one another, producing the symphony of good health. Abundant data support the importance of biodiversity in health, and its loss causes various inflammatory conditions, including asthma, allergic and inflammatory bowel diseases, type 1 diabetes, liver disease, obesity, and much more.[1, 2] I'll go into greater detail about why this is the case later this chapter when I explain why inflammatory foods, in particular, tend to lead to weight gain and digestive symptoms for so many. To reverse dysbiosis (the imbalance of microbial communities we discussed in Chapter 2), we need you to restrict highly refined inflammatory foods from your diet. Doing this will rebalance your gut ecosystem, cool off systemic inflammation, and help rebalance your blood sugar, insulin levels, and more.

Remember that the type of gut microbiota predominating in your gut is strongly influenced by what you eat. In fact, in a study recently published in the journal *Nutrition*, scientists stated that "diet has the most powerful influence on gut microbial communities in healthy human subjects."[3] The Western diet is a master manipulator of the intestinal microbiota and villain of friendly flora.[4] "About 75 percent of the food in the Western diet is of limited or no benefit to the microbiota in the lower gut," according to Stig Bengmark, MD, PhD, honorary visiting professor in the division of surgery and interventional science, University College London. "Most of it, comprised specifically of refined carbohydrates, is already absorbed in the upper part of the GI tract, and what eventually reaches the large intestine is of limited value, as it contains only small amounts of the minerals, vitamins, and other nutrients necessary for maintenance of the microbiota."[5] Radical amounts of unhealthy inflammatory fats and sugary foods adversely impact the profile of gut microbial communities very quickly.[6] The Western diet has been shown to promote dysbiosis and disrupt gut barrier function, permitting the seepage of gut bacterial–derived toxins into the circulation, thus causing systemic inflammation.[7] Western diets also reduce microbial diversity, a common thread in many chronic inflammatory diseases including obesity, metabolic syndrome, Crohn's disease, nonalcoholic fatty liver disease, and more.[8-10] Diets rich in proinflammatory omega-6 polyunsaturated fatty acids found in conventionally raised corn-fed red meat (which as we'll see are particularly high in the Western diet) are linked to intestinal dysbiosis and systemic inflammation.[11] Likewise, safflower oil, rich in omega-6 proinflammatory fats, decreases the Bacteroidetes phylum—a microbial shift associated with obesity in many studies.[12] A pivotal study showed that giving omega-3 fatty acids such as fish oil together with the omega-6-rich proinflammatory fats *prevented* dysbiosis and diet-induced weight gain.[13] These data (and more) bolster one of my cornerstone arguments: You can take the Western diet and toss it in the trash can!

The good news: By changing your diet, you change the overall terrain of your inner ecosystem, a crucial step in your progress toward weight loss and spectacular health.

There's only one slight downside to this approach—"collateral damage." We don't yet have a way to pinpoint and eliminate *only* the strains of gut bugs contributing to your weight gain and ill health. Despite the work in animals and humans, science still hasn't provided insight into the specific organisms that *consistently* cause weight gain. Yes, there are trends and patterns, and dysbiosis is clearly a critical factor in fostering weight gain—but we as a scientific community currently lack the ability to selectively target a phylum or species of dysbiotic organisms with antimicrobial interventions. Intense efforts continue to map the human gut microbiome, yet, for now, we lack the ability to identify which organisms are responsible for metabolic dysregulation in a given individual. For instance, the ecosystem of gut microbes of an individual may have an overpredominance of a certain bacteria in the phylum Firmicutes, which is associated with obesity in mice and in some human studies. However, the specific species of gut microbes and their metabolites (the chemicals they make) that contribute to weight gain may differ from person to person. Although technologies exist to identify bacterial metabolites—this field of study is called metabolomics—scientists still lack the sophistication to identify or deliver targeted therapies to eliminate "the community of bad bugs" causing weight gain.

The fact is that some of your healthy flora will die off during Phase 1. There's no way around that. Your flora are composed of a matrix of communities of commensal "friendly" organisms and potential pathogens, all of which are fed by what you eat. Research has taught us that fat-forming bad bugs tend to thrive on inflammatory fats and sugary foods. That's why we'll limit these foods in this phase. However, when you're dealing with ecosystems as complex as your gut microbiome, changes like these can have broad effects across the numerous microbial populations in the ecosystem. As we discussed in Chapter 1, the gut ecosystem includes fungi and viruses (outnumbering bacteria by 10 to 1), whose contribution to health, let alone obesity, is unknown. Dietary patterns alter the intestinal microbiota both functionally and ecologically—that means the communities change, their activity in the body changes, and the biochemicals they make also change. Remember, for example, that gluten-free diets can reduce the amount of bifidobacteria—a healthy strain of bacteria—in your gut. Yet I'll ask you to go gluten free on Phase 1. Why would I recommend a diet for 30 days that may put at risk some of the friendly flora at home in your GI tract? Well, there are several reasons.

First, you'll be cutting off the food supply of microbes that thrive on sugary proinflammatory foods, which helps shift the communities of your gut ecosystem away from dysbiosis. Less dysbiosis means the good strains of friendly flora in your gut can reclaim their proper place in the gut microbiome and do their job of promoting a lean metabolism more easily and efficiently.

On Phase 2 of the Gut Balance Revolution meal plan, I'll show you how to expand these populations of friendly flora once we've tilled the soil. Of course, this is only one example. Many other strains of detrimental microbes depend on foods we'll limit in this phase, so you're looking at an overall upgrade, diversification, and rebalancing of your gut microbiome.

Second, it's important to rev up your metabolism during Phase 1 by reducing the glycemic load of the foods you eat. This has a broad array of important metabolic effects—some of which we've already discussed, some of which we'll examine in greater detail in this chapter.

For example, if you're eating the Western diet or the standard American diet (SAD), radically reducing your sugar intake is a critical step to achieve optimal weight and life-long health. Most Americans eat what some doctors have called "pharmacological doses" of sugar, wreaking havoc on the body by setting off a cascade of negative biochemical effects leading to systemic inflammation, blood sugar imbalance, insulin resistance, metabolic syndrome, and, ultimately, type 2 diabetes and many other chronic illnesses. Phase 1 will help you begin to address these kinds of problems.

Finally, when it comes to rebalancing and diversifying the gut microbiome, there are just three possibilities.

1. **Change the way you eat and live.** This is the best way I know to rebalance your gut microbiome, and it starts with tilling the soil of your gut, creating a "clean slate" in which healthy flora can be planted. This is our objective during this phase of the program.

2. **Add in tons of prebiotic and probiotic supplements and/or foods and hope they outcompete the weight-retaining microbes.** Probiotics are great for some individuals but not all, and once the soil of your gut is ready for them, they can be an excellent adjunct to this type of program. But just eating a bunch of probiotic foods or taking supplements tends not to work nearly as well as tilling the soil and setting the stage for this "reseeding."

3. **Prescribe antibiotics that kill off bacteria.** These medications do exist, but they're like the nuclear option for gut microbiome health problems. They're only necessary (or even desirable) when no other options are available, and there are consequences that must be carefully considered when going this route. These medications kill off massive quantities of bacteria—not bothering to differentiate friend from foe. Antibiotics of any kind (especially ones this powerful) have negative long-term consequences for gut microbiome health and raise concerns for causing obesity, as we saw in Chapter 2. For some health conditions, antibiotics may be necessary, but it's always best to try more benign interventions first.

I strongly prefer option 1 in most cases. Yes, there will be *some* collateral damage. Yes, you'll kill off a few health-promoting microbes along the way. But remember that we're

The Three Fs That Help
Your Friendly Flora Flourish

Most diets take a fairly one-dimensional approach to what you eat, insisting that you "eat this, not that." But a healthy diet for humans can contain a very broad array of foods, and cultures all over the world have flourished on everything from acorns, mesquite, and fish (the Pima) to goat's milk and blood (the Maasai), so there's no magic formula for how every human should eat.

But there *are* some "foods" traditional human cultures simply didn't have access to, and we really shouldn't be eating them either. These are the sugary, starchy, highly processed foodlike substances that make up the majority of the Western diet and take up most of the real estate in your local supermarket. So we'll forget these on this program, as I'll explain in a moment.

Putting aside these obvious foodlike substances that send our metabolism out of balance (Coca-Cola and Cracker Jack, anyone?), I do have guidelines regarding what will help you and your friendly flora flourish under various circumstances. These aren't as black and white as the "eat this, not that" advice commonly reported in the news, but they're a good benchmark for how to eat in order to lose weight and get healthy. That's why on this program I decided to take the "Three F" approach to eating:

- **Favor.** These are the healthy, whole foods that will support your inner garden. They'll constitute the majority of your diet in a given phase.

- **Few.** You can simply reduce your intake of certain foods; you don't have to eliminate them entirely. So for each phase, I've called out the foods you will want to limit but not necessarily exclude.

- **Forget.** Some foods you want to omit entirely, at least until you get to Phase 3 and allow yourself an occasional break. Even then, you'll want to stay away from some things we call "food" that simply aren't, and you may find you don't want to eat these products anymore even on your days off from the program.

It's important to note that the Three Fs change from phase to phase. Pay special attention to the charts on pages 241–256, where all this is outlined in detail, especially if you decide to make your own meals during the program.

The Gut Balance Revolution meals have been built on these principles, so you can just follow the appropriate meal plan exactly as designed and easily stay on the program. I'll talk more about the meal plans, the foods lists, and how to use them in Chapter 11. We've managed to create some *spectacularly* delicious recipes while sticking to precise nutritional guidelines. I think you're going to love them.

preparing the soil for the good flora for your garden. When you till a piece of land to prepare it for a crop, a few good plants may get dug under, but you accept this sacrifice for the greater good of the garden you're creating. The same holds true for your inner garden.

To prepare the soil of your gut, we'll *forget* certain foods altogether and eat *fewer* of a class of foods that causes gastrointestinal distress to flourish and may lead to further dysbiosis if your inner ecosystem is out of balance. We'll *favor* the healthy, whole foods your good gut microbes and your body prefer.

Now let's dive into more details about what's allowed in Phase 1, what you need to reduce, and what to eliminate altogether. It's easier to start at the end and talk about what foods you'll want to forget for the next 30 days, so we'll begin with that.

Forget Foods That Promote Dysbiosis, Inflammation, Blood Sugar Imbalance, and Insulin Resistance

During Phase 1, we'll omit a number of foods that cause disruptions and imbalances in your gut ecology, cause your blood sugar to spiral out of control, set off inflammation

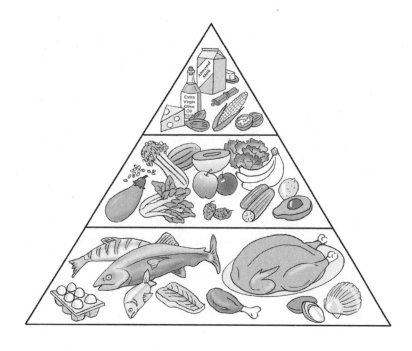

The Gut Balance Revolution Phase 1 Food Pyramid: This figure prioritizes the foods to eat during Phase 1, the reboot phase. Foods that are limited are at the top of the pyramid (i.e., gluten- containing foods and oils). Fruits and vegetables that have a relatively low to moderate FODMAP content (greens, squash, cucumber, berries) are placed in the middle of the pyramid. High-protein foods such as poultry, eggs, and fish, which are to be eaten in abundance, are at the base of the pyramid.

throughout the body, and generally wreak havoc on your metabolism, your waistline, and your overall health. Eliminating these foods is your first and most important step in tilling the soil of your gut and rebooting your metabolism.

You'll find the complete list of foods to eliminate in the Forget column of the Phase 1 food plan, starting on page 241. For now, let's review a few of these foods to highlight exactly how detrimental they are to your health.

Sugar

The average American eats 150 pounds of sugars (total caloric sweeteners) annually. In 2000, 66 pounds of beet and cane sugar and 87 pounds of corn sweeteners were consumed by Americans.[14, 15] That's a lot of sugar. To get a sense of just how that stacks up, consider that before the Industrial Revolution, humans consumed about 20 teaspoons of sugar per person per year; in Paleolithic times, that amount was as little as 2 teaspoons.[16, 17] Recent reports by the World Health Organization (WHO) and the Centers for Disease Control and Prevention (CDC) find that Americans currently consume an average of 15 to 20 percent of their daily calories from added sugars–that's about 300 to 400 calories a day based on a 2,000-calorie diet.[18, 19] This is particularly problematic in light of the fact that the WHO now recommends that no more than 5 percent of our daily calories should come from added sugar.[20] This means the average American eats three to four times more sugar than he or she should every day. These new WHO recommendations came on the heels of research attributing increased risk of cardiovascular disease mortality to excessive sugar consumption.[21] The American Heart Association concurs with the WHO and recommends that women consume no more than 100 calories a day from added sugars and men no more than 150 calories a day (1 teaspoon of sugar = 17 calories).[22]

Researchers at the Division for Heart Disease and Stroke Prevention of the CDC examined the National Health and Nutrition Examination Survey database, which contains information on some 11,733 individuals who, between the years 1988 and 2010, consumed 25 percent of total calories from sugar.[23] They found that this excessive sugar consumption *tripled* the participants' risk of cardiovascular disease mortality compared to those who consumed less than 10 percent of their calories from sugar.[24] Prior linkages have connected high sugar intakes to type 2 diabetes, obesity, fatty liver disease, stroke, and other adverse health conditions.[25] The study's researchers stated: "Our findings indicate that most US adults consume more added sugar than is recommended for a healthy diet."

Can anyone say "understatement"?

What are considered added sugars? Just cruise down the middle aisles of your local grocery store and look at the labels of processed foods–they are loaded with added sugars. The following list* provides some samples. Understand that these sugars and syrups are *added* to foods or beverages when they are processed or prepared. This does not include naturally occurring sugars such as those in milk and fruits.

- Anhydrous dextrose
- Brown sugar
- Confectioners' (powdered) sugar
- Corn syrup
- Corn syrup solids
- Dextrose
- Fructose
- High-fructose corn syrup (HFCS)
- Honey
- Invert sugar
- Lactose
- Maltose
- Malt syrup
- Maple syrup
- Molasses
- Nectars (e.g., peach nectar, pear nectar)
- Pancake syrup
- Raw sugar
- Sucrose
- Sugar
- White granulated sugar

*Source: choosemyplate.gov/weight-management-calories/calories/added-sugars.html

It's quite a list—and it doesn't even cover every possible form of sugar you'll find in your supermarket. No wonder some doctors say we're consuming pharmacological doses of sugar in amounts that impact our biochemistry. But how does it affect us?

1. **It imbalances our blood sugar.** When we consume immense doses of sugar, our blood glucose levels become elevated. Stable blood glucose is a hallmark of good health, so this by itself is reason enough to limit sugar intake.

2. **It leads to insulin resistance.** In response to all this sugar, our pancreas releases a substantial amount of insulin to usher the sugar into our cells, where it can be metabolized and converted into energy or stored as fat. When the influx of sugar exceeds metabolic needs, that sugar is packed away as fat on your butt, hips, thighs, tummy, and everywhere else you don't want it. As the fat cells grow, they become resistant to insulin's effects over a long period of time. Your body then requires more insulin to properly maintain blood sugar levels and provide cells with energy. This is a key component of metabolic syndrome and can eventually lead to type 2 diabetes.

3. **It inflames the body.** Sugar in significant quantities is inflammatory, and systemic inflammation is intimately related to chronic illness and fat gain.

4. **It promotes glycation.** When your blood glucose is elevated for long periods of time, the excess glucose irreversibly binds to proteins in your body, which then clump together into advanced glycation end products (AGEs). These molecules can lead to neuropathy and other health problems.

5. **It upsets gut microbial balance.** Harmful microbes such as clostridium, enterococcus, and other species in your gut *love* sugar.[26] Plus, inflammatory fats, so high in the

Western diet, work as a partner in crime with sugar, creating even more disruptions in gut microbial balance.[27] When you eat too much of these foods, noxious bacteria thrive, which can lead to gastrointestinal dysbiosis and all the problems that come with it.

The bad news about sugar doesn't end there. Another recent study found that eating large quantities of fructose rapidly leads to gut-derived endotoxemia and liver damage, even in the absence of weight gain.[28] This is particularly interesting to our discussion here for several reasons. To understand why, you need to know something about fructose.

Fructose is a kind of sugar that used to be found most often in fruit. It's a monosaccharide—a simple sugar—and some people are intolerant of it even in fruit, as we'll see when we discuss the FODMAPs group of highly fermentable foods.* For most folks, however, fruit is a perfectly safe way to consume this sugar. Fruit isn't the culprit. In fact, there are loads of studies showing that a diet rich in fruits and plants prevents many chronic diseases and cancers. Whole fruit is also loaded with fiber, which slows the release of monosaccharides into the bloodstream without the massive surge in insulin release triggered by other forms of added sugars. We're seeing concurrent epidemics of nonalcoholic fatty liver disease (NAFLD) and obesity worldwide, with excessive consumption of refined sugars (not fruit) as the leading cause.[29] So who's the bad actor in this drama of sugar, weight gain, and the far-reaching health consequences that come along with it? Enter the dragon—high-fructose corn syrup (HFCS).

HFCS: No Worse Than Table Sugar—Or Is It?

For decades, there's been a raging controversy about high-fructose corn syrup.† On one side stands the National Corn Growers Association, claiming that HFCS is no worse than table sugar. On the other side stand doctors and scientists concerned that this supersugar may adversely impact human health more severely than table sugar.

Evidence is mounting that there's real cause for concern about HFCS. Fructose consumption has increased in recent decades, especially due to increased consumption of sweetened beverages and processed foods with added fructose.[30] In fact, from 1980 to 2000 the consumption of cane sugar stabilized while the consumption of corn sweeteners has increased more than 50 percent during the same time period.[31, 32] HFCS intake has been associated with pathologies such as NAFLD.[33, 34] In fact, a recent study has

---

* For this reason, we will be limiting the types of fruits allowed in Phase 1. It's not because they are unhealthy; rather, it's because they are high in FODMAPs that are highly fermentable by gut bacteria, causing uncomfortable digestive symptoms, and some may cause imbalances in the composition and biodiversity of the gut microbiome. See all the details in the section on FODMAPs on page 61.

† Plain corn syrup can be used to enhance the appearance of foods, but it's often combined with white table sugar because it's not very sweet due to a large composition of glucose. The addition of "unbonded" or "free" fructose to corn syrup gives it an incredibly sweet taste so there's no need to add table sugar.

shown that individuals with NAFLD who were placed on low-fructose/low-HFCS diets experienced improved liver function, more balanced liver chemistry, and enhanced cardiometabolic markers.[35]

A meta-analysis of 3,102 articles linked HFCS intake to features of metabolic syndrome: high resting blood sugar, hypertension (high blood pressure), and abnormal cardiovascular lipid profiles.[36] These and other studies about the impact of fructose on liver health are only a few in a growing body of research that suggests HFCS, like table sugar, is detrimental to our health and our waistline. But why?

As its name suggests, HFCS is corn syrup chemically altered so that it is particularly high in *free* fructose and glucose monosaccharides, which are readily absorbed into the bloodstream. In contrast, table sugar has *equal* fructose content to HFCS, but the fructose is bound to glucose as sucrose, a disaccharide that requires enzymes to break it apart before it can be absorbed into the bloodstream. The free fructose form is what gives HFCS a supersweet taste and allows food chemists to use much smaller quantities of it than they would table sugar to achieve the same level of sweetness. This provides food companies a low-cost way to add sweetness to food, pushing their profit margins higher, along with your blood sugar level and waistline.

It's this trait—intense sweetness for a fraction of the cost—that's led to HFCS being a popular additive in processed foodstuffs the world over. Since 1975, it's found its way into everything from soda to bread to breakfast cereals to canned beans, condiments, "yogurt," and even some commercial pickles—potentially detracting from their health-promoting probiotic effect (recall that some gut pathogens thrive on sugar). The result: Most Americans are eating a high-fructose diet. Could this be one of the reasons the national waistline has ballooned out of control since the 1970s despite an overall lower caloric intake?

While there's ongoing debate and a ton of finger-pointing between the table sugar and HFCS camps, the truth is that they're both capable of causing a metabolic storm of inflammation and obesity when overconsumed. Head-to-head studies show that they're similarly noxious to our body and need to be limited in our diet.[37] Sugar-sweetened beverages are problematic because they're a source of many of our ills and account for a large portion of calories in today's youth—in a dose-response fashion, the more youngsters consume, the more problems they have.[38] One study reported that nearly 94 percent of children ages 3 to 5 years consumed sweetened milk products, 88 percent consumed fruity drinks, 63 percent consumed sodas, and 56 percent consumed sports drinks and sweet tea.[39] Remember, the dose makes the poison. When dealing with a poison, keep the dose down!

How does all this sugar impact the gut microbiome and intestinal health? It isn't pretty. Back in Chapter 2, we discussed endotoxemia, the process by which gut-derived bacterial toxins find their way into your bloodstream. Certain gut bugs produce lipopolysaccharide (LPS), a critical component of their cell walls but a substance that isn't very good for us. You see, your immune system is particularly sensitive to LPS. We don't

What About Diet Sodas?

The first thing people ask me when they hear my take on sugar is, "What about diet sodas and artificial sweeteners? They're okay, right?" In a word, no!

Evidence has been piling up against artificial sweeteners in general and diet sodas in particular for some time now. For example, a new study out of The Johns Hopkins Bloomberg School of Public Health shows that overweight people who drink diet sodas tend to consume *more* calories overall—approximately 194 additional calories daily.[40] This research confirmed the observations of scientists at the University of Toronto's Department of Nutritional Sciences, who observed 3,682 overweight participants in a study recently published in the journal *Obesity*.[41]

How could this be? Well, people who make the switch to diet drinks appear to eat more to compensate for the caloric deficit, as if their body weight set point has been moved upward. But why? A possible reason is that diet sodas may trigger appetite. It appears that the combination of carbonation and aspartame synergizes and elicits powerful signals from reward centers in the brain. This increased activation of reward regions may trigger hunger responses, as we discussed with sugar.[42] Research out of Salerno, Italy, demonstrated that the presence of carbonation itself reduces the neural processing of sweetness perception, which could lead to the consumption of *more* sugar.[43] Carbonation and its adverse impact on digestive hormonal reflexes, along with taste signals in the gut and brain elicited by aspartame, may all be involved in the increased caloric consumption associated with diet sodas.

To make matters worse, there have been questions about aspartame and other sweeteners since their creation, including some concerns that they may be carcinogens.[44] A study with profound implications recently published in the journal *Nature* linked the use of noncaloric artificial sweeteners (NASs) such as saccharin, sucralose, and aspartame to the development of diabetes—the condition that they were designed to avert and combat—thus their use for "weight control" is now fraught with deep concerns. Interestingly, these scientists linked the underlying root cause of the deleterious effects of the NASs on blood sugar dysregulation resistance to disruption of the gut microbiome. They were even able to confer glucose intolerance to otherwise healthy, germ-free mice via fecal transplants and normalize blood sugar via antibiotics.[45] In fact, there's evidence that aspartame disrupts the stability of the gut microbiome, another reason to advise caution.[46]

Glucose, on the other hand, reduces postconsumption hunger and increases satiety signals by inducing gut hormones that make you feel full while reducing the appetite-stimulating hormone ghrelin.[47] My suggestion: Stay away from artificial sweeteners. They aren't good for you, and you won't find them on this program.

know exactly why, but we do know that when it senses LPS, the immune system sets off a massive inflammatory reaction.

Excess fructose consumption in primates has been linked to gut-derived endotoxemia. The LPS released by the gut bugs in this process is eventually absorbed into the liver's circulation, injuring the hepatic tissues and causing fat accumulation,[48] which may be the causal link between HFCS consumption and NAFLD. This is the same mechanism we discussed in Chapter 2, where we learned that when high-fat Western diets were fed to animals, gut-derived endotoxemia, type 2 diabetes, and inflammation-related metabolic diseases emerged.[49]

Whether we blame HFCS or table sugar, they are *both* overconsumed in the form of highly refined carbs and junk food, which have in large part created the diabetes and obesity epidemic. HFCS and table sugar have been shown to drive hyperinsulinism, increased fat accumulation, excess belly fat, obesity, and related diseases. Both HFCS and table sugar increase appetite while free glucose reduces appetite![50] These sugars also work on the reward-pleasure centers in the brain via the release of dopamine, suggesting they may be addictive.[51, 52]

What a win for the fast-food industry. They fill us up with supersize sodas loaded with table sugar and/or HFCS. We become hungrier, consume more high-fat junk food filled with HFCS, and unknowingly become addicted. All this goes to show that the interrelationships between what you eat, gut microbial imbalances influenced by your diet, and the resultant systemic inflammation (which leads to weight gain) are a profound set of interlocking puzzle pieces that need to be addressed to lose weight and to address the obesity epidemic in our society.

If you're interested in learning more about excess sugar consumption, I recommend *Fat Chance* by Dr. Robert Lustig, one of the premier experts on the problems with fructose, and *Salt Sugar Fat* by Michael Moss, a journalist who has exposed why the food industry dumps obscene quantities of sugar, salt, and fat into virtually all the food it makes. The bottom line: We eat way too much sugar, and we need to kick the habit to reboot our gut microbiome, rev up our metabolism, lose weight, and get healthy. You won't find much sugar on this program, and it will be particularly limited in Phase 1.

Starchy Carbs

Sugar isn't the only dietary demon in the American way of life. A close second is sugar's cousin: refined starchy carbs. This includes bread, bagels, pasta, cereal, crackers, cookies, and cakes made from refined grains depleted of fiber and nutrients; white potatoes (think french fries); white rice; and just about any processed food in the middle aisles of your supermarket. These foods are sugar in disguise. Your body barely knows the difference–they're converted almost immediately to sugar after you eat them, and they set off all the same biochemical and gut microbial reactions.

This is why, especially in Phase 1, I ask you to keep your total carb load very low: no more than 50 grams a day. But don't *count* carbs or calories (as you would in most other weight-loss programs); that's not necessary as long as you follow the food charts and meal plans in Chapter 11. But you do need to be aware of why I'm asking you to make this change.

Fifty to 60 percent of the standard American diet is carbohydrates–and I'm not talking veggies here, folks. I'm talking chips and soda–starchy carbs and sugar. Low-carb diets have been shown to burn fat in the short term, likely because reducing your carb load helps rebalance your hormones (especially insulin), reduces inflammation, and starves out dysbiotic bugs in your gut–all very good things when it comes to getting rid of unwanted weight. On the flip side, traditional low-carb diets nonselectively "starve" good gut microbes, including fat-burning bifidobacteria–leading to the aforementioned collateral damage. As you will see, the Gut Balance Revolution keeps the carb count low during Phase 1 while expanding the biodiversity of the gut microbiome and minimizing collateral damage to the good gut microbes.[53]

Other low-carb plans put you in a state called ketosis, which means that certain cells in your body begin to use ketones (or ketone bodies) as their primary fuel source. I mention this because some folks worry that going into ketosis is dangerous–quite the opposite. Research has shown that ketogenic diets are a very effective method for kicking off weight loss and are safe for healthy individuals for up to 6 to 12 months (and perhaps longer, although they are unsafe for people with preexisting kidney problems).[54] The mechanisms underlying the effects of ketogenic diets on weight loss are still a subject of debate, but they may include the following:[55, 56]

- Dr. Robert Atkins's original hypothesis suggested that weight loss was induced by losing energy through excretion of ketone bodies, which are appetite suppressants. More recent science supports the principle that protein increases satiety and reduces appetite, meaning you naturally eat less overall.[57, 58]

- As you eat more protein, energy production shifts toward protein oxidation, which is inefficient. It is "more expensive" for the body to burn protein than sugar or fat for energy. This means more calories are burned as you metabolize your foods.

- Ketogenic diets seem to have an impact on the appetite control hormones leptin and ghrelin.[59]

- Fat production (lipogenesis) is reduced while fat-burning (lipolysis) is increased, and the overall efficiency of your fat-burning machinery is enhanced.[60]

- To get the glucose it needs, your body shifts to gluconeogenesis (which just means it creates glucose from the protein you consume). This has a higher "metabolic cost" than eating straight carbs or sugar, meaning your body burns more calories (even at rest) when you shift into ketosis.[61, 62]

Furthermore, low-carbohydrate diets can improve insulin resistance and glucose levels, reduce hemoglobin A1c, and improve glucose uptake in people who are overweight and/or suffer from type 2 diabetes.

There's even evidence that ketogenic diets can reduce small-particle LDL (one of the more dangerous types of cholesterol), lower triglycerides, and increase HDL ("good" cholesterol)—all wonderful effects for cardiovascular health.[63]

While some people experience an initial period of fatigue and lethargy (typically lasting a few days up to a week), these diets ultimately help improve cognitive impairment, mood, and energy in people who are overweight.[64, 65] And ketogenic diets are increasingly being shown to have therapeutic value for uncontrolled seizure disorders and possibly brain tumors.[66, 67]

In the long run, these generic super-low-carb ketogenic diets do have some problems, as we discussed in Chapter 3. They tend to lead to an increased body weight set point and yo-yoing if you stay too low carb for too long. However, I designed the Gut Balance Revolution program so that you won't stay in ketosis for more than 30 days. The overwhelming majority of people are perfectly safe going into ketosis for this amount of time or even longer, and the research clearly indicates that going into ketosis for this time period supports weight loss and may have other benefits such as anticancer and neuroprotective effects and improved sports performance.[68] Additionally, ketogenic diets have not been shown to promote osteoporosis or liver dysfunction, a concern that some people have about these types of diets.[69]

One caveat: If you have kidney problems, doing Phase 1 as outlined in this book isn't for you. In this case, I recommend you work with a physician in your community who is familiar with the concepts in this book and who can help you adapt the diet to your needs.

For the rest of you, eating low carb for the first month of the program will reignite your metabolism and help rebalance your blood sugar levels and gut microbiome. It's healthy and safe, and there are loads of delicious low-carb foods (see the recipes in this book if you don't believe me!). So get the sugar and starch out of your diet and see how you feel.

Later, when we get to Phase 2, we'll selectively reintegrate some of these foods and strategically increase your carb load gradually. In other words, you don't need to stay on this low-carb part of the program forever—just long enough for your body to reset itself using the healing power of whole foods.

Inflammatory Fats

Fats have long been a vexing issue in nutrition. For many years, we were taught, incorrectly, that fats are intrinsically evil and that low-fat diets were the holy grail of weight loss and wellness. Over time, this "low-fat" view has come under increasing scrutiny, and the fat myths most of us once believed have been dispelled by research. For example, a pivotal randomized clinical trial recently observed that a moderate-fat diet was an effective part of a weight-loss plan and was associated with improved lipid-related risk factors and fasting insulin levels.[70] In a meta-analysis published in 2010, scientists reviewed data from 21 studies that included nearly 348,000 participants and came to the conclusion that "there is no significant evidence for concluding that dietary saturated fat is associated with increased risk" of coronary heart disease or cardiovascular disease.[71]

So it's clear: Myths about fat simply don't hold up under scrutiny. Fat is not inherently bad. In fact, it's necessary for your survival. You could live without carbohydrates—you wouldn't be happy, but you would be alive. Without any fat in your diet, you'd perish. We need fats for optimum cellular membrane health and for a healthy nervous system. Your brain is 65 percent fat. The complications of essential fatty acid deficiency are legion.[72] Why would you deprive yourself of something so essential?

The simple answer is that you shouldn't. But that doesn't mean you should go out and eat fat with abandon. The real story about fat is too complicated for sound bites, and we scientists don't know as much about it as we'd like to think. What's the optimal intake of fat for the human body? What are the upper limits we can eat while still remaining healthy? What *types* of fats should we focus on? Which should we avoid? This is where the water gets muddy. However, there are a few things we are reasonably certain about.

Fat comes in basically two flavors: inflammatory and anti-inflammatory. You've probably heard a lot about omega-3s, omega-6s, omega-9s, and so forth. These distinctions are important enough to explore a bit. What the numbers represent is the carbon atom on which a double bond is formed. Omega-3 fats such as alpha-linolenic acid (ALA), eicosapentaenoic acid (EPA), and docosahexaenoic acid (DHA) are fundamental to human health. Omega-6s are mainly (though not entirely) inflammatory fats, extremely prevalent in the Western diet, as we'll explore shortly. Omega-9s are anti-inflammatory in nature but less common. They can be found in foods like avocado, squid, olive and sunflower seed oil, almonds, and several others.

A few foods contain only one type of fat—fish, high in omega-3s, are a good example. For other foods, the story is more nuanced. Some omega-6s, such as those in borage oil, black currant seed oil, and evening primrose oil, are healthy anti-inflammatory fats.[73] Others, such as corn oil, are unhealthy inflammatory fats. Should you avoid *all* foods that contain omega-6s? Not necessarily. What you really want is to have a good balance between inflammatory and anti-inflammatory fats. You can't eat food and eliminate *all* the inflammatory fats—it just won't happen. It's the ratio between the two that's important. And it's this ratio that is wildly out of balance in the modern Western diet.

The ideal ratio between inflammatory and anti-inflammatory fats is a perfectly balanced 1 to 1. Currently, we eat a diet that's 20:1 to 50:1 in favor of inflammatory fats.[74] By now, I'm sure you realize why that's a problem.

Where did all of these inflammatory fats come from? From the hydrogenated oil, soybean oil, cottonseed oil, corn oil, "vegetable" oil (a combination of the others), and other

What About Animal Fat?

Research on animal fat is lagging. On the one hand, it's been shown that diets high in conventionally raised red meat contribute to weight gain, cardiovascular issues, and certain cancers. We now know that this is likely due to the high levels of inflammatory fats in these animals—plus the fact that conventionally raised red meat is laced with antibiotics in sufficient levels to alter the gut microbiome and contribute to obesity. Studies in mice have shown that when given equivalent amounts of antibiotics as are found in our meat supply, mice become fat. Could this be one reason humans are facing an obesity epidemic? More research is needed.

On the other hand, grass-fed animals raised on pasture are more widely available than they used to be, and some evidence suggests that these animals are higher in healthy, anti-inflammatory fats than their conventionally raised counterparts. Unfortunately, no research has been done proving whether or not shifting from conventionally raised to pastured animals impacts long-term weight, the gut microbiome, or health.

Based on evidence, I've elected to keep red meat to a minimum on this program and focus on lean protein sources that we know support optimal weight and health, including seafood, skinless white meat chicken, and vegetable sources such as tofu.

If you're going to eat red meat, stick with pastured sources, as they may be higher in healthy fats, and they're typically free of antibiotics.

---

inflammatory fats poured into all of the processed foods we eat. These poor-quality fats set off systemic inflammation, causing you to pack on fat and setting the stage for every chronic disease in the book. And remember the many experiments in mice and humans we reviewed in Chapter 2 showing how a Western diet high in inflammatory fats shifted the gut microbiome toward a less diverse and less healthy ecological community. We'll dramatically limit these inflammatory fats in this program, and for good reason: They're bad for your inner ecology and overall health.

At the end of the day, it's not how *much* fat we consume that gets us into trouble (I'm including myself—remember I was nearly 300 pounds as a teenager!), it's those high glycemic proinflammatory foods that wreak havoc on your blood chemistry and gut microbiome.

EAT FEWER FODMAPS

Possibly the most important class of foods we'll address in Phase 1 is FODMAPs. Remember that FODMAP is an acronym for fermentable oligo-, di-, and monosaccharides and polyols. Reducing your intake of these foods is critical to the success of this program.

Saccharide is simply another word for sugar. So oligosaccharides, disaccharides, and monosaccharides are all forms of sugar. They're short-chain carbohydrates. Monosaccharides have one sugar molecule; disaccharides have two sugar molecules, and so forth. Polyols are sugar alcohols—a sugar molecule with a molecule of alcohol appended to it. Sugar alcohols can be found naturally in some foods, but the place they're most commonly found is in certain artificial sweeteners, such as xylitol, mannitol, and sorbitol.

These foods are highly fermentable, and they're not well absorbed in the small bowel—they pass from your stomach through your small intestine and into your large intestine mostly undigested and unabsorbed. The degree to which they're digested varies from person to person. For example, some people don't produce enough lactase—the enzyme needed to break down lactose (a disaccharide) in milk products. Other people have fructose (an oligosaccharide) transport defects, causing malabsorption of this sugar and creating a feast for their gut bugs. Fructans and galacto-oligosaccharides are polymers of sugars (fructose and galactose, respectively) that require bacterial enzymes for their digestion, so they're usually processed in the large bowel unless you have an overgrowth of bacteria in the small bowel (aka SIBO—more about this later). Because these highly fermentable foods pass to the large bowel either undigested or only partially digested, they can cause several problems.

First of all, your gut microbiota *love* to eat FODMAPs—they're like fast food for your flora. They gobble them up, ferment them, and produce gases like hydrogen, carbon dioxide, and methane. Gas is bad enough, but FODMAPs can lead to more serious problems. You see, your body naturally tries to dilute small, concentrated doses of undigestible

Where's the Fiber?

No question about it: Fiber is one of the most important foods you need for long-term health and optimal weight. It helps you feel full, it's fabulous food for your flora, it helps with stools, and it "scrubs" your intestines. Most health organizations recommend getting at least 25 to 35 grams of fiber a day. Unfortunately, Americans aren't getting anywhere near this much fiber in their diet—their average intake is only 15 grams per day, and only 5 percent of Americans consume the daily recommended intake.[75]

Despite this, I'm recommending that you limit your fiber intake during Phase 1. We'll enhance fiber intake in Phase 2, along with prebiotic foods (foods that selectively feed your friendly flora) to diversify your inner garden once you've tilled the soil and it's ripe for planting the seeds of a healthy gut microbiome.

carbohydrate molecules by forcing water into your GI tract. This can lead to a host of uncomfortable symptoms, including gas, bloating, pain, loose stools, and more.

This is compounded if you suffer from a condition called small intestinal bacterial overgrowth (SIBO), which occurs when the microbial communities in your small intestine are overabundant and harbor a mix of gut bugs that resembles the flora in your colon. This can happen for many reasons, such as when the valve separating your colon and your small bowel doesn't close properly[76] or if gut bugs aren't being cleared from the small bowel from lack of small intestinal movement, lack of stomach acid or pancreatic enzymes, and many other reasons.

You can imagine why this may cause problems. When you have SIBO and you eat lots of FODMAPs, the gut microbes now in your small intestine feast on these carbs and cause even more gastrointestinal distress from gas and bloating.

In my experience–remember Ted's case history from Chapter 1?–there's an intimate relationship between gut dysbiosis (including but not limited to SIBO), weight problems, gastrointestinal symptoms, and chronic conditions like irritable bowel syndrome (IBS). And I've noticed that obesity seems to predispose people with these conditions toward a poorer prognosis.[77] I've treated many patients for SIBO using a revolutionary low-FODMAP diet, which improves the condition.[78] In patients who have SIBO and who are also overweight to obese, weight loss has been a bonus on this diet. My personal experience parallels the research.

Science has demonstrated a link between SIBO and obesity.[79-82] A recent study noted that 41 percent of obese patients suffered from SIBO.[83] A 2008 study revealed that SIBO prevalence is higher in obese patients than in the normal population, concluding that "in morbidly obese patients, bacterial overgrowth prevalence is higher than in healthy subjects and is associated with severe hepatic steatosis."[84-86] It's been accepted for a decade that GI symptoms like gas, bloating, and flatulence are more prevalent and intense in overweight people.[87-89]

Another study reported a positive association between body mass index (BMI), abdominal pain, and diarrhea.[90] And it's been shown that factors that directly impact the gut microbiome (such as diet, physical activity, and body weight) influence the propensity of digestive symptoms. These observations were later corroborated by a study done on children, in which exercise, diet, and weight loss helped reverse IBS symptoms in those who were overweight.[91] Taken together, these reports confirm the higher prevalence and severity of functional digestive symptoms in overweight individuals. And they linked the observed higher prevalence of SIBO in the overweight to abnormalities in small bowel transit. Surprisingly, gastric transit has been found to be accelerated in overweight people, meaning carbs are dumped quicker into the bloodstream and there is little time for the body to send satiety signals from the gut to the brain to stop eating.

This has led Dr. Anthony Kalloo of Johns Hopkins to strategically apply intragastric Botox injections to slow down the hurried stomach in the overweight.[92]

Studies have also illustrated a complex interrelationship between SIBO and type 2 diabetes. Remember that imbalances in your gut microbiome can contribute to the development of type 2 diabetes–and vice versa. For example, diabetic neuropathy can adversely impact the nerves in the small bowel that govern your whole gut transit time–the time that it takes food to move through your GI tract (aka your "gut clock" and "cleansing wave," which we'll discuss in more detail in Chapter 10).[93]

Does this mean that if you're overweight you definitely have SIBO and/or a gut movement disorder? Not necessarily. But if you experience flatulence, gas, and bloating after meals–particularly high-starch or sugary meals–you may well have the condition. Even if you don't, it's highly probable that your gut microbiome is out of balance if you're overweight.

In either case, reducing your FODMAP intake helps reduce these symptoms.[94] By limiting these highly fermentable short-chain carbs and sugary foods that your gut bugs love to eat, you'll severely limit the food supply of these misplaced microbes and reduce their infestation of the small intestine, leaving your inner garden freshly tilled and ready to be seeded and fertilized in Phase 2.

It's important to understand that not all FODMAPs are inherently bad for us. In fact, some FODMAPs–like asparagus and artichokes–are superfoods in the right contexts, as they selectively feed the beneficial bacteria that bolster our metabolism. But if you suffer from weight problems or SIBO–or *both*–you need to initially *reduce* your intake of these foods for a short time, which will improve digestive symptoms.

For this program to be effective, you need to *reduce–not eliminate*–FODMAPs. Feeding with a limited amount of healthy gut microbiome–friendly FODMAPs has been shown to improve biodiversity.[95] The amount of FODMAPs you can consume and still remain healthy is individual, and over time you may experiment with the amount of these foods in your overall diet. For Phase 1, I recommend consuming a diet that is low in FODMAPs, as this plan will fit the most people. See the Phase 1 food plan on page 241 for my specific guidelines on what to leave out of your diet during this part of the program. Or, to make it easy on yourself, just follow my delicious, gut-balancing daily meal plan: It has been specifically tailored to optimize your FODMAP intake.

If you're interested in a more detailed discussion on SIBO, check out my book *The Inside Tract*. If you want to know more about FODMAPs, I strongly recommend *The Complete Low-FODMAP Diet* by Sue Shepherd, PhD, and Peter Gibson, MD. They're the leading world experts on the science of FODMAPs, and the book is a treasure trove of information on these tricky sugars.

Next, two special FODMAPs we'll leave out of Phase 1: gluten and dairy.

Gluten

Technically, gluten isn't a FODMAP. It's a protein found in many high-FODMAP grains, including wheat, rye, and barley, which are a special kind of oligosaccharide called fructans. Fructans are chains of fructose molecules with a glucose molecule at the end. As mentioned earlier in this chapter, these molecules cannot be digested by the human body. Only your gut flora can help you eat them, and they're a rich source of food for gut bugs. When your gut microbiome is imbalanced or gut bugs are misplaced (i.e., in the small intestine), overeating these foods can exacerbate these problems—so we'll limit them in Phase 1.

Even if you don't follow the health section of the newspaper or aren't up on the latest in nutritional science, you've certainly seen the growth of the gluten-free section in your supermarket. We're inundated with antigluten messages, and for some people gluten *is* a problem. But the story about gluten is more complex than the media would have you believe.

I've seen many people come through my clinic with adverse reactions to gluten. As a GI specialist, I'm well aware of the problems gluten causes to the inside tract—especially the small intestine—for people who have an all-out autoimmune reaction (celiac disease) or a sensitivity to the substance. About 3 million Americans are diagnosed with celiac disease, though some research suggests it may be more common than this. Dr. Peter Green, an expert on the disorder, has called it a "hidden epidemic." The data on gluten intolerance are more difficult to ascertain, as it can present as a host of symptoms that people may not connect to diet. Suffice it to say, millions of Americans have problems with gluten. I'm pleased to see a growing awareness about these problems, as it offers people who suffer from these issues much-needed affirmation.

That said, gluten isn't the one and only cause of chronic illness and weight gain in America. Not everyone is sensitive to it. And there are *no data* proving that going off wheat or gluten itself for the long term will assist with weight loss. Going off cookies, crackers, bread, and pasta—yes, this is associated with weight loss. Going off gluten, not so much. After all, there is plenty of unhealthy gluten-free junk food (refined and processed grains such as cookies, crackers, bread, pasta, and so on) on the market! And a long-term gluten-free diet presents challenges in maintaining adequate niacin, folic acid, calcium, zinc, and fiber intake.[96] Plus, there's some evidence that eliminating gluten from your diet if you're not sensitive to it could have adverse effects on your gut microbiome—particularly your levels of bifidobacteria, which foster a healthy, lean metabolism.[97, 98]

Finally, remember that at the end of the day, gluten-free cookies, crackers, cakes, bread, and pasta are still just cookies, crackers, cakes, bread, and pasta. Eating them in excess isn't healthy, doesn't do your gut microbiome any favors, and doesn't substitute for the whole, healing foods you need to achieve optimal weight and thrive.

Dairy

Milk products are high in calcium and most are enriched with vitamin D, two critical cofactors for a strong skeletal structure. They also appear to support weight loss–a number of studies show an association between calcium, vitamin D, and dairy intake and maintenance of a healthy weight.[99-102]

Fermented dairy products are high in the friendly flora you need to rebalance your gut microbiome. As you'll see in Phase 2, I'll encourage you to add plenty of probiotic-rich dairy that helps diversify the mix of friendly flora in your gut microbiome. Foods like yogurt and kefir are critical in that part of the program. If you tolerate dairy well, these can be among the most healing and helpful foods in your diet.

On Phase 1, however, we'll eliminate dairy because it's high in FODMAPs, and the sugar it contains may be rapidly fermented by gut bugs, causing gas, cramping, and even fertilization of these nasty critters. In Phase 2, we'll reintroduce dairy, mainly in a highly therapeutic probiotic form to help you reverse dysbiosis and lose weight.

Calcium and Lactose Intolerance

Dairy is the most bioavailable form of calcium in our diet. So how can you get adequate calcium if you're lactose intolerant? This can be tough, but here are some nondairy sources to consider.

Green vegetables, such as the superfoods kale, Swiss chard, and greens, are loaded with calcium. So are beets, almonds, beans, buckwheat, figs, kiwifruit, miso, potatoes, cocoa, soy, sesame seeds, and tahini. But you need to eat a lot of these foods to receive enough calcium to meet the Dietary Reference Intakes (DRIs) recommended by the USDA and the Institute of Medicine.[103] And foods that are high in fiber—or, more critically, those high in dietary phytates and phosphorus—may block calcium absorption (important to remember if you are trying to get adequate calcium from nondairy sources).

Take spinach, for example, one of the vegetables highest in calcium. One cup of cooked spinach has about 245 milligrams of calcium,[104] but not all of it is absorbed, since spinach (like many of the foods listed) is high in oxalic acid, which binds dietary calcium, preventing its absorption in the gut. You'd need to eat 5 to 6 cups of spinach daily just to meet the DRIs for calcium. That's more or less true for the rest of the veggies mentioned above.

So if you're lactose intolerant, increase the amount of these veggies in your diet and consider a high-quality calcium supplement. Dr. Sue Shepherd, who discovered the low-FODMAP approach, recommends supplementing calcium (see page 340 for specific guidelines) for those on the diet for more than 30 days.

Some people are intolerant to dairy, which contains several components that people can be sensitive to—the most common culprits are lactose, a FODMAP, and casein. Lactose is the only disaccharide in the diet that causes people problems, and the reason comes down to how much lactase (the enzyme that digests lactose) you make. If you make too little lactase, you can't digest lactose properly and are "lactose intolerant." However, this is a pretty one-dimensional term, as levels of lactase expression and the degree of intolerance vary widely. Remember, the dose makes the poison. Someone with lactase production deficiencies may tolerate a low dose of lactose products such as Cheddar cheese but become ill when eating whole milk or ice cream.

Casein is a protein in dairy products that produces symptoms in some people in similar ways gluten does. Tolerances vary, so discovering what works for you and your body is key to any long-term healthy eating plan.

As with gluten, reactions to dairy are highly individualized. And as always, the dose makes the poison in lots of cases. Some can't handle any at all. Others may be able to consume a little dairy. And for still others, dairy may not present a problem. It all depends on you. One final word: If you're dairy sensitive or intolerant, don't worry. There are plenty of nondairy probiotic-rich foods to focus on in Phase 2.

FAVOR FOODS THAT REV UP YOUR METABOLISM

So far, we've discussed lots of foods you *can't* eat during this phase of the program. At this point, you may be wondering what you *can* eat during Phase 1! Don't worry—there are plenty of delicious, healing, whole foods we'll focus on for this phase.

Talking about these healing, whole foods is my favorite part of the plan. As disciplined as this style of eating may seem, it's actually *not* about deprivation at all. It's about honoring your role as caretaker of the ecosystem inside of you and nourishing that inner garden with foods that will help it heal. When it heals, you heal, and you lose weight along the way as a perk. So reward yourself with the gift of good health by favoring these foods on Phase 1.

Appetite-Reducing Protein

Looking for a delicious appetite-reducing food that naturally builds fat-burning machinery in your body without causing huge surges in your blood sugar and insulin levels? Protein is precisely such a food. When you stick to sources free of inflammatory fats, it's among the healthiest foods you can eat. Here's why.

Lean, high-quality protein (such as wild, line-caught salmon or cod or American farm-raised tilapia; skinless poultry; eggs; wild game; and healthy vegetable sources like nuts and tofu) is extremely satiating—it naturally reduces your desire to eat. Studies have repeatedly shown that people who increase their protein intake reduce their overall caloric consumption due to protein-induced satiety.[105-108] Protein is by far the most satiating macronutrient,[109] making it a perfect place to start improving your diet for a weight-loss program like this.

This has been proven by studies at Maastricht University, which showed that increasing dietary protein promoted weight loss by increasing energy expenditure and inducing satiety.[110-112] It's likely one reason higher-protein, lower-carb diets tend to work so well, especially in the induction phase–they make you feel full longer and help you burn more calories. Here are more specifics on how it works.

Eating protein affects fullness-related hormones and gut peptides, including ghrelin, glucagon-like peptide 1, insulin, cholecystokinin, and peptide YY.[113] It also increases thermogenesis–the amount of calories you burn just by digesting your food. It takes *a lot* of energy to break down and oxidize protein, and even more to convert protein to sugar through the process called gluconeogenesis. So eating protein increases your overall metabolic rate while at rest. You burn more calories even while sitting around as your body spends energy to break down the protein in your diet.

The scientists at Maastricht demonstrated this in a groundbreaking study in which 113 people consumed a very low-energy diet for the 4–week induction, resulting in a 5 to 10 percent loss of excess body weight. Then these subjects were followed for 6 months postdiet to see if they could maintain their reduced weight. The subjects were randomly assigned to groups receiving a standard diet or a diet containing 30 grams of additional protein a day.

Both groups lost a similar amount of weight during the low-energy portion of the induction phase of the program. But the group who ate more protein in the maintenance phase (after the low-energy induction phase) preserved more weight loss and kept more inches off their waist. These people lost 7.5 percent of their body weight and were able to keep it off longer than the nonprotein group. Researchers concluded that these results could be explained by increased satiety, enhanced thermogenesis, increased sleeping metabolic rate (the rate at which you burn calories in your sleep), and improved fat oxidation.[114] Similar findings have been replicated many times in different trials by other scientists.[115, 116, 117]

The takeaway: When it comes to weight loss, maintenance is where it's at. That's what distinguishes this program. Many diets allow you to lose a few pounds for a while, but when the diet is over, you're more likely than not to gain them back and then some–pushing your body weight set point ever higher. Increasing your protein intake appears not to have this rebound weight-gain effect, an impressive fact indeed.

The type of protein you eat may produce different effects on appetite, satiety, and metabolism. Two types seem to stand head and shoulders above the rest in terms of their ability to reduce appetite: fish and whey protein.[118] Fish appears to have this effect by increasing blood levels of tryptophan, an amino acid that's a precursor and signaling molecule for serotonin (the "happy and full" neurotransmitter), which is involved in satiety.[119] And whey protein apparently not only has an impact on appetite hormones but also produces superior insulin responses and provokes a lower rise in blood glucose than other forms of protein.[120] Dairy and eggs can also be highly satiating.[121, 122]

Consider the recent meta-analysis comparing high-protein–low-carbohydrate diets, like Atkins, with high-carbohydrate–low-fat diets, such as the plan of Dr. Ornish.[123] Weight loss was significantly greater with the high-protein diets in studies lasting up to 6 months, although the differences *weren't* significant in studies spanning 12 months. There are many reasons why these effects are short lived—compliance, compensatory mechanisms, effects on the gut microbiome, and more. This further supports the fundamental precepts on which the Gut Balance Revolution is built: a short-term ketogenic diet followed by a gradual shift toward a more Mediterranean style of eating. The rationale is clear: Ketogenic diets help induce weight loss in the short term. In the long term, they are hard to maintain and may have some negative effects on the gut microbiome depending on which carbs are being permitted. Thus, gradually shifting from a very low-carb diet to a more Mediterranean style of eating (Phase 3) seems to be the key for long-term sustainable weight loss, as we'll discuss in Chapter 8.

Where's the Beef?

Given all this positive news about protein, you may be wondering why there's no red meat in the meal plans. Unfortunately, there's ample evidence that red meat (at least the hormone- and antibiotic-laden and GMO-corn-and-soy-fed type commonly found in the American marketplace) and processed meat products (like hot dogs) are associated with weight gain. Numerous studies have associated increased red meat consumption with obesity and reduced intake with improved adiposity, body weight, markers of metabolic syndrome, and inflammatory markers.[124-129] These foods are loaded with inflammatory fats (conventionally raised animals are much higher in omega-6 fatty acids) and antibiotics—which, at doses present in meats, can lead to weight gain in mice and possibly in humans.[130]

The Gut-Heart Connection

Red meat and processed meat products have also been associated with colorectal cancer—which has been increasingly linked with gut dysbiosis as a risk factor.[131] Furthermore, profiles of metabolic by-products of gut bacteria have been recently reported to help identify those with colorectal neoplasia.[132] Recent evidence also shows that disruption of gut microbiome balance caused by diets high in animal protein may be the hidden link between red meat and cardiovascular disease.[133-135] How could gut microbiome imbalance impact your heart health? To figure this out, Dr. Stanley Hazen from the Cleveland Clinic took a novel approach. He bought a George Foreman grill and started cooking up steaks and giving them away for free to hungry students. He then measured

Protein: How Much Is Too Much?

The Gut Balance Revolution is a *short-term* higher-protein ketogenic diet (Phase 1) coupled with measures to resolve dysbiosis (Phase 2) and maintain optimal weight, gut microbiome balance, and total health for life (Phase 3).

Tempted to maintain a high-protein diet for 6 months or more? There may be consequences. Groundbreaking research reported in the journal *Cell Metabolism* linked protein intakes with age and mortality in 6,381 Americans over the course of an 18-year study conducted in the United States and Italy.[136] Those ages 50 to 65 who reported a high protein intake had a 1.5-fold increase in overall mortality (analogous to the risk imposed by cigarette smoking as an independent risk factor) along with a fourfold increase in cancer death risk in the following 18 years. Among those whose protein source was heavily plant based, including nuts and legumes, the risk of death from cancer or any cause was negated. These data, along with other mounting evidence, support my recommendations about limiting antibiotic- and hormone-laden red meats, which have many cancer-related associations.

Mouse studies were performed in tandem to correlate findings in humans to mechanisms involving the growth hormone receptor (GHR)/insulin growth-factor-1 (IGF-1) involved in cell repair and proliferation, which also has the potential to support tumor cell progression, obesity, and aging. The study reported that high-protein diets in mice promoted progression of breast cancer and melanoma through GHR/IGF-1 signaling. In humans, those having high levels of GHR/IGF-1 further increased the risk of cancer and all-cause mortality in the high-protein group. The science offers a clear caution to those whose weight-loss and maintenance solution is a long-term high-protein diet.

Some doctors have expressed concern about the theoretically detrimental effect of high-protein diets on calcium balance and bone health. According to the acid-ash hypothesis, eating meat (especially red meat) creates an acidic environment in your blood, sending your pH out of balance and causing your body to "steal" minerals from your bones to buffer the acid in the meat and balance your blood pH. While it's theoretically plausible, evidence doesn't yet support it. In fact, the data paradoxically show that dietary protein increases bone mineral mass and reduces incidence of osteoporotic fracture due to calcium repletion.[137-139] So this isn't a factor I'm concerned about, especially on a 30-day ketogenic diet program.

One legitimate concern is that heavy consumption of sulfur-containing amino acids can cause a loss of nephron mass, an indicator for renal failure. That's why people with kidney insufficiency or failure shouldn't follow this diet but should consult their physician to adapt this program to their individual needs.

the students' blood for levels of a compound called trimethylamine N-oxide (TMAO). High levels of this compound correlate with an increased risk of atherosclerosis and cardiovascular events. Based on previous research he'd done in this area, Dr. Hazen guessed that these students had higher levels of TMAO because they were meat eaters. Why would meat eaters have higher levels of TMAO? It seems that those who eat meat regularly become very efficient at converting the L-carnitine in red meat to TMAO. But how did he know this metabolic shift had anything to do with changes in gut microbial balance?

To find out for sure, he took a group of the original volunteers and asked them to take a broad-spectrum antibiotic for 2 weeks and then repeat the test. On follow-up, the amount of TMAO in the group that took the antibiotic was much lower. His conclusion, corroborated in follow-up studies: Eating lots of red meat led to a *proliferation of gut bugs*, creating chemicals that increase the risk of heart disease.

On the flip side, those on a strict vegan diet, who eat no red meat for at least a year, do not produce TMAO, perhaps because this prebiotic-rich diet favorably shifts the gut microbiome away from production of TMAO and cuts down on one of its sources, L-carnitine. Another possibility is that red-meat eaters tend to consume other unhealthy foods (aka junk food) as part of the Western diet that cause dysbiosis, thus providing a source of TMAO, and underconsume items that improve gut microbial biodiversity and are prebiotic in nature (like nuts, fruits, veggies).

This idea that the Western diet can rapidly *and* adversely shift the gut microbiome has now been reproduced and published in the journals *Science* and *Nature*–two of the most highly regarded scientific publications.[140, 141] Exactly which bugs proliferate varies from study to study. But the core point here is simple: The way to someone's heart is through the gut microbiome.[142] Eating junk is like putting a dagger through the heart!

The research is clear: Eating too much conventionally raised red meat pumped full of antibiotics and high in proinflammatory omega-6 saturated fats imbalances your gut microbiome. For all these reasons and more, I've elected to eliminate conventionally raised red meat from Phase 1. You don't have to keep it under wraps forever–pasture-raised lean red meats are reintroduced in Phase 2. For now, though, shift your attention to healthy sources of protein such as eggs, fish, whey, and poultry raised without antibiotics or hormones.

Anti-Inflammatory Fats

The low-fat dietary dogma of the 1980s and '90s is being questioned. Reducing your total fat intake isn't nearly as important as balancing the types of fats you eat. The Gut Balance Revolution is not a low-fat diet. It's a *low–inflammatory fats* diet. There's a big difference.

Instead of the inflammatory oils that constitute most of the fat Americans consume, we will focus on anti-inflammatory alternatives that fight chronic illness and help you lose weight. The two most important fats we will focus on in this program are:

1. **Extra-virgin olive oil (EVOO).** It's hard to overstate the health benefits of EVOO. A 2010 Spanish study found that the cardiovascular protective effects and other health benefits of the Mediterranean diet may largely be due to olive oil.[143, 144] Investigators looked at individuals who were genetically prone to inflammation and cardiovascular disease and provided them either no dietary intervention or the Mediterranean diet with a high intake of EVOO or nuts. After 3 years, those who followed the Mediterranean diet program with EVOO had the greatest reduction of body weight. What in EVOO provides its benefits? One of the active ingredients is oleocanthal, which has been found to have similar anti-inflammatory effects to nonsteroidal anti-inflammatory medications such as ibuprofen.[145] This is one reason EVOO is a staple of the Gut Balance Revolution. There's also solid data for the use of the Mediterranean and even the Baltic Sea diet for overall health and for weight maintenance—see details in Chapter 8.

2. **Canola oil.** This unsaturated fat is higher in omega-3s and healthy omega-6s than any of the other commonly used cooking oils in the Western diet. Studies show that the aminolevulinic acid in this oil may reduce your blood pressure, balance cholesterol, and fight off inflammation.[146] Canola oil not only improves cardiovascular risks (blood lipids, inflammatory markers) but also improves insulin sensitivity.[147] The only downside: Much of the canola oil on the market is genetically modified, which I typically recommend avoiding. In any event, it should only be used in high-heat cooking, which you won't be doing much of during Phase 1.

These and the other fats allowed on this program will fend off the inflammation that keeps your gut microbiome out of balance, causes pounds to pile up, and leads you down the road to chronic illness. These healing fats are a core part of this program, and I encourage you *not* to do a "low-fat" version of this diet. The total amount of fat you consume will be well within healthy limits, and it will help cool off your body while melting away pounds. This is one reason low-fat diets are *not* successful in the long term. You are starving your body of the very essential anti-inflammatory fats that you need to fight inflammation and prevent disease. Yes, the calories in/calories out approach to weight loss makes it look attractive to cut calorie-expensive fat from the diet, but in the long term, this is counterproductive.

Healing Carbs

Carbohydrates are among the healthiest foods on the planet. I'm not talking about cookies, cakes, crackers, rice, potatoes, and their ilk. I'm talking about low-glycemic fruits and vegetables packed with healthy phytonutrients that heal your body and nourish your gut microbiome. There may be no easier way to improve your overall health than to increase the amount of fruits and vegetables you eat each day. Good evidence shows that increasing your intake of veggies reduces your risk of heart attack, stroke, and more. For example, the Harvard-based Nurses' Health Study—one of the largest and longest nutrition studies ever—shows that people who ate more than eight daily servings of vegetables were 30 percent less likely to have a heart attack or stroke.[148] No one ever became overweight or ill by eating too much kale and raspberries. In fact, these are highly therapeutic superfoods included throughout this program.

There's only one tiny caveat to the "fruits and veggies are the healthiest foods on the planet" argument: Some fruits and veggies are high in FODMAPs. Remember, that doesn't mean they're unhealthy. They're highly fermentable and help bacteria grow—and some are selective for friendly flora (called prebiotics), which we'll discuss in Chapter 6. Suffice it to say that we need to minimize these whole foods–based FODMAPs for a short time while your inner garden is being rebalanced.

On this phase of the program, we'll load up on the veggies and some fruits, but we'll stick to those that are lower in FODMAPs. As long as these low-FODMAP vegetables aren't breaded, creamed, or fried, they're allowed on the program. But we'll especially favor low-FODMAP fruits and veggies that nourish your body while giving your gut microbiome a chance to *reboot* itself. For details on which fruits and veggies to favor and which to eat fewer of, see the Phase 1 food chart starting on page 241.

A Few Other Dietary Tips for Phase I

Just a few more notes, then you're on your way to tilling the soil of your gut microbiome and losing weight.

Soups

I love soup, and not only because it reminds me of home. Good data show it supports weight loss because it increases satiety.[149] To understand why, you need to know about a concept called energy density.

The energy density of foods is defined as the amount of energy per unit weight of food. Adding water to foods influences energy density, because it adds weight without calories. Soup has quite a lot of water but very few calories (unless it is cream based), so it's low on the energy density scale. This is important, because low–energy density foods have been shown to reduce weight, lower BMI, and reduce overall caloric consumption. Scientists now believe this is why eating a salad or a soup before a meal tends to reduce your overall food intake. The low–energy density soup or salad satiates you without adding too many calories, so you consume less food over the course of the meal, particularly when the soup includes a vegetable puree.

In one study, scientists covertly added pureed veggies into various soups, then compared the energy intake of those who got the veggie puree against a control group who ate the same soup without the puree. The vegetable puree group naturally ate about

202 fewer calories daily than their peers who ate the puree-free soup. Good news for those who want to lose weight.

Warm, filling, nourishing soups will keep you satisfied for hours, so you'll find many outstanding soup recipes in the meal plans in Chapter 11. I encourage you to indulge in these nourishing, comforting, healing, weight-loss-supporting dishes.

Water

The average human is 60 to 75 percent water. Every one of the cells in your body depends on water for life and health—yet many of us don't drink enough. Make sure you're hydrated by drinking a minimum of 64 ounces of water daily. Carbonated beverages shouldn't replace water, as they may lead to the consumption of more food. So avoid carbonated water and stick with plain, flat, filtered tap water.

There's evidence that increased water consumption benefits weight-loss efforts. Investigators at the Berlin School of Public Health systematically analyzed the world's literature on this subject and found that 11 studies met their strict criteria for review.[150] Those dieters who consumed more than 1 liter of water a day were found to lose more weight than those who drank less. And those who drank 2 cups of water before a meal lost 4 pounds more than those who didn't. The mechanisms by which water consumption improves weight loss are unclear.

The School Nutrition Association in 2010 reported that in the United States a stunning 30 to 40 percent of daily calories is consumed as beverages, with 144 calories of high glycemic soft drinks and fruit juices.[151, 152] A can of regular soda contains about 140 calories of added sugar—about 7 percent of total daily energy needs, based on a 2,000-calorie diet. The report showed that water accounted for only 35 percent of US beverage consumption. Swapping zero-calorie water for high-calorie, sugary beverages is a good way to jump-start weight loss.

Snacks

Developing a healthy relationship with food means eating when you're hungry. Sometimes, that means having a meal; other times, it means having a snack. Tune in to your hunger signals and try to follow them to guide your eating. I've incorporated snacks into the meal plans, but to give you a better sense of how and when to snack, here are some guidelines.

1. **Eat three meals and two snacks.** This is a good guideline, not a hard-and-fast rule. The key is to keep your appetite and blood sugar from moving wildly up and down like a roller coaster. Most of us can do this by sticking with three squares and one or two snacks in between.

2. **Don't graze.** Snacking and grazing are different things. It's fine to have a small snack between meals to stabilize your blood sugar and reduce your appetite. Eating small amounts of food all day long is *not*. This just keeps your blood sugar and

insulin levels elevated throughout the day, setting off negative hormonal and metabolic effects. So snack, but don't graze.

3. **Go for a handful of low-FODMAP nuts and fruits**. Here's how to make the easiest, most nutritious gut-microbiome-balancing snack in the world: Consult the Phase 1 food charts on pages 241–256. Select your favorite low-FODMAP nuts (mine are walnuts). Grab a piece of your favorite low-FODMAP fruit (I love blueberries). Enjoy!

Alcohol

The question comes up in my clinic all the time: *Can I drink alcohol? Just a little red wine?* No doubt a little alcohol can be one of the joys of life, and good data have clearly shown that red wine, in particular, can help people live healthier[153] and longer.[154, 155] But add a little more and all kinds of negative consequences occur, including an imbalanced gut microbiome.[156] So avoid alcohol for 30 days in Phase 1. We'll add it back in during Phase 2.

Coffee

More than 60 percent of Americans drink coffee, most for that early-morning boost or to overcome the afternoon slump. But does the beverage have any health benefits? *Yes.* There are so many health benefits that coffee is now recognized by many as a superfood. In fact, I list coffee as a superfood for Phase 3, where I discuss all the latest research about its health benefits.

This is good news, because most of us don't want to give up our morning cup of joe, but it doesn't quite tell the whole story about the coffee bean. While there's evidence that coffee is healthy, excessive amounts may lead to significant problems, including acid reflux and other GI symptoms, insomnia, anxiety, aggregate arrhythmias, and high blood pressure.

So if you keep coffee in your diet, drink it in moderation—no more than one or two cups daily. Skip the cream and sugar and opt for a dash of anti-inflammatory and fat-burning cinnamon, cocoa powder, or nutmeg instead. Organic decaf is okay, too, if you prefer it. The organic processing averts exposure to potentially harmful organochemical solvents.[157]

One final note on coffee: If you rely on it to get through your day, you may want to rethink this policy. In many cases, coffee is used to compensate for a sleep debt, and as we'll see in the lifestyle section in Chapter 10, lack of sleep is strongly associated with—and is a possible cause of—weight gain, obesity, and a host of health problems. We shouldn't need stimulants to get through the day, and you'll find you don't need to when you rebalance your gut microbiome.

There's quite a bit to digest in this chapter (yes, the pun is intended). But there's a way to make it easy on yourself: Just stick to the Gut Balance Revolution meal plans and recipes in Chapter 11. These meals follow rigorous nutritional guidelines, they're easy to make (most take as little as 15 minutes), and they are so scrumptious you can even invite your foodie friends over to partake. Losing weight and getting healthy have never been more delicious.

What You Can Expect During Phase I

Phase 1 is designed to help you till the soil of your gut microbiome and kick-start your metabolism. Follow these steps to lose weight and feel healthier. It won't happen overnight, but it will happen. This phase will begin the process of rebalancing your gut microbiome, reduce systemic inflammation, help rebalance your blood sugar, banish chronic symptoms you've experienced for years, renew vigor, and set the stage for lifelong vibrant health.

The first few days may be hard. That's normal. Some people experience "withdrawal symptoms," including irritability, grumpiness, fatigue, headaches, and possibly others. This is more likely to be a problem if you've been eating a lot of carbs and drinking lots of coffee and if your inner garden is more like a cesspool. If that's the case, you have the most to gain by sticking with this plan. For most people, these symptoms begin to fade after a few days, and from there on out their energy increases, their symptoms decrease, and they lose weight.

No one can guarantee how much weight you'll lose in the first 30 days of any diet as individual responses will vary. I'm comfortable saying many of you may lose as much as 15 pounds after the first month on the Gut Balance Revolution. It could be more for some, less for others. Everyone is different. Biochemical individuality and personalized medicine will, in my opinion, be the hallmark of 21st-century medicine. The goal is not to lose as much weight as fast as you can. Programs that promise that tend to fail in the long run. It's far more important to achieve a slow, sustained burn, where you see a steady drop in weight, an increase in energy, and a reduction in symptoms over time.

So don't focus too much on the numbers. I'm all for weighing yourself, but don't obsess about it. Focus instead on how your clothes fit, how your belly feels, and how energetic you feel. Pay attention to symptoms that disappear and how your overall body and brain perform. These are the real signs that your gut microbiome is healing. The weight loss will come.

LOOKING AHEAD

That covers all the dietary basics for your first 30 days on the program. But before we move on to Phase 2, I want to take all of this a step further by teaching you about a few superfoods that will supercharge your success on Phase 1. That's what the next chapter is about.

CHAPTER 5

Rev Up Your Metabolism with Dr. Gerry's Top 10 Superfoods for Phase 1

"Let medicine be thy food, and food be thy medicine." These words of Hippocrates, the father of Western medicine, are as true today as they were when first spoken more than 20 centuries ago. In fact, growing evidence shows that certain "superfoods" support weight loss and optimal health, while other foods (like sugar and processed carbs) are metabolic poisons that hamper weight loss and contribute to chronic illness. While there's no standard definition of a superfood, most agree that they constitute special, nutrient-rich foods that provide disease-fighting properties and are especially good for overall health and well-being.

I not only want you to lose weight on this program. My dream for you is much bigger than that. I want you to achieve optimal health, rebalance your gut microbiome, build resilience, and protect yourself from the chronic illness epidemic that ravages America today. That's why on each phase of the program, I ask you to focus on integrating into your diet some key superfoods that will rev up your metabolism, help you heal your body, and nourish your inner ecosystem. For each of the three phases of the Gut Balance Revolution, I'll highlight my top 10 favorite superfoods, plus award some honorable mentions. These foods are featured in the gut-balancing meal plans in Chapter 11. In Chapter 4, I provided a Phase 1 food pyramid to help you visualize the preferences and priorities of foods and in your diet. I'll do this for each phase. Favor these superfoods, and your gut microbiome (and your health!) will thank you for it.

I. EGGS

No food has gotten such an undeservedly bad reputation as eggs. Fear of this food evolved in the 1980s, when doctors were concerned that the cholesterol in eggs might increase overall cholesterol levels in the body. As it turns out, this idea was never founded on scientific principles; it became a myth that was perpetuated for decades.

The effect of dietary cholesterol on blood cholesterol has never been clear. The kind of cholesterol found in eggs is different from that in the human body, so it's entirely possible eggs have zero effect on your cholesterol levels. Even if they did, we now know that the story behind cholesterol is far more complicated than we previously realized–raising total cholesterol isn't nearly as important a risk factor in heart disease as raising low-density lipoproteins (LDL) and a subclass of LDL called LDL pattern B. These lipoproteins contain relatively high amounts of cholesterol and are associated with an increased risk of atherosclerosis and coronary artery disease.

Eggs are actually a superprotein. They contain all nine of the essential amino acids your body needs to thrive. It's been shown repeatedly that people who eat eggs for breakfast feel fuller longer, reduce their overall daily caloric consumption, and lose weight. A study published in the *Journal of the American College of Nutrition* reported that overweight women who ate eggs rather than bagels for breakfast had greater feelings of satiety and a reduced appetite and consumed fewer calories throughout the day and for the next 36 hours.[1]

Two compelling studies from St. Louis University show that an egg breakfast is superior to a caloric and energy density–matched bagel breakfast. The first study, reported in 2005, compared egg (18.3 grams of protein) and bagel (13.5 grams of protein) breakfasts. The egg breakfast increased satiety and reduced energy intake at lunch, with no rebound increase in energy intake in the 24-hour period following.[2] In the second study, reported in 2008, scientists provided two groups of obese participants with an isocaloric breakfast consisting of either two eggs or a bagel for at least 5 days per week for 8 weeks. The egg breakfast group showed a 61 percent greater reduction in body mass index (BMI), a 65 percent greater weight loss, a 34 percent greater reduction in waist size, and a 16 percent greater reduction in percent body fat.[3]

A 2010 study, looking at blood chemistry, confirmed these findings in a randomized crossover design in which subjects served as their own controls. The results were shocking! Participants consumed fewer calories after the egg breakfast compared with the bagel breakfast, which carried over for the next 24 hours. Bagel consumers were hungrier and less satisfied 3 hours after breakfast compared with egg eaters. The bagel eaters had higher levels of blood glucose, ghrelin (a hunger-stimulating hormone), and insulin.[4] These findings suggest that eating eggs for breakfast results in stabilized glucose and insulin, a suppressed appetite (due to the ghrelin response), and reduced energy intake.

Think skipping breakfast is the solution? Think again! A study published in the *American Journal of Clinical Nutrition* looked at this issue to see if skipping breakfast was associated with alterations in appetite, food motivation and rewards, and snacking behavior in overweight girls. A 6-day randomized crossover study was performed on 20 overweight young women with an average age of 19.1 years. For their morning meal, they ate a high-protein breakfast or a normal-protein breakfast or none at all. On the 7th day, participants underwent biochemical testing and responded to questionnaires. The high-protein breakfast was associated with appetite suppression, lowered ghrelin, raised peptide YY (which lowers appetite), and even decreased evening snacking.[5] The normal-protein breakfast, while associated with better satiety than breakfast skipping, didn't alter appetite hormones as did the high-protein breakfast. The takeaway: Eggs are a superbreakfast loaded with protein and nutrients. Bagels are empty calories–bad carbs that turn quickly into sugar and spike insulin levels, which drives fat accumulation.

Studies consistently show that eating a protein-rich breakfast lowers appetite throughout the day. Your best bet is to eat more calories while you are physically active–so that egg breakfast offers a perfect combination.[6]

Do eggs have a role in the lunch menu? You bet! Eggs are an all-star protein source to consider at any meal or snack, as you'll see in your meal plans for all three phases. A 2011 study analyzed the results of eating three different lunches–an omelet, a baked potato, and a chicken sandwich. The omelet was found to be more satiating than the potato or chicken meal, and the energy intake at dinner was not significantly different between the three–there was no rebound increased consumption at dinner after a greater satiety response at lunch.

But the benefits of eggs aren't reserved to weight loss alone. They also support cardio-vascular function and brain health and protect your liver due to the high levels of choline and phosphatidylcholine they contain. Eggs are also good for your eyes, since they're high in two superstar eye nutrients, zeaxanthin and lutein. So embrace the lowly egg and reintroduce it to its proper place as a staple in your diet.

2. CHIA SEEDS

Looking for a plant food packed with healthy anti-inflammatory fats, high-quality protein, and fiber to help you feel fuller longer? Something loaded with antioxidants to protect against heart disease and type 2 diabetes, lower blood lipids, and possibly ease the inflammation of arthritis?[7, 8]

Look no further than the humble chia seed. Chia has been used as a medicinal food in Central and South America and across many cultures to prevent diabetes, obesity, and cardiovascular disease. Many studies support these traditional uses.[9-11] The chia seed is rich in omega-3 and anti-inflammatory omega-6 fatty acids, flavonols, and phenolic acids, which provide many health benefits. Chia oil is particularly high in polyunsaturated fatty acids (omega-3s), which account for its potent cholesterol-lowering effect.[12] A mere tablespoon of this powerful plant food packs a walloping 2,500 milligrams of omega-3 fatty acids, 4.5 grams of fiber, 3 grams of protein, and a boatload of phytonutrients. And it's one of the few seeds considered low FODMAP, so it's a perfect fit for Phase 1—yet it still has relatively high levels of soluble fiber, making it a top food for Phases 2 and 3 as well. Use ground chia in your morning shakes to up your intake of healthy fats. Sprinkle it on salads to add a little crunch at lunch. Chia is the gluten-free gem that's been used as a superfood to bolster the health benefits of breakfast bars, yogurts, cereals, salad dressings, and other products in the food industry.

3. CINNAMON

This beloved zero-calorie medicinal spice comes with a bevy of healthy benefits pertinent to weight control and the complications of being overweight.[13] One USDA study showed that as little as $1/4$ teaspoon of cinnamon daily lowered blood sugar, cholesterol, triglycerides, and LDL in type 2 diabetics.[14, 15] It's also a fat-burning powerhouse that boosts metabolism and has been proven to help your body block the absorption of glucose and enhance the action of insulin to clear sugar from your blood.

Cinnamon is one of the most powerful antioxidant spices and an anti-inflammatory agent that counteracts the effects of obesity. It's been shown to slow gastric emptying, which stabilizes blood sugar by slowing its transit into the small intestine, its principal site of absorption. Remember that overweight and obese people often have poor satiety mechanisms and faster gastric emptying of food, so they tend to dump loads of sugar into the bloodstream, inducing a surge of insulin release by the pancreas, which facilitates fat accumulation. So cinnamon is a clear winner for these folks. Research also shows that cinnamon slows the rate of gastric emptying and stabilizes aftermeal blood glucose in healthy subjects.[16] Adding 6 grams of cinnamon to rice pudding significantly delayed gastric emptying and lowered blood sugar levels after the meal—one reason cinnamon is an excellent addition to the diet for overweight individuals.[17-19]

Cinnamon is also a powerful antimicrobial agent that works against a number of pathogenic gut microbes, making this a top spice as a Phase 1 superfood.[20] So add cinnamon to your daily cup of coffee or sprinkle it on the low-FODMAP fruits allowed in Phase 1 for a tasty snack or luscious dessert.

4. BERRIES

Berries are my favorite sweet treat for Phase 1. They're powerful foods rich in disease-fighting polyphenols such as anthocyanins, flavan-3-ols, procyanidins, flavonols, ellagitannins, and hydroxycinnamates.[21] These compounds provide many cardiovascular protective benefits, including improved endothelial function, reduced blood lipids, decreased arterial stiffness, and reduced blood pressure.[22] These effects are particularly notable in cranberries, strawberries, and blueberries. Fermented blueberry products such as wine are strongly anti-inflammatory (enjoy it in limited amounts in Phase 2).

Blueberry juice has been shown to prevent obesity in mice due to the heart-healthy anthocyanins just mentioned.[23, 24] Blueberries are also low on the glycemic index, strongly anti-inflammatory, and even fight cancer![25, 26]

Blueberries can help you lose weight, too. A study with obese rats found that blueberry peel extract reduced body-weight gain and inhibited fat accumulation in these animals.[27] This had nothing to do with reduced food intake but rather occurred by downregulating fat-influencing genes–factors that included a key adipose cell transcriptional regulator (read: fat-maker signaling molecule) called perixosome proliferator-activated receptor.[28] So a few blueberries can actually send your cells and your genes messages that say, "Let's stop making so much fat."

Blueberries also inhibit fat cell growth and differentiation.[29] When rats with metabolic syndrome from eating high amounts of fructose (sound familiar?) were fed blueberry pomace, they lost weight and their leptin levels were reduced more than control groups'.[30] These effects are further supported by studies showing blueberry phenols have anti-diabetic effects and improve insulin sensitivity in obese, nondiabetic, insulin-resistant people.[31, 32] A similar antidiabetic effect has been described for bilberry extracts.[33]

Another perk of berries is their ability to favorably alter gut microbiome balance. They selectively inhibit the growth of some ferocious pathogens such as salmonella, staphylococcus, and listeria.[34] In particular, blueberry husks have a prebiotic effect–their fermentation by our friendly flora becomes particularly important for Phases 2 and 3. In fact, blueberries are a superfood for all phases. They are low in FODMAPs and have a low-glycemic impact, yet they're extremely anti-inflammatory, making them perfect for Phase 1. Their antimicrobial effects and prebiotic power make them awesome for Phase 2. And they're insulin sensitizing while stifling the growth of fat cells–and that's what we want in Phase 3.

Raspberries are another example of a low-FODMAP plant food that's high in fiber and phytonutrients while being rich in flavor. One cup of raspberries contains an amazing 8 grams of fiber–a dose your friendly bacteria will love. They're packed with vitamins and nutrients like calcium, magnesium, phosphorus, potassium, and vitamin C.

The anthocyanins that give the berries their beautiful color are COX-2 enzyme inhibitors–powerful anti-inflammatories shown to fight systemic inflammation, reducing C-reactive protein (a primary marker of inflammation) levels. The anti-inflammatory effects are so strong that a beneficial biochemical called ellagic acid found in red raspberries was able to protect animals from chemical-induced colitis (an inflammatory bowel disorder).[35] Raspberries also reduce blood sugar and insulin response when consuming other starches.[36] This gives you an edge in your fight against heart disease, type 2 diabetes, and weight gain. Try berries sprinkled with cinnamon and a little crushed chia seed for a spectacular superdessert or as part of the Blueberry Protein Smoothie on page 276.

5. GREEN TEA

After water, tea is the most frequently consumed beverage in the world. It's produced from the leaves of the *Camellia sinensis* plant, typically classified by degree of fermentation. Black tea (fermented) is predominantly consumed in Western countries. Oolong tea (partially fermented) is primarily consumed in southern China and Taiwan. And green tea (unfermented) is mainly consumed in Asia. All types of tea are rich in flavonoids. Catechins are the main flavonoids in green tea, while black tea mainly contains chemicals called theaflavins and thearubigins.[37] The polyphenols in green tea, such as epigallocatechin gallate (EGCG) and epicatechin gallate, which are responsible for its beneficial effects (including its antioxidant potential and antimutagenic capacity), are converted into thearubigins and theaflavins during the fermentation process that creates black tea.

Many studies link green tea to enhanced weight loss, plus a number of health benefits worth mentioning.[38] Green tea—along with another superfood, cocoa, and the new kid on the superfood block, coffee—provides cardiovascular protective properties including stroke prevention. The flavonoids and polyphenols in green tea improve endothelial function and lower total and LDL cholesterol as well as decrease the risk of stroke.[39, 40] Green tea extract reduces blood pressure, inflammatory biomarkers, and oxidative stress; stabilizes blood sugar; and improves parameters associated with insulin resistance in obese hypertensive patients.[41, 42]

When it comes to weight loss and fat-burning, green tea has a number of benefits that make it and black tea and coffee attractive superbeverages for a lean metabolism. The caffeine in green tea enhances energy expenditure and fat oxidation by activating the sympathetic nervous system, while the polyphenols counteract the reflex decrease in the resting metabolic rate that usually accompanies weight loss.[43]

Two meta-analyses evaluated 49 studies for the effect of green tea and its extracts on weight regulation. Overall, caffeinated green tea was found to promote and maintain weight loss.[44, 45] A third meta-analysis that evaluated 15 studies with 1,243 patients confirmed that caffeinated green tea was associated with enhanced weight loss, reduced waist circumference, and lower body mass index (BMI).[46]

How much tea should you drink for these effects? My recommendation: Shoot for two to three cups of caffeinated green tea daily.

Green tea appears to have a prebiotic effect, too—it helps support the growth of the fat-burning friendly flora. Green tea powder in combination with a single strain of *Lactobacillus plantarum* promoted growth of lactobacillus in the intestine and attenuated high-fat diet-induced inflammation.[47] Green tea catechins also decrease fat absorption and affect short-chain fatty acid production—by-products of fermentation that improve the health of your GI tract in a variety of ways and are involved in the regulation of satiety hormones, energy expenditure, and fatty acid oxidation.[48-50] In a clinical trial of 14 healthy volunteers, 1.3 cups of green tea was shown to improve satiety.[51]

Now, I'm not saying it's okay to have a Big Mac with fries—and a cup of green tea to neutralize your (un)happy meal. But I encourage you to use superbeverages like green tea, black tea, and even coffee as therapeutic drinks to melt the fat away. They have a powerful thermogenic effect, revving up your body's fat-burning machinery.

6. GINGER

Zingiber officinale, commonly known as garden ginger, is an important spice with myriad health benefits. This piquant spice has been used in Ayurvedic and traditional Chinese medicine since the inception of those therapies. Ginger is often referred to as the "universal remedy." What ancient medical practitioners knew instinctively about ginger is now being borne out by science.

Evidence suggests that ginger consumption has anti-inflammatory, antihypertensive, glucose-sensitizing, and stimulating effects on the gastrointestinal tract.[52] The rhizomes have been used for centuries for the treatment of arthritis, rheumatism, sprains, muscular aches, pains, sore throats, cramps, hypertension, dementia, fever, infectious diseases, catarrh, nervous diseases, gingivitis, toothache, asthma, stroke, and diabetes.[53] The anti-inflammatory and antioxidant effects of ginger are very strong—as powerful as common nonsteroidal anti-inflammatory medications (NSAIDs).[54, 55] The antioxidant activity of ginger extracts lasts even after boiling for 30 minutes at 212°F, indicating that the spice's constituents are resistant to thermal denaturation. So you can cook with ginger and still receive health benefits.[56]

The anti-inflammatory effect of ginger as a first-line agent in the treatment of rheumatoid arthritis (RA) was suggested in an animal model of RA. In the study, a ginger-turmeric rhizomes mixture was found to be superior to the drug indomethacin against RA severity and complications.[57]

You probably realize why this is important: Inflammation leads to weight gain and is a major contributor to just about all chronic illness. So cooling down the fire-promoting enzymes and biochemicals is priority number one for optimal weight and health.

Ginger may also reduce your body weight! The structural composition of gingerols is similar to the molecular composition of capsaicin (see Cayenne Pepper, page 86, suggesting it may have similar effects on weight loss. When gingerols are injected into the paws of animals, increased thermogenesis occurs,[58] probably because gingerols, like capsaicin, activate our "fight-or-flight" sympathetic nervous system that, in turn, increases thermogenesis and fat oxidation.[59] One study found that giving men grains of paradise, a species of the ginger family, activated brown adipose tissue and increased whole-body energy.[60] This is a critical point, as brown adipose tissue is one of two types of fat (the other being white adipose tissue) that is metabolically active, with white tissue supporting inflammation and insulin resistance and brown tissue supporting enhanced thermogenesis and energy loss by boosting metabolism. So the fact that ginger activates brown adipose tissue is a major perk.

An intriguing study from the Institute of Human Nutrition at Columbia University assessed the effects of a hot ginger beverage on energy expenditure, feelings of appetite and satiety, and metabolic risk factors in 10 overweight men in a randomized placebo-controlled crossover trial.[61] The results were impressive. Investigators reported ginger significantly increased the thermic effect of food (the process of heat production and release in the body–a form of energy expenditure), lowered hunger, lowered prospective food intake, and increased feelings of fullness. Additional studies are needed to confirm these findings.[62]

A recent study evaluated changes in body composition, blood pressure, lipid profile, and testosterone in 49 faculty, staff, and students participating in a 3-week low-energy dietary intervention (women ate 1,200 to 1,400 calories; men 1,600 to 1,800 calories).[63] The program consisted of a green drink superfood blend. In the second week of the study, a "cleanse" supplement loaded with anti-inflammatory nutrients was added.* This was replaced with prebiotic and probiotic supplements in week 3. The group lost an average of 8.7 pounds and as much as 14.2 pounds–well beyond that expected with a low-energy diet alone–yet another reason to give up the calories in/calories out rhetoric of the past. Even more important, total cholesterol, LDL cholesterol, and blood pressure were reduced, while both waist and hip circumferences diminished. Overall, the 13 men in this study also experienced an increase in testosterone. This study raised some eyebrows about the possible connections between accelerated weight loss, improvements in serum cholesterol, improved male sex hormone levels, and how all of this may be connected to the anti-inflammatory, gut microbiome restorative nature of the program.

Another interesting study compared the efficacy of ginger and orlistat on obesity management in male albino rats.[64] Orlistat is an FDA-approved medication used for promoting weight loss in obese individuals by interfering with the activities of the fat-digesting enzyme lipase made in the tongue, stomach, and pancreas. Inhibiting lipase causes fat to be excreted from the body instead of absorbed and stored, leading to weight loss but also to foul-smelling stools and other possible complications. In the study, ginger was shown to have a greater ability to reduce body weight than orlistat without inhibiting lipase. Ginger supplementation was also reported to significantly raise heart-healthy HDL cholesterol. In fact, ginger had a greater effect in increasing HDL cholesterol than orlistat. The ginger provided all of the benefits and none of the side effects.

---

* The "cleanse" contained magnesium, chia seed, flaxseed, lemon, camu camu, cat's claw, bentonite clay, turmeric, pau d'arco, chanca piedra, stevia, zeolite clay, slippery elm, garlic, ginger, peppermint, aloe, citrus bioflavonoids, and fulvic acid.

There are many gastroprotective effects of ginger worth mentioning, since many people who are overweight tend to suffer from digestive distress (refer to Chapter 4). Scientific studies have validated that ginger can be used as a home remedy to improve many of these digestive complaints, including constipation, dyspepsia, belching, bloating, epigastric discomfort, indigestion, and nausea. Ginger has also been shown to be effective in preventing gastric ulcers induced by NSAIDs.

In my digestive health practice, I've found ginger to be a wonderful tool for managing upset stomach and other digestive complaints. If you suffer from these symptoms, try adding a little ginger to your stir-fry. Or steep it in a cup of hot water for a delicious ginger tea. It will calm your stomach as it helps you burn fat.

7. AVOCADO

Avocados are one of the rare foods containing high amounts of healthy anti-inflammatory fats, a decent amount of protein, tons of healing phytonutrients, and a magnificent amount of fiber (11 to 17 grams per avocado!)—all in one convenient package, keeping you feeling fuller longer than many other foods.

Avocado oil is especially high in monounsaturated fatty acids (MUFAs) and very low in saturated fats. This superfood is particularly rich in an omega-9 fat called oleic acid, a MUFA that has been shown to quiet hunger. Additionally, MUFA-rich diets help protect against abdominal fat accumulation and diabetic health complications.[65] Clinical studies conclude that avocado consumption supports cardiovascular health in a number of ways, most prominently by its beneficial effects on serum lipids. Avocados can fit into a heart-healthy dietary pattern such as the Dietary Approaches to Stop Hypertension (DASH) diet plan and the Mediterranean diet, as emphasized in Phase 3. A randomized single-blind crossover study showed that as little as half an avocado a day may reduce hunger and increase overall levels of satisfaction. Scientists asked overweight adults to add approximately one-half a Hass avocado to their lunch meal,[66] which was found to significantly enhance postmeal satisfaction and reduce the desire to eat for up to 5 hours. Avocados also have a beneficial effect on blood cholesterol levels, likely due to the fruit's high beta-sitosterol levels, a chemical that blocks cholesterol absorption. Plus, they've been proven to benefit eye health because they're high in leutin and zeaxanthin, and the strong antioxidant content protects against skin wrinkling.[67, 68]

Probably the main reason people don't think of avocados as a weight-loss food is due to their caloric content. This idea is founded on the calories in/calories out theory of weight loss, which we now know is obsolete. When people eat avocados, they tend to consume *fewer* calories throughout the day because they feel fuller—a net gain. Spend a few calories on avocados and you'll save more calories in the long run. Mix up some guacamole or cut an avocado in half and add a little salt, pepper, and lime juice for a perfect flora-friendly snack.

8. QUINOA

Pronounced KEEN-wah, this helpful whole grain is underused (and unknown by many) in this country. Interestingly, it's been around since the time of the Incas, who called it the "mother of grains"–a name it no doubt deserves based on its nutritional profile. It's got a good dose of fiber (5 grams per serving) and has a low-glycemic impact. Quinoa is high in magnesium, which is a key regulator of energy and promotes good blood sugar control. It's also rich in potassium and iron, along with other key nutrients involved in energy production, such as riboflavin and manganese.

Gluten-free quinoa is one of the few whole grains low in FODMAPs, which is one of the reasons I've included it in this phase. This healing whole grain is also high in protein, another reason for its inclusion here. Another perk: It's filling. A study at the University of Milan showed that quinoa has a satiating effect–the highest among the gluten-free grains.[69]

Two cautions: First, quinoa is coated with saponin, a potentially toxic, bitter-tasting chemical.[70] So rinse it thoroughly before cooking–rinsing doesn't diminish the nutritional benefits of quinoa.[71] Second, be aware that this superfood is high in oxalates, which could be a problem for folks who tend to form oxalate kidney stones.

Throughout this program, I've tried to focus on "normal" foods you can find in any supermarket. Quinoa takes us a little off the beaten path, but it's becoming more widely available. Try adding it to your diet to replace other whole grains during this phase. Unless kidney stones are an issue for you, I recommend that you include this filling, wholesome grain in your Phase 1 meal plans and beyond.

9. CAYENNE PEPPER

Cayenne pepper is a member of the *Capsicum* genus of vegetables, along with chile peppers and bell peppers. This spicy pepper adds zest to tasty meals mainly through a family of compounds called capsaicinoids. The compound responsible for this hot taste is known as capsaicin. The amount of capsaicin in the chile pepper directly correlates with the sensation of heat–more capsaicin results in a hotter chile pepper. It also means a healthier chile pepper.

Capsaicin has loads of health benefits due to its anti-inflammatory and antioxidant capacity. Many studies document its cardiovascular benefits–it can lower triglycerides and cholesterol, decrease platelet aggregation, and enhance the body's ability to break up small blood clots.[72, 73] However, two studies show high doses in pill form may lead to myocardial infarction.[74, 75] Stay away from capsaicin supplements–take it in its wholefoods form instead. Again, the dose makes the poison!

Although many think of hot pepper as a cause of stomach ulcers, capsaicin actually prevents their formation. It's also an inhibitor of a molecule called substance P, which mediates pain in nerve endings.[76, 77] Studies have shown that topical application of capsaicin ointment improves pain relief in diabetic neuropathy, postherpetic neuralgia, and neuropathic pain.[78] Despite the popular use of capsaicin as a topical application for arthritis, there are conflicting data regarding its efficacy.[79] Capsaicin has also been reported to have anticancer properties.[80]

Chile pepper has long been associated with weight loss, and the data show that a little can help you burn away unwanted pounds.[81] Capsaicin lights up your fat-burning metabolism as few other spices can, in part because it triggers your stress hormone response system. When your sympathetic nervous system (also known as the fight-or-flight response) is activated, hormones called catecholamines, such as epinephrine and norepinephrine, are released into the bloodstream. This process increases thermogenesis, whereby fat is oxidized more effectively. That means your fat becomes fuel for your metabolic fire in as few as 20 minutes after eating cayenne.[82] Just eat a little chile pepper and, 20 minutes later, you're burning fat like a champ. This thermogenic effect isn't unique to capsaicin. As you may recall, we discussed enhanced thermogenesis and fat-burning when we talked about caffeinated green tea. The same is true for ginger, as well as a few supplements such as bitter orange and guar gum.[83, 84] Capsaicin also seems to promote satiety.[85] What a perfect combination for weight loss—burn more fat calories while feeling less hungry!

A recent meta-analysis identified 68 studies evaluating the potential role of capsaicin in weight management.[86] An impressive 13 of 15 trials reported an increase in postconsumption energy expenditure, 7 of 11 showed increased lipid oxidation and decreased fat stores, and 5 of 7 trials confirmed capsaicin's effect on suppressed appetite. However, the most impressive evidence for capsaicin's effects on weight loss showed an increased energy expenditure of at least 50 calories daily when cayenne pepper was used as an accent spice—that adds up to 5 to 7 pounds of fat loss a year just by adding a dash of this spice to one meal daily!

10. WHEY PROTEIN

Have you ever seen whey protein on a list of superfoods? Probably not. This food is undervalued by many, which is a shame. It's a superprotein if there ever was one.

Whey is a lactose-free milk-derived protein, typically well tolerated by those with lactose intolerance. It's also free of casein, the other dairy component that many are sensitive to. (Dairy product proteins are typically 80 percent casein and 20 percent whey.) This makes whey a safe form of protein for most folks who are dairy sensitive. But if you're one of the rare few who is sensitive to the whey component of dairy (or you simply don't like it), you might try a rice, hemp, or pea protein substitute.

Compared with other foods, whey protein contains the highest concentrations of branched-chain amino acids, especially leucine, which preserves fat-burning muscle for a lean metabolism.[87, 88] Administration of either an amino acid mixture or leucine alone has been shown to suppress food intake for up to 24 hours.[89] Studies in the elderly show that whey supplementation was associated with a decrease in adiposity (fat) and preservation of lean muscle mass.[90, 91]

Whey is a high-quality protein that promotes a sense of fullness and satiation after meals and decreases further food consumption. Whether it's more satiating than other protein sources is a matter of debate; there's literature in favor of and against its superiority.[92-95]

Whey protein also doubles as an immune system regulator because it's rich in anti-inflammatory chemicals called glycomacropeptides and beta-glucans. This is why whey-enriched formulations have been shown to improve the outcome of Crohn's disease in children.[96-98] When given to adult patients with Crohn's disease, whey improved intestinal barrier function as evidenced by diminished small intestine permeability.[99] As we learned in Chapter 2, many overweight people have imbalances in their gut microbiome associated with defects in gut barrier function similar to Crohn's disease. When these defects are serious enough, toxins from enteric bacteria can "leak" into your circulation, inciting a systemic inflammatory response, insulin resistance, and fat accumulation.[100] Whey protein heals the gut lining and cools down the inflammation, helping to reverse this problem.

All this raises a much larger discussion about dairy and its role in weight management. In the next chapter, I'll discuss how yogurt and kefir help you get and stay slim by seeding your gut microbiome with fat-burning flora. Whey protein can also be fermented to become a probiotic that repopulates the gut microbiome. Interestingly, a novel probiotic product has recently been developed based on a traditional dehydrated wafer once used in a Mexican dessert. To make it, they take sweet goat whey and ferment it with *Bifidobacterium infantis* or *Lactobacillus acidophilus*.[101]

There's no doubt about it. Whey is a superfood to keep in mind as a high-protein supplement that offers a host of health benefits and promotes slimness.

LOOKING AHEAD

After 30 days on Phase 1, it'll be time to reintegrate some of the foods we eliminated, seed your gut with the good bugs you need to thrive, and fertilize your inner garden so it can flourish again. This is what we'll do in Phase 2. That phase of the program is designed to reincorporate foods that are high in prebiotics and probiotics. These special foods will reinoculate your gut with healthy bacteria and further diversify your microbiome. Scientific evidence has connected probiotics and prebiotics to positive long-term weight and health outcomes. In the next chapter, we'll review these data, and I'll explain exactly how to add these foods back into your diet so that you can fully balance your inner ecosystem.

CHAPTER 6

Phase 2: Rebalance

RESEED AND FERTILIZE YOUR INNER GARDEN

Close your eyes for a moment. Picture a lush field of green populated with an endless array of beautiful wildflowers in every color imaginable. The flowers sway gently in the breeze as far as the eye can see. As you envision this scene, you touch on a deep quiet within, and a sense of profound peace washes over you. You feel relaxed, whole, and healthy.

This field is your inner garden, the ideal vision of the ecosystem deep within your gut. The grass and flowers that live there are the flora we'll plant in your gut during this phase of the program. Now that we've prepared the soil in Phase 1, it's time to reestablish a thriving gut microbiome that will help you achieve your ideal weight and optimal health. We'll do that by seeding and fertilizing your inner ecosystem during this part of the program. To do this, there are two simple but extremely important steps.

1. **Reseed your inner garden.** During this phase, we'll incorporate fermented foods such as yogurt, kefir, sauerkraut, kimchi, and others that are rich in healthy microbiota such as bifidobacteria. These probiotics have been shown to promote healthy gut microbiome balance and weight loss.

2. **Fertilize the friendly flora.** Your friendly intestinal flora need something to eat for your gut microbiome to thrive. That's why in Phase 2, I want you to add a class of fiber-rich, highly satiating complex carbohydrates called prebiotics into your diet. These foods are like Miracle-Gro for the friendly bacteria in your inner garden; they'll help reestablish harmony in your inner ecosystem.

Reseeding your gut with friendly bacteria and fertilizing them with prebiotics has a broad range of biochemical and metabolic effects that help you develop the lean metabolism you desire. The science increasingly shows that rebalancing your gut microbiome using the approach we'll take during this phase supports long-term weight loss.

I recommend that you stay on Phase 2 until you achieve your desired weight. By following this plan, you can expect a sustainable loss of 5 to 10 pounds of excess body weight per month as long as you are on Phase 2. Plus, inflammation will continue to be reduced throughout your body, your blood sugar and insulin levels will stabilize further, and you'll experience focused energy that lasts all day.

Okay, let's get started.

RESEEDING YOUR INNER GARDEN

Your first task: to cast seeds that will bloom in the lush, diverse inner ecosystem you need to achieve optimal weight and health. We'll do that by integrating numerous probiotic-rich foods into your diet.

Probiotics are live microorganisms that when consumed in adequate amounts have been shown to confer health benefits on the host. Growing research points to the important role of probiotics in favorably altering gut microbiome balance by increasing health-promoting bacteria such as lactobacillus, bifidobacteria, and others. This is critical, because your microbiota influence numerous biological systems that regulate the availability of nutrients, energy storage, hunger, fat mass, inflammation, and insulin sensitivity—which all play an important role in weight and health.

Research in this area has exploded in the last few years. More than 10,000 publications have reviewed the potential health benefits of probiotics. The vast majority of these were published after 2008, so we're in the midst of a gut microbiome renaissance—there's clearly enough data to strongly suggest that you should integrate probiotic-rich foods as a critical component of Phase 2 if you want to achieve long-term weight loss and lasting health.

We'll do this by diversifying the species of your gut microbiome instead of focusing on specific species or phyla of bacteria. In contrast to popular belief and television marketers, there's no single strain of bacteria, fungi, or yeast that works as a magic bullet to completely rebalance your inner garden and permanently shift you toward a lean metabolism. There are a few favorable species that seem to enhance overall health. But the data are varied, and the benefits are often strain specific.

For example, at least 200 studies have been done on humans and animals on the use of different lactobacillus species for weight loss alone.[1] This species is part of the phylum Firmicutes—the fat-forming bugs that took most of the blame in the early studies linking gut microbiome balance to obesity. It appears the story is a little more complicated than these early studies suggested.

In a recent meta-analysis of the lactobacillus data, scientists learned that different strains of lactobacillus seem to have different effects on weight regulation and overall health. For instance, in 13 studies that included 3,307 subjects (897 of whom were human), scientists found that *Lactobacillus acidophilus* seems to cause weight *gain.*

Do All Probiotics Help with Weight Loss?

◆ Myth: All probiotics will promote weight loss.

◆ Fact: Some probiotics work better than others. Be careful with single strains of lactobacillus for weight regulation. *Lactobacillus gasseri* (LG2055), *L. plantarum,* and *L. paracasei* promote weight loss.

In contrast, another well-designed study showed that consumption of fermented milk containing *Lactobacillus gasseri* (LG2055) was associated with significant weight loss, a lower waist and hip circumference, reduced subcutaneous and abdominal visceral fat, and improvement in metabolic markers compared to consumption of fermented milk without additional bacteria.[2] Fermented milk has many health benefits and helps shift the balance of your inner garden to support a lean metabolism.

Studies on *Lactobacillus plantarum* and *L. paracasei* show that these strains may shrink fat cells and reduce total body fat.[3, 4] Additional research has shown that various strains of lactobacillus decrease fat mass, reduce the risk of type 2 diabetes, and help mitigate insulin resistance.[5, 6] And these studies account *only* for research on one species of probiotics.

Hundreds of other studies have shown that modulating the gut microbiome using probiotics has a wide range of health effects that include:[7]

▤ Improving blood lipid patterns

▤ Reducing risk for hypertension

▤ Enhancing intestinal health and reducing risk of inflammatory bowel disorders

▤ Supporting the immune system

▤ Reducing risk of allergies and/or their symptoms

▤ Synthesizing and enhancing the bioavailability of nutrients

While there may be some relationship between specific strains of bacteria and health outcomes–such as the link between *L. gasseri* and weight loss–the important message is that the community of bacteria and their interaction are what produces health outcomes. Diversity is the key to inner ecosystem health–so that will be our goal in Phase 2. Animal studies in this area lend further support to the idea that rebalancing your gut microbiome by using probiotic-rich foods can lend a powerful helping hand in your journey to optimal weight. These studies have shown that simply administering probiotics without other dietary changes leads to weight loss, reduction in adipose (fat) tissue, reduced blood glucose, increased insulin and leptin sensitivity, and more.[8, 9] This has been my clinical experience as well. Consider Josephina, whose stubborn weight wouldn't budge until she tried probiotics.

THE GUT BALANCE REVOLUTION SUCCESS STORIES

Josephina

Josephina is a health-care provider in her mid-forties who found herself gaining weight uncontrollably. When she maxed out at 320 pounds, she could hardly carry on with her job and care for her family. She developed type 2 diabetes and experienced labored breathing whenever she exerted herself.

Desperate for help, she underwent gastric bypass surgery. Although she recovered well and looked and felt much better, she lost only 70 pounds, 41 percent of her excess body weight—but she knew she should've lost much more. (Data from seven studies and 1,627 patients undergoing this surgery show that the mean first-year weight loss is 67.3 percent.[10]) Josephina was disappointed that her results were so far below average.

That's when she began looking for help. I asked her some questions that led me to believe she was experiencing a common complication of gastric bypass surgery—small intestinal bacterial overgrowth, or SIBO. Remember from Chapter 4 that SIBO is a common result of obesity—that's why I recommend a low-FODMAP diet to curb symptoms and help shift the microbial terrain in the gut during Phase 1. Josephina's case was a little different. The altered anatomy from her surgery resulted in what doctors called a "blind limb"—a part of the intestine that diverts digested materials away from the digestive tract and into a short one-way tube. This part of the intestine lacks flow and is stagnant, and SIBO is a common outcome.

This reminded me of a game-changing study in which morbidly obese patients undergoing gastric bypass surgery were consequently diagnosed with SIBO through breath testing.[11] Researchers at Stanford University School of Medicine explored whether probiotics could accelerate weight loss in those who developed SIBO resulting from gastric bypass surgery. Forty-two subjects were randomly assigned to receive either 2.4 billion colonies of an undisclosed lactobacillus species or a placebo daily. The lactobacillus supplement resulted in a loss of 10 percent more excess body weight at 3 months, and the trend continued at 6 months of therapy. A significant reduction in SIBO was also observed. I shared the outcome of this study with Josephina and recommended she take a probiotic product with a mix of lactobacillus and bifidobacteria species. In a month, she lost 10 more pounds without changing her diet or level of physical activity and noticed that her gastrointestinal symptoms had improved markedly.

Choose the Right Chicken!

Remember that conventionally raised poultry is infused with antibiotics to promote growth by disrupting the birds' gut microbiome? A study on conventionally raised broiler chicken compared weight gain in those birds fed either antibiotics or probiotics or no additive to their diet.[12] Each of these three groups was subdivided into three more groups by whether their fat source was soybean oil (proinflammatory), free fatty acids (mix of pro- and anti-inflammatory fats), or standard feed.

The results are compelling. The birds fed antibiotics gained more weight than either the probiotics- or standard-fed birds. In fact, the probiotics made the birds lose weight. Plus, the type of fat used made a difference. The group that was fed proinflammatory soybean oil gained the most weight compared to those fed free fatty acids and standard feed. The birds that gained the *most* weight were in the group raised on *both* antibiotics and soybean oil, showing a synergistic interaction. That's why I recommend antibiotic-free poultry and grass-fed over corn- and soy-fed cattle.

We'll talk more about the specific ways probiotics tend to effect these changes later in the chapter, when I explain which of these foods to focus on during this phase. But first, let me introduce you to another class of foods to integrate in Phase 2: prebiotics—the fertilizer for your inner garden.

FERTILIZING YOUR FRIENDLY FLORA

When you plant a garden, you don't just throw some seeds down and hope they'll grow. You tend the garden, adding fertilizer as necessary so the plants can flourish. The same is true of your inner garden: You must be attentive to it and provide the food it needs to make it a healthy, diverse ecosystem.

One of your gut bugs' favorite foods is prebiotics. These are foods your human metabolism cannot digest but your good gut bugs absolutely adore. They're a class of soluble fibers that help your gut microbiome thrive. Many of these foods are the FODMAPs we reduced during Phase 1 of the program to help reverse any gut dysbiosis you may have been suffering from. Now that we've mitigated this gut dysbiosis by tilling the soil of your gut microbiome, it's a good idea to reintegrate some of these foods, enhance your fiber intake, and give your bugs the foods they need to thrive.

As with probiotics, prebiotic-laden foods correlate with weight loss and health gains. In a series of Belgian studies, researchers showed that giving people 5 to 20 grams of prebiotics per day altered gut microbial balance and led to reduced blood sugar, increased satiety, decreased hunger, and reduced fat mass.[13]

Yet another double-blind, placebo-controlled trial put one group on oligofructose (a prebiotic in the FODMAP family) and gave the other group a calorically equivalent placebo. The group receiving the prebiotics lost 2.2 pounds of body weight in 12 weeks without any other changes in diet.[14] Most of this weight was fat mass lost from the trunk of the body. (You know that belly fat you want to target? Well, this is how you do it!) The placebo group *gained* weight.* Both groups had the same amount of calories added to their diet, but the *type of calories*–the prebiotics–made the difference.

Need more proof? In a groundbreaking study, researchers provided a group of type 2 diabetics only 8 grams of the prebiotic inulin daily for 4 weeks, with no other changes to their diet. The group taking the inulin saw a "statistically significant reduction in blood glucose"–a stunning finding that reveals just how effectively food can be used as medicine. Indeed, data are emerging that suggest prebiotics should be considered as a treatment for metabolic syndrome.[15]

Why do prebiotics have such a powerful impact on weight and health? One of many reasons is that they influence the production of peptide (small protein) hormones in the gut called glucagon-like peptide 1 and 2 (GLP-1 and GLP-2), which are thought to play an important role in appetite, satiety, gut motility, insulin function, and many bodily functions. We'll go into more detail about GLP-1 and GLP-2 later in this chapter, but the short story here is that when you feed your gut microbiome the right way, they cause the gut to produce these peptide hormones that support your overall health–a pretty big score for prebiotics.

The best news: Providing prebiotics and probiotics at the same time, which is what we'll do in this program, may have even more profound health benefits. Studies have shown that taking prebiotics and probiotics together (aka synbiotics) produces a favorable metabolic profile of short-chain fatty acids (SCFAs) in addition to the other health benefits listed above.[16] These anti-inflammatory fats help your gut absorb water, help regrow healthy gut lining cells in the colon, and may provide defenses against colon cancer and inflammatory bowel disease. This is an important though not surprising finding. Seed your gut microbiome with health-promoting gut microbes–aka "friendly flora"–while providing them with their favorite foods so they can thrive, and you end up with a plethora of benefits as well as weight loss. The power of this ecosystems approach to eating never ceases to amaze me. I discovered this as a teen light-years ahead of the data, and it helped me *lose more than 120 pounds and keep them off for good!*

So how do you get these health benefits? Simply focus on the right foods in Phase 2 and forget or eat fewer of the foods that don't support the lean metabolism you deserve. Here's how to do that.

---

* The placebo contained maltodextrin, which comes from treated grain starch, primarily corn or rice starch. It can also come from wheat and potatoes. Though not a sugar, it still has a glycemic index of 130 by itself (table sugar is only 65). This starchy, high-glycemic "sweetener" in the placebo caused weight gain despite not adding more caloric energy.

What About Prebiotic and Probiotic Supplements?

You may be more familiar with prebiotics and probiotics in the form of supplements than in foods. These supplements can be a great adjunct to a diet and lifestyle change program, and as you'll learn later, they may help you rebalance your gut microbiome and lose weight more quickly and effectively. However, they're not necessary for you to complete this program. They're an optional step you can take if you choose.

It's important to know what to look for when choosing these products. For example, look for live mixed strains of probiotics—the number of colony-forming units (CFUs) in the product is important. So is locating products that are free of fillers, binders, and other toxic agents.

FORGET FOODS THAT SEND YOUR INNER ECOSYSTEM OUT OF BALANCE

During Phase 1, you did a lot of work to remove from your diet junky foods that send your gut microbiome and your metabolism out of balance. We got rid of sugar (in all of its subversive forms), starchy carbs (bread, pasta, potatoes, and so on), and unhealthy inflammatory oils (soy, corn, vegetable, and others). You learned why these substances are unhealthy and read about studies showing that the overconsumption of these products is correlated to weight gain and poor health.

In Phase 2, to achieve your health and weight-loss goals, I want you to continue abstaining from the most harmful forms of these foods. So continue avoiding the following:

- **Sweeteners.** As you'll see in the following section on the foods you can add back into your diet, during this phase of the program you may have limited quantities of certain sweeteners. However, I want you to continue avoiding the most egregious ones.

  - High-fructose corn syrup (HFCS).

  - Agave–it's high in FODMAPs.

  - Artificial sweeteners, including but not limited to the sugar alcohols: mannitol, xylitol, and sorbitol, which are also high in FODMAPs. Note that some "all natural" yogurts–a food critical in this phase–are allowed by the FDA to include artificial sweeteners, so make sure you read labels carefully.

  - Refined honey, which is among the top most insidious sweeteners of all time. It's high in fructose (a FODMAP) and it's overused. Steer clear of any refined honey, though raw honey is a different story. Good data show that a teaspoon or less per day of raw honey has positive effects on gut microbiome health–thus earning an honorable mention in the Phase 2 superfoods list. Don't overdo it, but if you're looking for something sweet in your coffee or whey protein shake, a little raw honey is just the ticket.

- **Sweet drinks**. This includes soda, fruit juices (they spike blood sugar and insulin levels and rate high on the glycemic impact index), vitamin waters (full of added sugars), and their ilk.

- **White flour and potatoes** (including products made with them). Avoid pasta, bread, cookies, crackers, cakes, and so on, as they're all high on the glycemic impact index and spike blood sugar and insulin.

- **Inflammatory oils**. While my restrictions on these are fewer than they were in Phase 1, you should still stay away from corn oil, lard, hydrogenated oil, palm oil, safflower oil, and a few others.

- **Gluten**. Barley, wheat, rye, and other grains that contain gluten are high in FODMAPs. Many people are sensitive to them, and you can use other less harmful whole grains to support your gut microbiome instead (such as quinoa). For now, stay away from foods high in gluten. Oats are another great option; they are high in prebiotics and benefit the gut microbiome, so their benefits outweigh the potential for gluten cross-contamination, which is a result of being processed in the same mill as gluten-enriched grains.

Depending on how much weight you have to lose, you may need to remove these foods from your diet for a few weeks, a few months, or even longer. After you've completed your weight-loss journey, arrived at your goal weight, and are in maintenance mode, you'll shift to Phase 3, when you can indulge in the occasional sweet treat, potato chip, or french fry without too many adverse consequences. Look for more details in Chapter 8.

But aside from an occasional treat, most of these products have no place in the human diet, and I recommend that you limit all of them for the long term. The preponderance of these foods is one of the leading causes of the overweight and obesity epidemics. If you want to embrace the Gut Balance Revolution and take a stand against the imbalanced food environment in which we live, I ask you to avoid these products during this phase. As with Phase 1, you'll find all the specifics on what to avoid in your Phase 2 food charts on pages 246–251.

ADD BACK A FEW OF YOUR FAVORITE FOODS

Phase 2 isn't all discipline and deprivation! You'll have much more flexibility in this phase than you did on Phase 1. The restrictions on FODMAPs are dramatically reduced, you can now have a little lean red meat and pork, and some select prebiotic-rich whole grains have been included due to their wonderful fertilizing effects on the friendly flora. Even the occasional pint of beer, glass of red wine, chunk of dark chocolate, and a few select sweeteners are allowed.

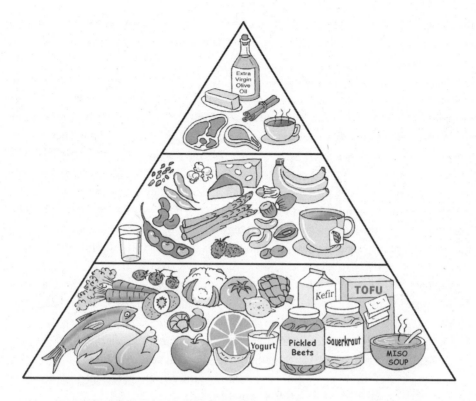

The Gut Balance Revolution Phase 2 Food Pyramid: This figure prioritizes foods in Phase 2, the rebalancing phase. Foods that are limited are at the top of the pyramid (i.e., lean red meats, butter, coffee, extra-virgin olive oil). Nuts, seeds, beans, green tea, and gluten-free whole grains are placed in the middle of the pyramid. Fruits, vegetables, fish, poultry, vegetable poultry soups, wild game, and fermented foods (such as pickled vegetables, sauerkraut, kefir, miso soup, yogurt, and kimchi) are at the base of the pyramid.

I specifically designed this part of the program in a way that would enable you to stick with it for longer periods of time without feeling deprived. This will allow those of you who have substantial weight to lose the dietary flexibility to achieve your weight-loss goals without falling off the wagon. So let's look at some of these delicious foods you can eat in moderation during Phase 2.

FODMAPS: THE DOSE MAKES THE POISON

During Phase 2, we reintegrate many, though not all, of the FODMAPs we eliminated on Phase 1. We'll keep out some of the major offenders like high-fructose sweeteners, high-FODMAP fruits (mangoes, pears, and others), gluten (like wheat, rye, barley), and a few other sources (sugar alcohols, for example). This will allow you to reduce your overall FODMAP consumption while still taking advantage of foods that provide health benefits but technically qualify as FODMAPs. A few of these FODMAP-rich foods–specifically, those high in prebiotics—are critical during Phase 2, and it's important to understand the relationship between prebiotics, fiber, and FODMAPs to fully recognize the rationale behind this program.

Many prebiotics qualify as FODMAPs. Of these, the fructans (inulin in particular) and oligosaccharides (such as fructooligosaccharides and galacto-oligosaccharides) are probably the most important. These foods are high in fiber, especially soluble fiber, which cannot be digested by the human gut alone—your gut microbiota must break these foods down for you. The good news: Your friendly flora absolutely love to eat this fiber. So once your gut microbiome is rebalanced, fiber-rich foods like these are a wonderful food source for your inner garden—a type of fertilizer that helps it flourish.

Fiber and the prebiotic effects of these foods have a wide range of health and weight-loss benefits as well. First, insoluble fiber is highly satiating. Because it dissolves in water and becomes a kind of gel in your gut, it gives you a feeling of fullness and reduces over-all hunger.[17]

The benefits of insoluble fiber show even more brightly, however, when we analyze them in terms of what they do for our inner garden and how this impacts our health and weight. These fibers are readily fermentable, so your good gut bugs love to feast on them. Research has shown that adding prebiotics to your diet increases the growth of commensal species like bifidobacteria, lactobacillus, and others. In fact, in order to be a prebiotic, these fibers by definition are required to stimulate the growth of bifidobacteria—called "the prebiotic effect."

For example, one study showed that increasing inulin-type fructans enhanced levels of bifidobacteria and lactobacillus in only a few days. These improvements in overall gut microbial balance disappeared in as little as a week after removing the prebiotic inulin from the diet.[18, 19]

Scientists have also demonstrated that prebiotics like oligofructose can alter as many as 102 different types of gut bugs in obese type 2 diabetic mice. These alterations were associated with reduced fat mass, increased lean muscle, improved glucose and lipid metabolism, reduced systemic inflammation, and more.[20] It's a long way from mice to men, but these finding are impressive, and they clearly illustrate that what we eat influences our inner ecosystem—which in turn impacts our health.

In fact, it's been repeatedly shown that prebiotics alter the overall terrain of the gut microbiome and lead to a reduction in inflammation, improvements in intestinal barrier function, and improved insulin sensitivity in both human and animal models.[21, 22] Why is this?

Many mechanisms are at play, but gut peptides are important actors connecting the pieces of the puzzle. We discussed two of these gut peptides in Chapter 2—glucagon-like peptides 1 and 2 (GLP-1 and GLP-2). A growing body of research shows that the release of these two gut peptides (along with a few others like peptide YY and ghrelin) is highly influenced by your gut microbiota. We think this has to do with the way your gut bacteria "talk to" your brain.

The amount of research about the bidirectional communication between the gut and the brain is rapidly expanding. These data are showing us that gut microbes are not only involved in the regulation of our metabolism but also trigger behaviors that ultimately influence our food choices. [23, 24]

Ultimately, when you feed your inner ecosystem prebiotics like inulin, oligosaccharides, and others, it seems to shift the overall balance of your gut microbiome in a positive way that leads to an increased release of peptides like GLP-1 and GLP-2–and that affects insulin levels, feelings of fullness, and more.

This has been well documented in the research. For example, in a recent Belgian study, scientists took a group of healthy volunteers and fed them 16 grams of inulin-type fructans a day for 2 weeks. GLP-1 and GLP-2 increased, the volunteers reported feeling fuller, they naturally ate less, and their glucose levels after meals (postprandial glucose) were reduced. But one of the most mind-blowing aspects of this study has to do with genetic expression.* These foods actually *reprogrammed* the body to reduce the size of fat cells in the volunteers involved in the study. [25]

Back to the Belgian study: Could it be that the prebiotics enhanced levels of healthy bacteria that then "talked to" the volunteers' DNA, saying, "Hey, would you mind reducing the size of this guy's fat cells?" More research needs to be done to tease out all the relationships, but this is a distinct possibility. (For a review of bacterial gene swapping, turn to pages 16–17 in Chapter 2.)

The bottom line: We need prebiotics to achieve optimal weight and health. In the previous phase, I asked you to dramatically reduce your intake of FODMAPs and soluble fiber. This was done to mitigate dysbiosis and reduce digestive symptoms such as gas and bloating to improve your quality of life as you shift the microbial terrain toward balance. Now that you've tilled the soil in Phase 1, it's time to refeed your gut microbiome with these healthy foods to rebalance your inner ecology and produce a lean metabolism. By enriching the biodiversity of microbial species in your gut, this new healthy network of symbiotes (go team microbes!) will provide a wide range of biochemical and metabolic benefits that support long-term weight loss and better health.

Remember that when it comes to FODMAPs, the dose makes the poison. Some folks can handle more than others, so listen to your own body and fine-tune this program to your needs. But the following guidelines for reintegrating FODMAPs in your diet should help.

- *Favor* **vegetables and beans high in prebiotics.** We'll talk more about these later. They include lentils, chickpeas, asparagus, artichokes, Jerusalem artichokes, and others.

---

* Inulin-like fructans are fermented by good gut bacteria into short-chain fatty acids, which activate cells via G-protein-coupled receptors (GPRs) such as GPR_{41} and GPR_{43}. The Belgian study showed that people eating this prebiotic-rich diet actually induced the expression of a gene called GPR_{43}, which is involved in determining how big fat cells are.

- **Eat a *few* whole grains and nuts**. More details to follow, but the short story here is that nuts–packed with omega-3 fats as well as prebiotics–are among the healthiest snacks you can eat, and there are good data showing select gluten-free whole grains (in moderation) support gut microbiome health and help you lose weight.

- *Forget* **high-FODMAP sweets, fruits, sugar alcohols, and glutinous grains**. This will reduce your overall FODMAP intake and eliminate foods that spike blood sugar and insulin levels and produce bothersome digestive symptoms.

Whole Grains for Health

Whole grains have a long history of inclusion in health programs and have been a dietary staple in many traditional cultures for millennia. But as Dr. William Davis describes in his best-selling book *Wheat Belly*, the source, digestibility, and gluten content of wheat has radically shifted over the years, creating a crisis of gluten overload and intolerance, with negative health effects.[26]

Wheat Belly is part of a cultural revolution telling us how we can add to our health by subtracting wheat from our diet–a sort of addition by subtraction approach. Dr. Loren Cordain's best-selling book *The Paleo Diet* delves into the history of Paleolithic hunter-gatherer people who didn't have access to the grains available today and explains how we can promote health by going back in time to the high-fiber anti-inflammatory diet of humanity's ancestors.

There's quite an audience for these low-grain diets. *Wheat Belly* had been a *New York Times* bestseller for 133 weeks as of the time of this writing. Furthermore, the *New York Times* best-selling book *Grain Brain* by Dr. David Perlmutter summarizes compelling data regarding how gluten-containing grains may begin a cascade of events in the gut, leading to a variety of neurobehavioral impairments and neurodegenerative processes.[27] And another researcher, Dr. Alessio Fasano, has published studies showing how gluten may break down the gut barrier defenses to initiate a chain reaction of downstream inflammatory events, possibly leading to autoimmunity.[28]

However, there are many critics who disagree with these folks and tell us that wheat and other gluten-containing grains are perfectly safe. So what's the real story?

The concerns of the low-carbers may have more than a grain of truth in them.

I was recently on Dan Rodrick's radio show on Baltimore's NPR affiliate, WYPR, discussing high-protein diets in weight loss and health.[29] Many of the callers were happy about their success with limiting grains and carbs, at least in the short term. This made sense to me, as the data show that low-carb ketogenic diets work in the short term, as discussed in Chapter 4. That's why I designed Phase 1 of this program as I did.

I agree that we're seeing more convincing data that there's a large population of people who are intolerant to wheat, and it's clear that for them, gluten can trigger a host of digestive symptoms.[30] In the gastroenterology literature, when wheat is given in the form of a capsule, it provokes symptoms in those with irritable bowel syndrome (IBS), and when it's restricted from the diet, symptoms improve.[31] Furthermore, glutinous grains are rich in FODMAPs and provoke symptoms in those with SIBO.

We're living in an era of consumer-driven gluten-free living, and science is trying to understand why so many benefit from gluten restriction. But much of the gluten-free dogma—and the products this new market has created—is misguided. After all, gluten-free cookies and cakes aren't healthy and don't deserve a place in your diet any more than their gluten-packed counterparts do.

For these reasons, I elected to keep gluten-rich grains out of Phase 1. A very low-carb program with limited grains for the first 30 days will help resolve SIBO, improve gut symptoms, and balance the microbial terrain. Unfortunately, there may be some collateral damage, as data show that a gluten-free diet can reduce the amount of important species of microbes like bifidobacteria, which play a critical role in gut immune function and weight regulation.[32] However, as previously cited, Halmos et al. reported that a diet low in FODMAPs enhanced gut microbiome biodiversity.[33] Thus, cutting out the junk and keeping some of the prebiotic FODMAPs will limit any compromise to the gut microbiome during Phase 1.

Now in Phase 2, we're reestablishing more healthy communities of gut microbes and refeeding them with prebiotic foods that help them thrive. Once this is achieved, most people can gradually introduce a modest amount of gluten-free whole grains in their diet without adverse consequences. In fact, these fibrous foods can be highly satiating and provide an important source of prebiotics (oligosaccharides). In the meal plans, you'll find nonglutinous whole grains for this purpose. As you'll see in the Phase 2 food charts on pages 246–251, amaranth, brown rice, buckwheat (also known as Japanese soba; not actually a form of wheat), popcorn, oat bran, quinoa, and teff* are all options for this phase.

Does that mean you should scarf down multiple bowls of brown rice or oat bran? Certainly not. Eating too many gluten-free whole grains can be problematic, as it can raise blood glucose levels. But in my experience, brown rice, quinoa, and the other gluten-free whole grains that I include in this phase aren't the type of foods people binge on.

As we'll see when we get to Phase 3, some of the best data we have show that diets that support long-term health and weight loss include some fiber-rich whole grains. So stick with the science and include a limited few healthy whole grains in Phases 2 and 3.

Go Nuts!

Aside from vegetables, it's hard to think of a group of foods more touted for its health benefits than nuts. These tiny, shelled tree fruits do indeed offer a bevy of benefits, not the least of which is their effect on your gut microbiome.

---

* Be careful with ordering teff when dining out, as many eateries (such as Ethiopian restaurants) do not make their own teff, and many vendors mix wheat with the teff. When in Washington, DC, or Baltimore, ask the owner of the restaurant Dukem (dukemrestaurant.com) for gluten-free teff 1 day in advance of your visit and she will oblige.

Nuts are probably most famous for their high level of healthy fats, especially the omega-3s. These fats may be one of the reasons people who eat nuts have such impressive health improvements. For example, an analysis of two massive health studies–the Nurses' Health Study and the Health Professionals Follow-Up Study–reviewed data on over 118,000 participants and found that the frequency of nut consumption was inversely correlated with all causes of mortality.[34]

Some nuts clearly demonstrate medicinal potential when added to your diet. For example, a study from India recently showed that people with metabolic syndrome who added a daily serving of pistachios reduced body fat, improved overall cholesterol levels, reduced inflammation markers, and even seemed to see a positive effect on fat-storing hormones like adiponectin.[35] All this from a simple nut–pretty impressive, right?

The positive health benefits don't stop there. A recent cutting-edge study shows that almonds and almond skins have a powerful prebiotic effect. Forty-eight volunteers were divided into two groups.[36] One group was given 56 grams of almonds (about 40 nuts) a day. The other group was given 8 grams of a commercial fructooligosaccharide supplement as a control. The group who ate the nuts saw a significant increase in bifidobacteria and lactobacillus and a reduction of other, potentially harmful species, such as *Clostridium perfringens*. A few nuts a day seem to help rebalance your inner ecosystem.[37]

Nuts have a number of health benefits that include promoting weight reduction. I will expand on the discussion of the health and weight-loss benefits of nuts in Chapter 9, when I discuss superfoods for Phase 3.[38] In the meantime, include plenty of nuts during Phase 2. One caveat: Don't go completely nuts on nuts–a little goes a long way. I kept a lid on nuts for Phase 1 since they have a relatively high carb load. Include them on Phase 2 and beyond, but be aware that overeating these healthy foods may undo your attempts to lose weight since they are energy dense. Keep it to one or two handfuls per day.

Where's the Meat?

A little lean, pasture-raised, grass-fed beef, bison, wild game, or lamb or some pastured pork can be a healthy addition to your diet. But look at all the modifiers in that sentence and compare it with the typical consumption of meat in this country. That may give you some sense of why I asked you to eliminate these foods during Phase 1 and why I strongly encourage you to limit them during the remainder of this program.

Americans eat way too much meat. If you've grown accustomed to 24-ounce rib eyes and half-pound burgers, don't go back to those habits now. A "little meat" means two to three weekly palm-size servings. Eating more meat than this has consistently been associated with weight gain, cardiovascular issues, and many other health problems. Recent evidence also shows disruption of gut microbiome balance caused by diets high in animal protein.[39]

Stick to a couple of small servings a week and you'll be fine. I *strongly* suggest you choose grass-fed and pastured sources. They're more expensive, but that will just motivate you to eat a little less. Animals raised conventionally in concentrated animal feeding operations (or CAFOs—another term for feedlots) are lower in healthy omega-3 fats and are pumped full of antibiotics that have serious detrimental effects on your gut microbiome and that recent data strongly suggest lead to weight gain.[40]

A TOAST TO YOUR MICROBIOME

I'd like to raise a toast to your gut microbiome, and in Phase 2, you can join in with a glass of beer or wine. These beverages, which have literally been with us since the beginning of recorded history (recipes for beer are among the earliest written documents), are perfectly healthy additions to the Phase 2 diet. As long as you keep your consumption to no more than one glass of beer or wine per day, these fermented beverages may even have some health and weight-loss benefits.

It appears that people who drink a light to moderate amount of alcohol have smaller waists than people who don't drink at all.[41] It's also been illustrated that moderate drinkers tend to gain less weight over time and have less abdominal fat specifically.[42, 43]

Red wine in particular is one of those foods that targets belly fat. We think it has to do with its relatively high levels of the antioxidant resveratrol, which modulates fat storage and may act directly on the fat cell itself.[44] A study published in the *Journal of Clinical Nutrition* concluded that resveratrol reduces the amount of fat cells generated by your body. That means it could be an excellent weapon in the battle of the bulge.

Some studies indicate drinking red wine with a fatty meal prevents the rise in blood lipids because the polyphenols in the wine block lipid absorption, improve cardiovascular metabolic markers, lower blood lipids, and prevent the activation of inflammatory pathways.[45] These same polyphenols also seem to have prebiotic effects—moderate red wine consumption may support gut microbiome diversity.*

Of course, you can't slam down a bottle of wine or drink multiple pints with your buddies. High alcohol intake (three or more glasses a day or more than eight in a week) has clearly been associated with weight gain and health problems. Chronic alcoholism shifts the healthy community of bacteria in the gut microbiome to a state of dysbiosis, which disrupts gut barrier function and can lead to endotoxemia and its legion of harmful consequences.[46, 47] On the flip side, moderate red wine consumption—one glass nightly—prevents endotoxemia and promotes the growth of bidifobacterium—another reason I've included it in Phase 2 and beyond.[48] Again—the dose makes the poison.

As long as you stick with these guidelines, I encourage you to enjoy a glass of this nectar that's been with us since ancient times. One final caveat: Drop hard liquor—it's been associated with increases in abdominal fat.[49]

---

* A glass of red wine contains only 1 milligram of resveratrol, and its health benefits may also be derived from its prebiotic influence on promoting microbial diversity.

FAVOR FOODS THAT DIVERSIFY YOUR GUT MICROBIOME: PROBIOTICS AND PREBIOTICS

Biodiversity is the hallmark of any healthy ecosystem. That's why, during this phase, you'll favor foods that enhance the biodiversity of your inner garden, rebalance your gut microbiome, and encourage the growth of bacterial communities that support your health. Specifically, we'll focus on foods with prebiotic and probiotic effects.

Foods containing probiotics will seed your inner garden with the friendly flora that help you thrive. Prebiotics are the fertilizer that helps seeds flourish, turning them into rich gut microbial communities that nourish and support you.

In the pages that follow, I'll discuss prebiotics in more depth, focusing specifically on prebiotic-rich vegetables. These are the foods you'll want to focus on as the fertilizer for your good gut bugs.

But first, let's talk a little about those gut bugs and how you can enhance and diversify them with fermented foods–the number one source of probiotics.

What Is Fermentation and Why Is It Important?

From a culinary point of view, fermentation is the act of transforming and preserving foods through the use of bacteria, fungi, and enzymes. Human beings have been fermenting foods for a very long time. Pottery shards from more than 9,000 years ago show residues of alcohol, suggesting that the tradition of fermenting foods is older than government, the written word, and possibly even civilization itself.

Virtually every culture in the world has a fermentation tradition, and it's easy to see why: Before refrigeration, fermentation was one of very few ways to preserve food. Of course, humans didn't invent this process–we stole it from nature. From a biological point of view, any process by which nutrients are converted to energy in the absence of oxygen (anaerobic metabolism) is considered fermentation. The outcome of this process is a combination of gases (like the bubbles in beer), acids (like lactic acid), and alcohol (all alcoholic beverages are fermented).

Fermentation is occurring inside you all the time. It's what your inner flora do. They take the sugars, carbohydrates, and soluble fiber you eat, ferment these substances, and convert them into other chemicals, from short-chain fatty acids to vitamin K and more. When we ferment foods, we're sort of "predigesting" them, changing their chemical composition before they've entered our bodies. We're also creating an environment in which probiotics–friendly flora that provide us with health benefits–can flourish.

It's interesting to consider that before microbiology even existed, cultures the world over had been actively "farming" bacteria by fermenting foods. (The word *culture* even refers to the act of intentionally cultivating living materials like bacteria, like a culture with which you inoculate yogurt, as well as to the beliefs, customs, arts, etc., of a society.) Humans have been practicing a rudimentary form of this science by actively encouraging the growth of particular strains of bacteria in their food for eons. Though primarily a method of preservation, by so doing these societies were garnering the health benefits of probiotics without even realizing what bacteria were or how they were involved in our health.

It's difficult to overstate the health benefits of eating fermented foods. They've been shown to regulate immunity, improve digestive function, and reduce inflammation. Recent evidence also indicates that they improve weight-loss outcomes and enhance metabolism in a variety of ways. And as you will learn, increasing your intake of fermented foods reduces your risk of chronic illness, including cardiovascular disease, type 2 diabetes, certain types of cancer, Alzheimer's disease, and more. They may even affect conditions like arthritis and allergies. We now know that these effects are largely due to the fact that probiotic-rich foods encourage the growth of healthy microbial species in your gut.

The health effects of lactobacillus and bifidobacteria–two of the more common strains of commensals found in fermented foods like yogurt, sauerkraut, and others– have been well documented. It's now well accepted that these friendly species of bacteria modulate processes like insulin resistance and inflammation that lead to weight gain.

For example, in one study, researchers took 45 people with glucose intolerance, gave half of them 10 billion colony-forming units (CFUs) of lactobacillus and the other half a placebo for 4 weeks. Those who got the lactobacillus showed a reduction in insulin resistance and inflammation.[50, 51]

In obese people, the administration of a single strain of lactobacillus has been shown to decrease fat mass and the risk of type 2 diabetes. This was illustrated in a study published in the *Journal of Pediatric Gastroenterology and Nutrition*.[52] In the study, 12 billion CFUs of *Lactobacillus rhamnosus* or a placebo was assigned to obese children for 8 weeks. Researchers noted that the probiotics ameliorated the progression of obesity and diabetes.

Exactly how these friendly flora achieve these effects is still being researched. However, some of the mechanisms we know are involved include:

- **Reduction in blood glucose and insulin, and increased insulin sensitivity.** These effects have been shown in study after study. One of the major players in this are the gut peptides GLP-1 and GLP-2.[53] Other factors may include alteration in satiety (meaning people who consume probiotics may eat less), the influence of probiotics on inflammation, and more.

- **Gut flora's interaction with the immune system and inflammation modulation.** We know your gut microbes "train" your immune system and thus have substantial influence on systemic inflammation. For a detailed discussion, see Chapter 2.

- **Reduction of leptin levels and increased leptin sensitivity.** Probiotics seem to influence hunger hormones like leptin and ghrelin–so when your gut microbiome is balanced, you tend to feel fuller and eat less.[54]

- **Altered activity in appetite centers of the brain (hypothalamus).** Your gut flora "communicate" with your central nervous system by enticing your intestines to release hormones that travel to your brain with peptides like GLP-1, GLP-2, peptide YY, and others, sending messages of fullness and satisfaction. The use of prebiotics in the treatment of neuropsychiatric disorders promoting mental health via the gut-brain axis is presently the subject of much research.[55]

- **Production of short-chain fatty acids.** Certain strains of bugs seem to produce more SCFAs than others. These important fats reduce systematic inflammation, help heal and repair the gut, and have other important health effects.

- **Absorption of lipids.** Remember from Chapter 2 that the amount of energy you harvest from your food and how fat is stored on your body are determined in part by your gut microbiome. When your inner ecology is in balance, fat absorption and deposition are managed more effectively.

- **Genetic influences that determine adipocyte size.** As we already learned, it appears that certain gut microbial communities "talk to" your genes, telling them how big your fat cells should be.

- **Increased production of conjugated linoleic acid (CLA).** This one is a little controversial. CLA is a healthy fat found in mammals. Certain strains of microbes (*Lactobacillus plantarum*, for example) produce more CLA. Substantial evidence links the production of this fatty acid to overall weight reduction in animal models.[56] To date, the human literature on this subject is mixed. But it still may be a mechanism by which gut microbes influence weight and fat gain.

These are only a few of the ways probiotics influence your ability to lose weight. There are many other connections, some of which are still being discovered by researchers. The bottom line is this: Probiotics have a profound influence on weight and health, and you can get more of these friendly bacteria by eating more fermented foods.

When you add more fermented foods to your diet, you don't need to pay too much attention to the exact species of bacteria you're ingesting. There is a broad range of probiotics in fermented foods, and focusing on any one of them simply isn't necessary. Remember, the name of the game is balance and biodiversity. Simply include more fermented foods in your diet and this is virtually guaranteed.

Learning how to ferment your own foods can be fun. It connects you to ancient traditions just as it offers a deeper understanding of the ecological relationships between you, your flora, and the world around you. That's why I've included recipes in Chapter 11 that will teach you how to ferment your own food. You'll learn how to make yogurt, kefir, sauerkraut, kimchi, and more.

You can purchase substitutes from the market if you don't have time to ferment your own foods, but please follow my recommendations on choosing the right types of foods. The "pickles" you buy in the store may not be "pickled" in the traditional sense. So make sure you read the next sections carefully if you are unable to cultivate your own ferments.

Even if you can't keep batches of fermented foods going all the time, I strongly encourage you to try making some of them from scratch. Cultivating probiotics in your home that you then consume to support your flora will create a more meaningful and profound relationship between you and your good gut bugs. It's a wonderful illustration of ecosystems at work, and it brings to light our multifaceted and nuanced relationships with the various ecosystems within and around us. Seeing these relationships will, I believe, give you further encouragement to keep your inner ecology balanced for life.

In the meantime, here are important notes to keep in mind when choosing fermented foods at the market. These foods come in two varieties: fermented veggies and fermented dairy products.

Fermented Veggies

Traditionally pickled vegetables are among the healthiest foods you can eat. They're packed with fiber and phytonutrients; because they're "predigested" their nutrients are more bioavailable;[57] and, of course, they're teaming with probiotics.

Unfortunately, the word *pickles* doesn't mean what it once did. Traditional pickles are prepared very simply: Take some veggies like cabbage, beets, or cucumbers. Shred, chop, or simply leave them whole. Add salt or brine (salt plus water). Drop in a little seasoning (dill, garlic, ginger, cayenne pepper, or just about any other spice you like). Cover them and let them sit in their own brine for 1 to 3 weeks or—in the case of kimchi or miso pastes—months or years. Bacteria from your hands and on the veggies themselves thrive in the anaerobic environment created by the brine, multiply like crazy, and transform the raw vegetables into pickles in the process. This is known as lactic acid fermentation; it's among the simplest and oldest forms of pickling on the planet. Sauerkraut, one of the simpler lacto-ferments, has been around for more than 2,000 years.

However, in our microbephobic culture, the word *pickles* is almost universally associated with vegetables drowned in mixtures of sugar, water, and vinegar and heated to high temperatures to kill off any bacteria. The result is a soggy, floppy product inferior in almost every way to the traditional pickle.

If you don't make your own pickled veggies at home, look for versions in your supermarket or health food store that were recently fermented and contain live cultures. These products will most likely be found in the refrigerated sections of your grocery store. Avoid the canned versions that have been sitting on the shelves and have long since lost any live probiotics. There are lots of pickled vegetables to choose from. Some examples are listed on the next page.

- Sauerkraut
- Cucumber pickles
- Pickled beets
- Pickled corn relish
- Pickled radishes
- Kimchi (which is a veritable superfood–see Chapter 7)
- Natto
- Miso
- Tempeh

These foods add a novel and delicious flavor to almost any meal. They can be eaten with omelets in the morning, as a substitute for salad in the afternoon, and as a delicious accompaniment to many dinners. For more ideas on how to use these pickles in your personal cuisine, check out the recipes and meal plans in Chapter 11.

Fermented Dairy Products

These are far more popular in America than fermented veggies. And of the fermented dairy products on the market, yogurt is king. On the surface, this seems great. After all, yogurt usually contains multiple strains of probiotics, including lactobacillus and bifidobacteria, both of which occur naturally in the milk of pastured animals like cows, goats, and sheep. So it can be a wonderful source of these friendly healing microbes.

Unfortunately, the yogurt in your grocery store has suffered a similar fate as many of the once healthy and delicious foods co-opted by modern food processing. First, it's *loaded* with sugar. You can hardly find a yogurt these days that doesn't come with an inch-thick disk of jelly buried in it. Many brands even contain HFCS and other powerful sweeteners that aren't good for your gut microbiome or your health. Many so-called "all-natural yogurts" are loaded with aspartame and other artificial sweeteners that have been associated with weight gain and other health problems.[58] All the sugar and artificial sweetener poured into most modern yogurt likely undo any health benefits brought about by the powerful probiotics it contains.

Another irony of modern yogurt production is that it's usually made from milk that's been put through ultra-high-heat pasteurization, which heats milk to 275°F, eradicating every microbe in the milk by sterilizing it completely. This bacteria-free milk is then inoculated with cultures of microbes like lactobacillus so that it can ferment into yogurt.

On the surface this seems crazy–kill off the bacteria only to add them back in? Well, the rationale goes back to the process of pasteurization. Milk, especially when it comes from cows raised in CAFOs, may contain microbes harmful to human health such as salmonella, E. coli, listeria, and others. Pasteurizing milk, especially at high temperatures, eradicates these bacteria.

Because of these issues, raw milk from local sources has become increasingly popular. Raw milk from grass-fed cows has been shown to have a higher content of omega-3 fatty acids (anti-inflammatory fats) and even CLA–which may promote weight loss.[59] At Johns Hopkins, a colleague surveyed a raw milk–buying community to determine whether raw milk consumption mitigated digestive symptoms provoked by pasteurized milk. The survey, completed by 153 of 265 members, showed that more than 20 percent reported gastrointestinal discomfort when drinking pasteurized milk, but 99 percent were able to consume raw milk without discomfort.[60] Those selling raw milk and the estimated 10 million American consumers of this controversial drink have come under tremendous scrutiny. Selling raw milk is actually illegal in half of the United States, so you may not be able to readily access it even if you want it.

In a recent report, the CDC notes that the rate of raw milk-associated illness quadrupled in 2007–2012 (13 annually) when compared to 1993–2006 (3 annually). These outbreaks mainly occur in states that are legally permitted to sell raw milk and their products (for example, cheese).[61] Among the dairy product-associated outbreaks that occurred between 1998 and 2011, 79 percent were due to raw milk products, and *most of those affected were children*, according to the CDC. For this reason, the CDC says that unpasteurized milk is 150 times more likely to cause foodborne illness than pasteurized products.[62]

Raw milk does have its dangers–I'm not a raw milk evangelist. However, the debate over raw milk illustrates our shifting attitude toward the bacteria around and within us. Consider the rates of *C. difficile* in hospitals as a counterpoint to these concerns about raw milk. In the last 10 years, rates of this potentially fatal form of infectious diarrhea have exploded, with 2.2 *million* cases recorded between 2001 and 2010.[63] Nearly 68 percent were contracted while a patient was in the hospital or under medical supervision–largely associated with antibiotic usage. Furthermore, antibiotic overusage has led to resistant strains called *superbugs*. There is a state-to-state national debate about whether or not we should be drinking raw milk while until recently there was barely a peep about a raging *C. difficile* epidemic that is becoming more resistant to treatment, along with superbugs threatening our health.* What is the number one cause of *C. difficile* infection? What is the number one overprescribed medication in the United States? You guessed it: antibiotics, which also appear to contribute toward our obesity epidemic.

For all these reasons, I encourage you to make your own yogurt if you can. You'll find recipes to fit your needs in Chapter 11. If you choose to buy yogurt, go with an unsweetened (plain) version. Look for local sources if you can. Definitely select yogurt from

---

* The Obama administration released a national 5-year strategy calling for a new presidential advisory council to make specific recommendations to the White House by February 2015. This strategy calls for a 50 percent reduction in the overall incidence of *Clostridium difficile* and in the number of methicillin-resistant *Staphylococcus aureus* (MRSA) infections by 2020. In addition, the president's Council of Advisors on Science and Technology (PCAST) released a 78-page report detailing practical steps the government can take to both track resistant germs and develop novel antibiotics to treat bacterial infections.

100 percent grass-fed animals if possible. I personally love White Mountain Bulgarian yogurt, which contains more than 90 billion CFUs of live cultures per serving.

You can also try alternative options like goat's and sheep's organic milk yogurt. And review the labels to make sure the product you choose contains live cultures (at least 1 million colony-forming units or CFUs per gram) and be careful about yogurts doused with added sugar. You can always add a little sweetener like maple syrup if you like.

The other major fermented dairy product in the American marketplace is cheese, which accounts for more sales than yogurt, although many Americans don't seem to realize it's a fermented product. Maybe that's because the American cheese standard–called American cheese–doesn't contain live bacteria. It's hardly cheese at all.

Cheese making is an ancient art, dating back at least 5,000 years and thought to have originated from nomadic herdsmen who stored their milk in sacks made from the stomachs of goats and sheep. The bacteria naturally occurring in the milk reacted with the lactic acid and rennet in the stomach linings, coagulated, fermented, and turned into cheese. Though it has been refined into a high art today, cheese makers still use this same basic set of processes to create cheese (though none that I am aware of store milk in stomachs!).

This kind of cheese–what we now call artisan cheese–is rich in probiotics. In fact, a brick or round of cheese is kind of a living thing that changes over time, its flavors becoming more complex as the bacterial communities it contains develop. Cheese makers are bacteria herders practicing a kind of microbial husbandry. And like fermented vegetables and yogurt, cheese making (and eating!) is a tantalizing example of what happens when the culture around us meets the cultures within.

However, "American cheese" is not such a product. In fact, it was intentionally developed to kill off the microbial communities in cheese. In 1912, a cheese peddler, James

What About Milk and Other Forms of Dairy?

Aside from fermented milk products, the only other dairy allowed in Phase 2 is butter—a healthy, delicious fat you can freely add to your diet at this stage. In fact, ghee is a probiotic form of butter that we highly recommend! Butter from grass-fed cows is best. Choose it if your budget allows. In turn, I'd like you to stay away from milk, cream, half-and-half, custard, and a few other forms of dairy. This will help keep your overall FODMAP count low and has the added benefit of eliminating a set of foods that many people are sensitive to. All the details on what forms of dairy are favored in Phase 2—and which forms you should forget—are in the Phase 2 food charts on pages 246–251.

Lewis Kraft, seeking to make cheese more "shelf stable," created a cheese that would keep for long periods so he could maximize his profits and minimize his losses from cheese spoilage. In the years that followed, food industry entrepreneurs would seek solutions for these problems in their own basement laboratories, just like Kraft.

After conducting experiments, he found that cooking cheese at high temperatures while stirring it constantly emulsified the fats within the cheese and created an easily pourable mixture that he could put into tins, seal, and keep long term. The key reason this "cheese" didn't spoil as quickly was precisely because he'd killed all the microbes by cooking it at high heat. Kraft cheese was born, and it became the flagship product for what would eventually be one of the biggest food conglomerates the world has ever seen.[64]

Today we see "cheese" in millions of processed food products the world over. Powdered cheese, cheese in a can, liquid cheese to shoot inside pizza crusts—the list goes on. These products aren't what I'd call cheese, and they're not what I recommend you include in your diet.

Instead, try adding artisan cheeses. These contain live cultures and are more readily available in supermarkets across America than they've ever been. Experiment with Edam, feta, fresh mozzarella, Brie, blue cheese, ricotta, fromage fraise (fromage blanc), and others. The options are virtually limitless, and these living foods not only add more probiotics to your diet but also enhance the flavor of a broad variety of dishes. So, say cheese! But steer clear of the processed type so typical in the standard American diet.

Of course, cheese and yogurt aren't the only fermented dairy products. You can also try kefir (a superfood I'll discuss in Chapter 7), sour cream, and others. Enjoy these fermented dairy products as a treat, and include them in Phase 2 to help rebalance your inner ecosystem.

Favor Prebiotic Plant Foods

We've already reviewed data showing why prebiotics are such an important part of your diet. They're the fertilizers your gut microbiome needs to flourish, and their benefits have been proven repeatedly in study after study. One question remains: Which prebiotics should you focus on?

Remember that you can include some gluten-free whole grains in your diet. Most of these have prebiotic effects, but don't overdo it, as they're high in carbs and can raise blood sugar—and that has myriad negative downstream metabolic effects. The same is true of nuts, some of which have prebiotic qualities.

So the prebiotics that I want you to favor most during this phase are fruits and veggies high in soluble fiber, plus legumes, a rich resource of prebiotics. These include but are not limited to:

- **Cherries.** Go for sour cherries if you can. They have a lower glycemic load, higher anti-inflammatory activity, and plenty of prebiotic fiber.

- **Berries.** You've already been eating these in Phase 1. Keep it up. Blueberries, raspberries, and others not only contain high levels of antioxidants but also have plenty of soluble fiber like pectin, which your gut bugs love to eat.

- **Bananas.** They're high in resistant starch and are prebiotic, so they feed beneficial bacteria. Try a firm, greenish banana—it tastes a little different and it's slightly higher in fiber and less sugary.

- **Asparagus.** This Phase 2 superfood is packed with healthy fiber your good gut bugs go mad for. See more on the amazing asparagus in Chapter 7.

- **Jerusalem artichokes.** Little known in America, this root vegetable is packed with inulin—the fructan that's been associated with so many impressive effects on the gut microbiome. Steam, peel, mash, and add a little butter to Jerusalem artichokes for a delicious prebiotic-rich alternative to mashed potatoes. Mashed cauliflower with a little butter is another wonderful alternative to potatoes, which leads me to the next class of prebiotics you should include in your diet . . .

- **Cruciferous veggies.** These include broccoli, cauliflower, collards, bok choy, Brussels sprouts, mustard, and kale. Cruciferous veggies are packed with prebiotic dietary fiber, shown to have significant influence on microbial communities in the gut.[65] They also contain a comprehensive profile of nutrients that support the liver, are high in antioxidants, and more. So go green and add plenty of these healthy veggies to your diet.

- **Beans.** The magical fruit. How come the more you eat of these superfoods, the more you toot? It's because your gut bugs are feasting on the galacto-oligosaccharides in them, fermenting the fiber, and releasing gas as a result. Beans are wonderful for the gut microbiome, they enhance satiety, they're easy to prepare, they're packed with phytonutrients, and they have many other health benefits we'll dive into in Chapter 7. Don't worry, you don't have to end up feeling embarrassed by including this magical fruit in your diet. There are ways to prepare beans that reduce their gaseous effects—I'll explain more later.

These are only a few of the all-star options of plant foods that are high in prebiotics. See the Phase 2 food charts on pages 246–251 for more ideas, and make sure to try the delicious prebiotic-rich recipes in Chapter 11.

That's all you need to know to succeed during Phase 2. Remember, if you want to make the program easy on yourself, just follow the meal plans and make the delectable recipes in Chapter 11. Your good gut bugs will absolutely love them. Your palate won't be disappointed either.

WHAT YOU CAN EXPECT DURING PHASE 2

This phase should be substantially easier than Phase 1, and that's a good thing because you're liable to remain on it longer. Any withdrawal symptoms you may have experienced in Phase 1 should be well behind you, and you'll be reintegrating enough foods in this phase to keep the diet interesting enough to keep you on the wagon. I designed Phase 2 this way because I want you to stay on it until you've achieved your desired weight.

You can expect a sustained weight loss of 5 to 10 pounds of excess body weight a month during Phase 2, so you may be on this phase for quite a while if you have substantial weight to lose. That's not a problem at all. Phase 2 is a healthy eating plan you can stick with as long as you like. If you ate this way for the rest of your life, you'd be getting all the healing foods you need to keep your body healthy and balanced. Since Phase 2 encourages the consumption of fermented dairy products, calcium supplementation to compensate for lack of intake of this mineral is not required.

Remember, the name of the game in Phase 2 is diversifying your gut microbiome and providing the fertilizer it needs to thrive. Of all the foods we've discussed in this chapter, pay special attention to the prebiotics and probiotics. These will nourish your inner ecosystem, empowering it to help you lose weight and stay healthy.

Once you've achieved your goal weight, you can transition to Phase 3, a more Mediterranean-style diet that allows you to indulge in the occasional treat while still helping you maintain your weight loss for the long haul. Look for details on how this works in Chapter 8.

LOOKING AHEAD

Now that you understand the principles of Phase 2, it's time to look at our superfoods for this phase. As you can probably guess, lots of them are the prebiotics and probiotics you need to seed and fertilize your inner garden. But I have a few surprises in store for you, including a fermented dairy beverage whose name literally means "good feeling," an ancient Indian spice that will help you burn fat and turn down systemic inflammation, and a fermented condiment from the ancient Near East. Include these superfoods in Phase 2 and your inner garden will flourish like never before.

CHAPTER 7

Dr. Gerry's Top 10 Superfoods for Phase 2

The superfoods for Phase 2 are filled with prebiotics and probiotics, though I have thrown in an anti-inflammatory spice and a pungent fermented condiment for good measure. No doubt a few of these will be familiar to you, but I think you'll be surprised by some of them. Include plenty of these foods in your Phase 2 eating plan and you'll burn more fat while enjoying the benefits of a health-promoting biodiverse gut microbiome.

I. OATS

Oats are the most nutrient-rich superstars in the cereal kingdom. The bran of oats is particularly high in fiber and is a good source of protein. One serving—just $1/4$ cup—of oat bran contains 4 grams of protein and 3.6 grams of dietary fiber.[1] Although the carb content appears high at 15.6 grams per $1/4$-cup serving, the rich, nonabsorbable fiber content keeps the *net* absorbable carb content to just 12 grams. The benefits of satiation, along with the prebiotic effects, make oats a weight-loss superfood. A serving of oats contains nearly the entire Recommended Dietary Allowance (RDA) of manganese—a trace mineral involved in bone health, blood sugar regulation, and more—and a good dose of vitamin B_1, copper, biotin, and other nutrients. One of the key features of whole grain oats is their negligible impact on blood sugar levels and gentle stimulation of insulin. It's a good carb to include in your weight-loss arsenal!

Oats originated in Asia, and the modern oat is a descendant of the wild red oats that were classically grown there. In Asia, oats were used medicinally. When they were brought to the West, they were thought of only as food for animals, specifically horses. Indeed, whole oats can't be digested by humans and are used solely as animal fodder.

Hulled oats, cleaned and toasted–called oat groats–are a wonderful food source for people. The Scots were among the first Europeans to add oats to their diet, and steel-cut oats (which I strongly recommend) are sometimes called Scotch oats to this day. Steel-cut oats are simply oat groats cut into several pieces. They retain more of the bran than rolled oats, and the bran is where the action is when it comes to the prebiotic effect of this superfood.

Oat bran is a powerful prebiotic. Bran is the part of a whole grain from which fiber comes. Oat bran is special because it contains a particular kind of fiber called beta-glucan, shown to reduce cholesterol levels and risk of cardiovascular events.[2,3] This relationship between increased dietary fiber and reduction in heart disease has been repeatedly corroborated. For example, in one study, researchers followed 10,000 people over 19 years and found that those who ate the most fiber had 12 percent less heart disease and 11 percent less cardiovascular disease.[4] A meta-analysis published in the *American Journal of Clinical Nutrition* showed even more impressive results–those with the highest fiber intake suffered 29 percent less cardiovascular disease compared to those with the lowest.[5]

The effects of oats on blood sugar levels, type 2 diabetes, and obesity have also been studied. Oats are digested slowly, so they keep blood glucose more stable over time. Their fiber also helps you feel full, leading to your eating less–and if you have them for breakfast, you'll feel full later into the day. This effect goes back to beta-glucan, which is a soluble fiber, so it soaks up water and creates a kind of gel in your intestines.

Oat bran is high in magnesium, a mineral that plays a role in blood sugar control and insulin secretion. An 8-year trial involving 41,186 women showed a fascinating relationship between oat intake, magnesium levels, and incidences of type 2 diabetes.[6] Women who ate whole grains rich in magnesium had a 31 percent lower chance of developing type 2 diabetes compared to those who had a magnesium-poor diet.

Oats seem to enhance immune response,[7] they may protect against breast cancer,[8] and they can help prevent and reverse childhood asthma.[9] Some doctors even suggest that their health-promoting activities are equal to or greater than those of fruits and vegetables.

Oats are gluten-free grains, although conventionally grown and processed oats have problems with cross contamination and may contain some gluten–which may become problematic if you are known to have gluten intolerance or celiac disease. If so, I am recommending you continue to avoid gluten and consume certified gluten-free, organic, steel-cut oats. For those without a gluten sensitivity, the issue of potential cross contamination is less crucial; if you can afford the additional cost, purchase the organic steel-cut oats, as they are free from gluten cross contamination.

Oats have helped me tremendously on my own weight-loss journey. Here's a tip that's worked for me: Cook some steel-cut oats, add a little unsweetened (plain) yogurt or kefir and a dab of 100% pure maple syrup or raw honey, and you've got a powerful gut microbiome-balancing superbreakfast that will help you burn fat (and protect your heart, immune system, and more) all day long.

Honorable Mention: Raw Honey

I asked you to avoid honey in Phase 1 due to its rich fructose content (38.5 grams per 100 grams of honey) and high glycemic impact. As a general rule, I ask you to *limit* raw honey in Phase 2 as well. Keep it to about a teaspoon at a time, and don't use it as a sugar substitute—use it in precious limited quantities as a superfood. But ample evidence shows that raw honey has positive effects on gut microbiome health.

There is also evidence that honey has antimicrobial effects against gut pathogens such as *E. coli* O17:H7, *Pseudomonas, Proteus, Enterobacter,* and other bugs we want to keep in check for a healthy gut microbiome. Raw honey, a prebiotic due to its rich oligosaccharide content that promotes the growth of bifidobacteria,[10] also limits growth of pathogenic biofilms. Honey has anti-inflammatory, antioxidant, immunoregulatory, and antitumor properties.[11, 12] It both contains and raises levels of nitric oxide in tissues, which improves healing, enhances antibiotic functions, and protects the nervous and cardiovascular system.[13] In addition, it has antibiotic effects[14] and positive effects on:

- Allergies[15]
- Bone health[16]
- Burns[17]
- Common cold[18]
- Diabetes[19]
- Leg ulcers[20]
- Skin care[21]
- Wound healing[22]

You may wonder why we're devoting so much time to discussing honey if it's so restricted in the meal plans. Remember the mantra—the dose makes the poison! Treat honey as a superfood, not a sugar substitute. Use it in tiny amounts in tea or coffee or as a sweetener for your shakes.

Note that high heat inactivates the propolis (waxy resin) and hence the antimicrobial activities of honey. True raw honey retains these properties and is often available at farmers' and organic markets. Look for organic or wild, nonpasteurized honey for all the gut-balancing benefits that will help melt those calories away.

You can also try manuka honey, made in New Zealand from the nectar of manuka flowers (*Leptospermum scoparium*). In 2007, the FDA approved a medical-grade manuka honey, sold as Medihoney, for treating wounds and skin ulcers.

An important note: **Don't feed infants honey.** On rare occasions, honey products may be contaminated with *Clostridium botulinum* spores and toxins, toxic to infants.

2. ASPARAGUS

Asparagus is the weight-loss tree of choice. Its small thin stalks, considered a delicacy for more than 2,000 years, are shoots that, left uncut, would grow into a small tree. Mature asparagus is inedible, but the delectable immature shoots are packed with health benefits.

For starters, asparagus is high in inulin–the prebiotic fructan we've been discussing throughout Phase 2. So it's an ideal food source for healthy microbial communities like bifidobacteria, lactobacillus, and others. The other major inulin contenders are Jerusalem artichoke and chicory root, both of which are more difficult to find in the American marketplace.

Its prebiotic effect alone is enough to recommend asparagus for this program,[23] but its benefits don't end there. It's rich in saponins, a class of phytonutrients repeatedly shown to possess a variety of biological properties, such as being antioxidant, antihepatotoxic, antibacterial, anti-inflammatory, immunoregulatory, and anticancer agents.[24-26] They also reduce blood pressure, balance blood sugar, and reduce body fat levels. Natural medicine clinicians often recommend asparagus to reduce ankle swelling.[27]

Asparagus, an antioxidant powerhouse,[28] is one of the few foods besides cruciferous vegetables containing a meaningful amount of glutathione–a powerful antioxidant that reduces fat-promoting inflammation and oxidative stress throughout the body. One serving provides the RDA of vitamin K, substantial amounts of folate and vitamin B_1 (which play a critical role in the regulation of homocysteine, an amino acid that can increase the risk of cardiovascular problems when it gets too high), vitamin C, vitamin E, and many other health-promoting nutrients.

The best thing about asparagus? It's easy to prepare. Steam it, grill it, roast it. Add a little olive oil, salt and pepper, and lemon. You and your good gut bugs will enjoy a feast!

3. BEANS

Beans are among the few foods that receive the support of virtually every major health and wellness organization on the planet. The American Diabetes Association,[29] the American Heart Association,[30] and the American Cancer Society,[31] to name a few, recommend two to three servings of beans weekly to reduce the risk of a wide variety of chronic illnesses, from type 2 diabetes to cardiovascular disease to cancer.[32,]

What makes beans such a powerful superfood? One element is their combination of fiber and protein. One serving provides about 15 grams of protein and between 11 grams (kidney beans) and 17 grams (adzuki beans) of fiber per cup.[33] This one-two punch of protein and fiber has a wide range of health benefits.

First, they stabilize blood glucose levels. Fiber and protein move through your digestive tract slowly, so they're converted to sugar slowly, which is precisely what you want to lose weight and get healthy. Fiber also reduces the uptake of cholesterol, and high-fiber diets have been associated with a reduction in both cholesterol and heart disease.[34] The gut microbiota may play a role in determining the risk of cardiovascular disease, so the prebiotic properties of soluble fibers in beans may protect against heart disease by favoring the growth of good gut bugs.[35]

Additionally, the fiber in beans is a wonderful food source for your good gut bacteria. When your friendly flora eat the mixture of fiber in beans, they seem to produce more butyric acid, which the cells in the lining of your colon use for various activities. This keeps the lower part of your digestive tract healthy and supports a perfect environment for a thriving inner ecosystem.

Beans are also rich in important antioxidant and anti-inflammatory compounds, yet another reason researchers believe they protect against chronic illness.[36] They contain high levels of saponins, just as asparagus does, and they also have three important anthocyanin flavonoids: delphinidin, petunidin, and malvidin–phytonutrients with both anti-inflammatory and antioxidant properties.[37] Their anti-inflammatory properties are so powerful that they can increase healthy colonic biomarkers and attenuate experimental colitis.[38]

These extraordinary plant foods even contain alpha-amylase inhibitors, chemicals that reduce the activity of the alpha-amylase enzyme (aka starch blockers).[39] That's important because this enzyme is involved in the rapid breakdown of food into simple sugars. By slowing down its activity, beans give you another edge against the blood sugar roller coaster you need to avoid to achieve long-term health and optimal weight. But is there proof that these firecracking leguminous plants can help you lose weight?

A 2014 study determined that a bean-rich diet that was high in fiber while low in absorbable carbohydrates enhanced satiety and promoted weight loss.[40] In the study, 173 obese women and men were randomized into either a high-fiber bean-rich diet providing 35.5 daily grams of fiber for women and 42.5 grams for men, or a low-carbohydrate diet. After 16 weeks, the difference in weight loss between the two groups (bean-rich 9 pounds, low-carb 11.4 pounds) was not statistically significant. However, the low-density lipoprotein (LDL) cholesterol and total cholesterols (atherogenic lipids) were significantly lower in those on the bean-rich diet compared to the low-carb diet. Another study in 2011 evaluated 32 obese subjects randomly assigned to one of two calorically equivalent, energy-restricted diets for 8 weeks: a legume-free diet or a legume-based diet.[41] The legume-based diet involved 4 weekly servings of lentils, chickpeas, peas, or beans. The legume-rich diet was associated with a significantly greater weight loss than the legume-free diet. Plus, the high-legume diet was associated with reduced proinflammatory markers and with improved cardiovascular profile (lipid profile and blood pressure).

These studies blow a hole in the low-carb-for-life approach to keeping the weight off. Our body needs good fibrous carbs to thrive–the survival of our friendly flora that sustain our livelihood requires fiber.

There *is* a downside to beans. They may increase flatulence. To avoid this problem, simply soak dried beans for a few hours, which has been shown to reduce two of the components that lead to gas: raffinose and stachyose.[42]

Canned beans are fine if you're tight on time. Rinse them well before eating and make sure you stick with salt-free versions–salt them to taste yourself. Presalted beans tend to be very high in sodium. I prefer cooking with presoaked dried beans, as the flavor and texture are better, and there's evidence they may retain higher quantities of the important phytonutrients that protect your health and your waistline.

4. KALE

Along with its cousins broccoli, bok choy, cabbage, mustard, Brussels sprouts, and collard, kale is the descendant of a wild cabbage plant that originated in Asia Minor. These plants are all called cruciferous vegetables, from the Latin word for "cross-bearing," which makes sense if you've ever seen the yellow cross-shaped blossoms these plants produce.

Cruciferous vegetables are a superfamily of foods, so powerful that some doctors recommend eating as much as four or five 2-cup servings weekly. And though it's hard to choose just one of these superveggies, recent research suggests that kale deserves a special place of recognition among its brethren. That's because it contains 45 different flavonoids–phytonutrients known for their anti-inflammatory properties. This is a stunning variety of flavonoids in a single food, and I'm not aware of any other vegetable containing as many. Of the flavonoids in kale, kaempferol and quercetin hold the spotlight.

A hundred calories of kale also provides 350 milligrams of alpha-linolenic acid, a healthy omega-3 fat contributing to the plant's anti-inflammatory properties. And it has more than 1,180 percent of the RDA of vitamin K, a key nutrient deeply involved in regulating the inflammatory process. That's a lot of anti-inflammatory muscle for one plant.

Research shows that kale may mitigate your risk of colon, breast, bladder, prostate, and ovarian cancer, probably due to its high levels of glucosinolates, a set of compounds that provide anticancer activity.[43] Kale also reduces blood levels of cholesterol, supporting heart health. The mechanisms by which it does this have been well documented. Bile, made in the liver using cholesterol as one of its primary building blocks, is needed to digest fat in the foods you eat. Once it's made, it's released from the liver and stored in the gallbladder. The gallbladder then delivers bile as needed to help you digest fat. Nutrients in kale bind to these bile acids in the gut, allowing them to pass through the digestive system and out through your bowel without binding to fat, forcing the liver to tap into your cholesterol store to make more bile, thus lowering overall cholesterol levels.

Kale lowers cholesterol so effectively that it was recently compared with a cholesterol-lowering prescription medication called cholestyramine, which reduces serum cholesterol using the same method outlined above. Steamed kale was found to be 42 percent more effective than the drug cholestyramine.[44]

5. MISO

Miso is made by steaming soybeans, mashing them, adding salt, and then inoculating them with *koji*–a traditional Japanese rice-based starter culture that typically contains high levels of the fungus *Aspergillus oryzae*. This mixture is then allowed to age and ferment for a few months to a few years. The resulting paste is a microbial paradise that you can use to rebalance your inner ecosystem by adding it to soups, salads, and stir-fries. Made from soybeans, miso provides many of the health benefits you get from beans while packing a probiotic punch at the same time–a spectacular one-two combination for gut microbiome health.

The Salt Problem and Obesity

Most everyone knows that too much sodium is a bad thing for cardiovascular health. Keeping sodium consumption in check is one of the biggest challenges facing those of us who dine out for work-related or social functions, because restaurants are notorious for adding salt to optimize food taste and create thirst to spike beverage sales.

Too much sodium in your foods can translate to big-time health problems, and lowering consumption to the CDC's and American Heart Association's recommended guidelines of 1,500 to 2,300 milligrams daily lowers blood pressure, stroke risk, cardiovascular risk, and mortality from ischemic heart disease.[45, 46] "Nearly everyone benefits from reduced sodium consumption," said Janelle Gunn, a public health analyst in the CDC's division for heart disease and stroke prevention. "Ninety percent of Americans exceed the general daily recommended sodium intake limit of 2,300 milligrams, increasing their risk for high blood pressure, heart disease, and stroke."[47]

So if this is a book about your gut and weight loss, why all the sodium coverage? Well, believe it or not, high sodium intake in adolescents has been linked to—you guessed it—being overweight! In a study reported in the journal *Pediatrics*, adolescents' sodium intake was as high as adults' and more than twice the guidelines of the American Heart Association.[48] High sodium intake was correlated with adiposity and inflammation independent of total caloric intake and sugar-sweetened soft drink consumption. And some data link sodium intake to heightened levels of inflammatory conditions, such as tumor necrosis factor-alpha.[49,50] High-salt diets have been linked to tissue inflammation and worsening of autoimmune disease. Sodium-restricted diets have been shown to lower inflammatory markers prior to changes in blood pressure.[51]

Ultimately, what does all this mean? Sodium intake appears to be linked to inflammation, which has been strongly linked to obesity. In putting together a program to reduce inflammation and promote weight loss and good health, I took the CDC's dietary guidelines for sodium content into account.

One criticism of miso has been that it's high in salt, and excess sodium can be a contributing factor to high blood pressure and cardiovascular conditions. But recent Japanese studies may indicate that there's nothing to fear from miso. In one study, researchers fed one group miso and a second group an equivalent amount of table salt. These two dietary alterations had very different effects. The high-salt diet increased blood pressure. The diet that included the same amount of sodium in the form of miso had no effect at all. Some studies have shown that miso may have a cardioprotective effect; in one large trial involving 40,462 participants, intake of miso reduced the risk of cerebral infarction, a major type of stroke.[52]

The process of miso fermentation seems to further enhance the nutritional profile of this superfood. For example, isoflavones in soy have come under recent scrutiny due to their impact on estrogen levels and the resulting health consequences that may ensue. The primary fungus used in miso fermentation, *Aspergillus oryzae,* seems to break down two of the more dangerous of these isoflavones: daidzein and genistein. The fermentation process also appears to create antioxidant compounds such as ferulic, coumaric, and kojic acids (among others), which may provide this food's anticancer activity.

Traditionally, of course, miso is made into soup, and no doubt this is among the most delicious ways to consume it. There's only one downside to eating miso as soup: You kill off some of the good bacteria by heating it. One way to minimize this is to avoid boiling miso soup, which most chefs recommend anyway simply to retain its nuanced flavors. Try to keep the soup below 120°F to retain its microbial cultures, though this is difficult without monitoring the pot with a thermometer.

A different approach is to add fresh, uncooked miso to salad dressings. This is a delicious way to incorporate the fresh miso paste that will give your inner garden the seeds it needs to flourish.

6. YOGURT

Fermenting milk to make yogurt was first done by Balkan nomads in the Middle East, who used this technique to preserve the milk from their animals as they roamed. Yogurt can be made from the milk of any ruminant animal, including sheep, goats, and cows. Cow's milk yogurt is by far the most popular in this country, but I encourage you to try yogurt from sheep and goats as well—they all have a different flavor and texture.

One of the best probiotic foods is live-cultured yogurt, especially handmade at home—it can contain up to 100 times as many live cultures per serving as store-bought varieties. I especially like goat's milk yogurts and cheeses, as they are particularly high in probiotics like *Streptococcus thermophilus, Bifudus, Lactobacillus bulgaricus,* and *L. acidophilus.* Your good gut bugs are telling your brain, "Yum—please make some for us to feast!"

Yogurt containing live cultures has been shown to decrease total cholesterol while increasing HDL, the healthy cholesterol you want more of. In one study, Iranian women

Honorable Mention:
Other Fermented Soy Foods

While we're talking about fermented soy products, let's take a moment to bring some other soy-based superfoods to your awareness and palate.

Tempeh is a probiotic food derived from fermented soybeans. The primary probiotic in tempeh is *Rhizopus oligosporus,* which produces a natural antibiotic against enteric pathogens (pathogens produced inside the body), as well as phytase, an enzyme that helps break down phytate acid, which increases the absorption of minerals. Fermented soy paste reduces visceral fat accumulation.[53] Plus, since tempeh isn't salted, it's suitable for people on a low-sodium diet.

Natto is made from fermented soybeans; it contains the bacterial strain *Bacillus subtilis*, which gives this food its characteristic stringy consistency. In addition to being a probiotic source containing soy, natto contains the enzyme nattokinase, which dissolves dangerous blood clots.[54] The protein and other nutrients in soybeans become more digestible after they're broken down by bacteria or mold, and that's why fermented bean products like tempeh and natto don't cause the flatulence associated with beans.

Soy itself may impart an antiobesity benefit. Several nutritional intervention studies in animals and humans indicate that soy protein consumption reduces body weight and fat mass in addition to lowering plasma cholesterol and triglycerides.[55] In animal models of obesity, soy protein limits or reduces body fat accumulation and improves insulin resistance, the hallmark of human obesity.[56] In obese humans, dietary soy protein also reduces body weight and body fat mass in addition to reducing plasma lipids. A head-to-head trial of calorically equivalent soy milk to cow's milk showed that there was no difference in the weight-reducing benefits.[57]

who consumed 10 ounces of yogurt a day for 6 weeks saw total cholesterol drop while HDL increased.[58] Researchers feel the reason may have to do with sphingolipids—healthy fats naturally occurring in yogurt that play a key role in cellular signaling. A recent study from India also showed that 2 cups of yogurt weekly reduced the risk of hip fracture.[59] The healthy bacteria in yogurt also help metabolize food more efficiently and produce higher levels of short-chain fatty acids—those healthy fats that are important for proper intestinal functioning.

These benefits only scratch the surface. The list is constantly expanding, especially since the first global summit on the health effects of yogurt was held in 2013.[60] For example, cultured milk and yogurt have been linked to a reduced risk of developing colorectal cancer and to preventing antibiotic-induced diarrhea,[61] improving digestive symptoms,[62] improving dental health,[63] preventing osteoporosis, lowering the risk of heart attack, and decreasing blood pressure.[64]

Studies have also shown that regular consumption of yogurt can reduce your risk of developing type 2 diabetes.[65] A recent analysis compared 11 years' worth of food journals from 3,502 people and found that those who regularly ate yogurt were 28 percent less likely to become diabetic.[66] Most scientists agree this is related to two components in yogurt: protein and probiotics. Yogurt is relatively high in protein, which is digested slowly, helping keep blood sugar stable over time. Greek yogurt is thicker and particularly high in satiating protein. A word of caution for those with a known sensitivity to casein–Greek yogurt is nearly 100 percent casein, as the whey is strained out to enhance thickness. While I couldn't find any head-to-head studies of Greek yogurt to conventional yogurt regarding satiety, metabolic parameters, or weight loss, I do recommend this form to patients who desire an appetite-curbing snack. Try it with berries, such as highly fibrous raspberries, and some nuts. There are now manufacturers of organic Greek yogurt.

The healthy probiotics in yogurt seem to further support its blood glucose balancing effects. The microbes in yogurt regulate the passage of food through your gut. Steady digestion is important for blood sugar regulation, as it keeps food from being digested too quickly (which can spike blood sugar and insulin) or too slowly (causing blood sugar and insulin to dip too swiftly after meals).

Studies suggest that dairy in general supports weight loss, and fermented dairy seems to be particularly useful in this regard, probably because the whey protein in dairy regulates satiety. Although the energy intakes for yogurt and other fermented dairy products such as cheese and milk are similar, yogurt produced the greatest suppressive effect on appetite.[67] Some interesting proof: A study of 212 Korean women found that those who consumed at least one daily serving of yogurt weighed less.[68] Another Korean study demonstrated that consumption of a specially formulated yogurt (NY-YP901) improved blood lipids and cardiovascular markers and induced weight loss in obese individuals with metabolic syndrome.[69] In yet another study, yogurt consumption was found to decrease body weight and postmeal hunger. Investigators found that those consuming yogurt had higher levels of the gut-derived hormone glucagon-like peptide 2, which suppresses appetite.[70] Other research shows that substituting the same quantity of calories of yogurt for other foods preserves lean muscle mass while augmenting fat loss, improving waist circumference, and reducing fat gain.[71]

One of the most compelling studies on the influence of yogurt on weight comes from Spain, where many people consume yogurt as a dessert. Investigators from Seguimiento Universidad de Navarra evaluated 8,516 men and women prospectively during a 2-year period as to yogurt consumption and outcome. Those who consumed more than seven servings (125 grams per serving) per week of yogurt (full fat) were associated with a lower incidence of overweight or obesity in comparison to those whose consumption was low (less than two servings weekly).[72] Moreover, this association was even stronger in those who were regular fruit consumers–typical of the Mediterranean lifestyle that forms the foundation for our Phase 3. The fruit likely provided a prebiotic effect to bolster the probiotic weight-reducing effect.

These effects seem to span age ranges from young to old, so most everyone can benefit from yogurt. One study attempted to improve constipation in elderly individuals by feeding them yogurt. While the yogurt didn't appear to improve constipation, it did help the participants lose significant body weight.[73]

I have a bias toward the probiotic cultures in yogurt, which are a big part of what makes it a superfood for weight loss because it restores your gut balance. But the healthy bacteria in this fermented milk product are not the only things that provide health benefits, so let's look at a few other important components of yogurt.

Yogurt is loaded with calcium and vitamin D. There are data showing that calcium and vitamin D may influence weight balance. In one study, women burned more fat and calories when they had 1,000 to 1,400 milligrams of calcium per day. And in a study of 218 obese-to-overweight postmenopausal women with vitamin D insufficiency, those who supplemented with vitamin D and attained sufficient serum levels lost more weight, reduced their waist circumference, and dropped more body fat.[74] So it's certainly possible that vitamin D and calcium provide fermented dairy products with additional weight-loss prowess.

Remember that today's milk is far from perfect because it contains antibiotics, hormones, pesticides, and other foreign substances or potential contaminants. We avoided milk products in Phase 1 due to their high FODMAP content and the fact that the fatty acid profile of conventional milk products is on the proinflammatory side. So why bring milk products back into Phase 2 and beyond?

Well, unless you're lactose intolerant, fermented milk products promote a healthy gut microbiome and appear to facilitate weight loss. It's also interesting to note that yogurt is lower in lactose than milk. As milk is fermented by these friendly bacteria, they digest part of the lactose. Even those who are lactose sensitive can eat yogurt in some cases–more so if it is homemade. Experiment with it, tune in to how your body reacts, and see if it works for you.

Not only does consumption of dairy products and their milk proteins increase satiety and reduce food intake, but it decreases blood glucose response when consumed alone or with carbohydrates.[75] And the fatty acids found in these products, particularly the conjugated linoleic acid (CLA), may support weight-loss attempts. (Refer to page 106 in Chapter 6 for a refresher on CLA.)

Remember that most industrial yogurt is first pasteurized and then inoculated with specific strains of bacteria–a process that works but that may produce suboptimal amounts of "live" probiotics. That's why I recommend you make your own yogurt and other fermented milk products. Use organic milk whenever possible, as it's typically

What About Fat-Free Dairy Products?

Is fat-free, or skim, milk as good as whole milk for reducing appetite? That controversy continues to rage in the medical literature. Even nutrition experts from Harvard say that there's a quicker blood sugar response to fat-free milk, as the fat in whole milk slows down the entry of milk sugar (lactose) into the small intestine, where it's absorbed.[76] There is ample evidence that fat-free dairy provides no additional benefit for a healthy weight status over regular-fat products.[77, 78]

If you've been convinced that fat-free milk products are healthier, you may think me mad for suggesting whole milk over fat-free in your tea and cereal. You may wonder if whole milk increases the risk of cardiovascular disease.

A recent study put things in perspective. Investigators examined the association between the type of dairy and the risk of having a myocardial infarction (heart attack). Bottom line: Overall, milk, cheese, and yogurt are inversely associated with cardiovascular disease (CVD) risk.[79] A meta-analysis of more than 600,000 multiethnic adults found no difference between full-fat or low-fat dairy consumption (less than 200 grams/daily).[80] This dose-response meta-analysis of prospective studies indicates that milk intake is not associated with total mortality but may be *inversely* associated with overall CVD risk. A Dutch study that was prospective and observational confirmed these retrospective conclusions about total dairy intake lowering CVD risk in those without preexisting hypertension and noted that only those who consistently consumed ice cream and butter lost this protective effect. These investigators also reported that only fermented dairy products are to be associated with a lower risk of stroke.[81]

antibiotic free and may be higher in healthy fats. Grass-fed cows have higher levels of CLA and more anti-inflammatory fat profiles.

There are now machines that make it simple to prepare your own yogurt at home. These can be a convenient addition to your kitchen. You'll find an easy recipe for yogurt in Chapter 11.

If you choose to purchase yogurt, look for brands containing live cultures with at least 1 million CFUs (colony-forming units).[82] The National Yogurt Association developed a Live & Active Culture seal to help consumers identify products that meets its standards for significant amounts of live and active cultures. Refrigerated yogurt products containing at least 100 million cultures per gram and frozen yogurt products containing at least 10 million cultures per gram at the time of manufacture may bear the seal. The store-bought yogurt with the highest cultures, according to New York City nutritionist Dr. Loren Marks, is White Mountain organic Bulgarian yogurt, containing 90 billion CFUs per serving (whitemountainfoods.com/Products.html). It goes wonderfully with fresh Turkish or Mission figs (not dried, which is loaded with sugars)—a nice prebiotic!

7. KEFIR

The word *kefir* derives from the Turkish word *keif,* which denotes the good feeling one has after drinking this fermented milk product.[83] Kefir looks like a runny yogurt or thickened milk and has a slight sour taste and smell. It originated in the Caucasus Mountains between the Caspian and the Black Seas. The people there seem to have preferred fermenting camel's milk to make kefir. Today, it's most commonly made from cow's and goat's milk.

Kefir is among the simplest fermented products to prepare at home. All you do is find a few kefir grains, drop them in milk, store the mixture out of direct sunlight for 1 to 2 days, stirring it occasionally–and, voilà, you have kefir.

The kefir grains themselves are one of the most fascinating microbial communities around. They are a SCOBY–an acronym that stands for "symbiotic colony of bacteria and yeast." The kefir SCOBY is an ecosystem in its own right that involves at least 10 to 20 different strains of bacteria and yeast, including lactobacilli, *Leuconostoc, Acetobacter,* and *Saccharomyces.*[84] During fermentation, the grains increase in size and number and are either left in the fermented milk or recovered and reused.

Multiple studies have shown that kefir has a wide range of health benefits.[85] Several studies demonstrated that kefir and its constituents have antimicrobial, anticancer, and immune regulation activities[86] and many others.[87] It improves gut microbiome balance through its powerful probiotic effects. This is probably one of the reasons it's known to protect against gastrointestinal diseases. For example, bacterial strains from kefir cultures reduce intestinal inflammation and ameliorate symptoms in those who suffer from colitis.[88] It also appears to help with lactose digestion in adults who suffer from lactose intolerance.[89]

The anti-inflammatory properties of kefir are impressive. Studies have revealed that it reduces cytokine production, mitigates mast cell degranulation, and reduces the production of IgE in people who suffer from allergies.[90] So if you suffer from the spring sneezes, drink up! Plus, preliminary evidence in animal models shows that it may be a key agent in the fight against cancer due to its antitumor properties.[91]

Historically, kefir has been recommended for the treatment of digestive conditions, hypertension, allergies,[92] and heart disease.[93] This superfood may even block cholesterol assimilation, reducing overall blood levels.[94] Kefir has anti-fat-forming effects that may, in part, explain the benefit of fermented milk in fighting obesity in one clinical trial.[95]

Kefir is high in vitamin K_2, thiamin, B_{12}, calcium, and a host of other vitamins and minerals–each of which adds to its superstar status among fermented dairy products.

Try making kefir at home and adding it to cooked steel-cut oats with a few blueberries for a delicious breakfast your inner flora will thank you for.

8. KIMCHI

Kimchi, the iconic food of Korean culture, is a natural but powerful probiotic. It's made in homes and restaurants across the country and served as a side dish with virtually every meal. The result is a mind-boggling array of kimchi in the world. If you've ever been to a Korean restaurant and been presented with dozens of small dishes filled with wonderful ferments of every shape, size, color, and consistency, then you may have some sense of how many different kinds of kimchi Korean culture has produced. But even for those of us who are fans of this cuisine, it's stunning to consider that 167 distinct styles of kimchi have been documented, and there may be even more, given regional and household differences in recipes.

The health effects of kimchi would take up a book in their own right.[96] So here we'll focus on *baechu*, a spicy Korean sauerkraut made from Chinese cabbage. The same fermentation process–lactic acid fermentation–is used for both sauerkraut and *baechu*, but unlike sauerkraut, *baechu* typically incorporates radish, red pepper, ginger, garlic, and a host of other vegetables and spices. This amalgamation creates health benefits greater than the sum of the parts.

Baechu is high in vitamin C, the B-complex vitamins, and minerals like sodium, calcium, potassium, and others. It typically has lots of capsaicin–the healthy, anti-inflammatory constituent of peppers we learned about in Phase 1.

A good deal of research has been done on the effects of kimchi on weight loss, and the results are stunning. In rats, kimchi normalized and sustained a healthy body weight.[97] How is that possible? Well, kimchi is actually like a superfood *within* a superfood! It contains Korean red-pepper powder or *kochukaru*, a thermogenic that may be partially responsible for kimchi's fat-burning effect.[98] Remember when we discussed the fat-burning effects of peppers in Chapter 5? Well, the capsaicin is almost certainly one of the reasons for the fat-burning potential of kimchi.

Rats aren't the only creatures that lose weight when kimchi is added to their diet. It works on people, too. In a study of obese women, one group engaged in 1 hour of exercise per week. The second group exercised and took a kimchi supplement (3 to 6 grams of freeze-dried kimchi daily). Those who took the kimchi capsules lost an impressive amount of weight–approximately 22 pounds over the course of 12 weeks. They saw significantly greater improvement in their body mass index (BMI), visceral fat, and triglyceride levels compared to the women who didn't receive the kimchi.[99]

Another study showed that fresh, fermented kimchi (not freeze-dried) has even more powerful effects. In this study, researchers encouraged overweight and obese subjects to eat kimchi regularly. When participants did so, they not only had a reduction in weight and BMI but their overall body fat percentage dropped, they experienced a decrease in waist-to-hip ratio, blood glucose stabilized, fasting insulin dropped, and leptin levels improved.[100] These researchers concluded that adding kimchi to the diet may reduce the risk of metabolic syndrome, cardiovascular disease, and type 2 diabetes.

There's also good evidence kimchi improves cholesterol profiles. In a recent study, researchers reviewed the effects of daily kimchi consumption on the lipid parameters of 102 adult Korean men between the ages of 40 and 64.[101] They found that eating kimchi increased HDL and reduced LDL; the preference for hot taste correlated with a reduction in systolic blood pressure, indicating that the capsaicin in the red pepper has antihypertensive properties.

Additional research suggests that kimchi may have anticancer properties[102] and modulate immune system function.[103] Kimchi has impressive antimicrobial activities against bad bugs such as *Bacillus subtilis*, *Escherichia coli*, *Salmonella enteritidis*, *S. paratyphi* and *S. typhi*, *Staphylococcus aureus*, and *Shigella boydii* and *S. sonnei*. Overall, kimchi is the one-stop superfood for protecting your health.

You can make your own kimchi at home or buy it at the supermarket. If you choose to purchase it, select a brand containing live active cultures. The jar should fizz when you open it, a sure sign that the friendly microbes you desire are alive and well.

9. TURMERIC

Turmeric, along with the other spices discussed throughout this book, may provide the best model for the food-as-medicine approach to halting the vicious cycle of obesity and inflammation. This bright yellow spice is most well known as one of the primary ingredients in curry. Americans are probably more familiar with it as the agent that makes ballpark mustard a bright yellow. Turmeric has an exotic floral fragrance, which may be why it was used as a perfume in biblical times.

Turmeric has long been used in Chinese and Indian medicine systems to treat ailments ranging from flatulence to chest pain to menstrual difficulties. Modern science is showing that it does, indeed, have some serious pharmacological capabilities. In fact, its primary active agent, curcumin, has anti-inflammatory properties as strong as prescription medications like hydrocortisone and over-the-counter painkillers like ibuprofen.[104] But while these medications can lead to ulcer formation and liver damage, curcumin has no such adverse effects.

Its anti-inflammatory action makes curcumin an excellent adjunct to treatment for a broad range of inflammation-based illnesses such as osteoarthritis, nonulcer dyspepsia (abdominal discomfort), inflammatory bowel disease, and rheumatoid arthritis; it may also be useful in preventing cancer and heart disease.[105, 106] As we discussed in Chapter 2, chronic low-grade inflammation may underlie much of the pathology contributing to the health risks associated with obesity. Given the amount of information on turmeric's health benefits, let's look into its potential for helping you keep the weight off and why I chose it as a superfood for the Gut Balance Revolution approach to a lean metabolism.

Curcumin has been shown to reduce intestinal inflammation, improve gut barrier function, and decrease the translocation of harmful bacterial by-products from the gut into systemic circulation (endotoxemia). Plus, it calms down the inflammatory and immune responses–important to a number of intestinal conditions as well as obesity.[107]

In fact, a number of studies performed on laboratory animals support the contention that curcumin improves the loss of body weight, increases basal metabolism, blocks adipogenesis (fat creation), facilitates the regression of fat cell mass, and reduces inflammatory markers.[108-110]

Inflammation is one of the villains driving the overweight and obesity epidemics in this country. It disrupts critical pathways involved in energy metabolism and injures a vast array of systems, producing many complications throughout the body.[111] Therapies that reduce inflammation can help derail the vicious cycle of weight gain and chronic illness.

Fat cells, of course, aren't simply innocent bystanders when you gain weight. They not only grow in size but produce and release proinflammatory, fat-forming molecules called adipokines (fat cell–derived cytokines) that have a broad array of deleterious effects on metabolism. They also influence the hormones leptin and adiponectin, which are directly involved in energy metabolism.

Leptin is secreted by your fat cells; circulating levels of it are directly proportional to the amount of body fat you have. When you become obese, your body becomes resistant to the actions of leptin (a condition called leptin resistance), which leads your fat cells to secrete even more of it. This not only causes you to feel hungrier (leptin stimulates appetite) but also further inflames your body. Studies demonstrate that leptin has proinflammatory effects that promote obesity,[112] and it's also been recently linked to disruptions in the intestinal barrier, already compromised in the development of obesity. Put simply, gaining fat sets off a vicious hormonal cycle encouraging your body to pack on ever more fat. Not a pretty picture.

What does all this have to do with turmeric? In cell cultures, curcumin prevents the damage to the intestinal barrier by leptin.[113] Curcumin supplementation lowers leptin levels while raising serotonin and tryptophan, all of which enhances satiety and lowers appetite.[114] Curcumin improves insulin resistance[115] by increasing adiponectin. Adiponectin, involved in insulin sensitivity, lessens inflammatory responses and influences numerous other metabolic pathways. When you're overweight or obese, you're most likely deficient in adiponectin because inflammation inhibits its secretion by fat cells. This contributes to insulin resistance. In obesity-engineered mice, adiponectin intervention can reverse insulin resistance. That curcumin increases your blood levels of this important hormone naturally is an impressive feat indeed. Additionally, curcumin blocks a key pathway in the inflammatory cascade called nuclear factor kappa B, or NF-κB. NF-κB controls the transcription of DNA involved in regulating immune responses, inflammation, infections, and other related processes.

But the good news doesn't end there. Curcumin prevents the damaging effects of blood sugar on tissue systems called glycation (the process by which glucose binds to proteins and interrupts enzyme systems and/or lipids and can compromise the integrity of cellular membranes).[116] Curcumin regulates key factors involved in fat cell gene expression, signaling, proliferation, and differentiation; fat cell programmed death (called apoptosis).[117, 118] (By the way, ginger–a Phase 1 superfood–has similar effects to curcumin on a cellular level, which is why these two related spices are primo to use for fat-burning.[119])

Curcumin is also good for cardiovascular health, and it helps modulate lipid metabolism. In fact, it acts much like statin medications–with none of the risks. It inhibits lipid synthesis and storage and stimulates fatty acid degradation. It also lowers bad cholesterol.[120] There's evidence that long-term intake of curcumin suppresses the growth of atherosclerotic lesions just as well as the statin medication lovastatin in mice fed a high-cholesterol diet.[121]

Similar findings can be seen in trials on humans. A study published in the *Indian Journal of Physiology and Pharmacology* gave 10 volunteers 500 milligrams of curcumin a day for 7 days. After only a week, their blood levels of oxidized cholesterol (one of the primary markers of later heart disease) dropped a whopping 33 percent.[122] Meanwhile, their overall cholesterol dropped 11.63 percent and their HDL increased by 29 percent.[123] Turmeric may also protect your brain. Studies have shown that it boosts immunity in Alzheimer's patients, removing amyloid plaques that are indicative of the disease.[124]

Perhaps the best thing about this healing spice is that it's so easy to incorporate in your diet. Buy a bottle of turmeric and experiment. Add it to whole grains and eggs; sprinkle it on chicken or pork before sautéing. You can even mix it with yogurt and make a delicious basting sauce for meats. This spice knows no bounds in terms of culinary applications, and its healing properties should ensure its place in your spice cabinet.

10. VINEGAR

The first writings referring to vinegar date back to about 5000 BC, when the Sumerians of Babylonia used ferments from unattended grape juice as a cleaning agent. If they hadn't let it sit so long, they could have had a nice glass of wine instead! Over the ages, historical figures have found clever uses for this strongly acidic fermentation by-product.[125] The first medicinal use of vinegar was ascribed to Hippocrates, the father of modern medicine, who used vinegar beginning around 420 BC to sterilize wounds, and he advocated that patients drink it for medicinal benefits. Drinking vinegar is mentioned in both the Bible and Talmud. During the Black Plague in Europe and on the battlefields of World War I, vinegar was used to clean wounds and save lives. In traditional medicine, vinegar has been used to treat a wide range of disorders from dropsy to poison ivy, from croup to stomachache and even diabetes.[126]

In a recent study published in *Diabetes Care,* vinegar was shown to have positive effects on insulin sensitivity in folks with insulin resistance.[127] Researchers found that vinegar may have physiological effects similar to the medication metformin, a drug given to diabetics to increase insulin sensitivity. There's also some evidence that the acetic acid in vinegar slows the passage of food down your digestive tract, making you feel fuller longer.

From the French *vin aigre* for "sour wine," vinegar is the result of alcohol (or other solutions of fermentable sugars) being exposed to oxygen, allowing the growth of *Acetobacter,* which ferments the alcohol into acetic acid. It was once believed that real vinegar couldn't be made without a mother of vinegar–a SCOBY not unlike the one in kefir (though it more closely resembles the disklike SCOBY of kombucha). While a mother of vinegar will expedite the process, it isn't needed. Simply leave wine, cider, sake, or any one of a number of other concoctions out on the counter and you'll eventually end up with vinegar. Wine produces wine vinegar, cider produces cider vinegar, and so forth.

Vinegar, like the other probiotic superfoods we've considered, is a paradise for healthy bacteria. Unpasteurized vinegar (that's what you want to look for) contains a great number of vitamins and minerals. In fact, some vinegars may have as many as 50 critical nutrients, including those that come from the original fruit or wine from which they were fermented.

In the 1970s, apple cider vinegar was promoted as a popular weight-loss agent, especially among bodybuilders, though there were no formal studies showing its efficacy. Other cultures have adopted the practice of using vinegar as a weight-loss agent. North African women, for example, have used apple cider vinegar to achieve weight loss for generations.[128] However, a recent report of a Moroccan 15-year-old female with dental erosion from the daily consumption of a glass of *undiluted* apple cider vinegar raises a red flag for the injudicious use of this ferment.

But it's not just North Africans who use vinegar to control weight. *Kurozu,* black vinegar produced from unpolished rice, is a popular weight-loss product in Japan, where fermented rice vinegar is also used for hyperlipidemia and even cancer.

There may be something to this folk tradition. Research reported in the journal *Lipids in Health and Disease* found this traditional fermented beverage blocked lipid absorption from the gut by inhibiting the pancreatic enzyme lipase.[129] These investigators showed that kurozu shrinks fat cells. A Japanese-based study showed similar results. Vinegar intake at both 1 or 2 tablespoons daily was shown to reduce body weight, body fat mass, and serum triglyceride levels in obese subjects.[130]

A recent study from the University of Malmö in Sweden provides some clues as to why vinegar may improve satiety and facilitate weight loss. Doctors there developed a well-designed study in which diabetics with gastroparesis–slow stomach emptying–drank very diluted vinegar (2 tablespoons in a glass of water) for 2 weeks, then switched to plain water for another 2 weeks. The results showed that the vinegar further delayed gastric emptying. As we learned in Chapter 4, gastrointestinal motility abnormalities have been observed in those with obesity.[131] And it's been observed that obese individuals experience accelerated gastric emptying, which hastens the delivery of sugars from food into the bloodstream—stimulating more fat-forming insulin. Vinegar, by delaying and slowing down gastric emptying, may promote a sense of fullness for longer periods and help balance blood sugar. Only a clinical trial, however, will verify this observation.

Another study that may support the folk-medicine use of vinegar for weight loss comes from a recent report in the journal *Food Chemistry.* It showed vinegar produced by tomatoes suppressed fat cell differentiation and fat accumulation in obese rats.[132]

As a side note, the acetic acid in vinegar may play a role in facilitating weight loss above and beyond its probiotic effect.[133]

Go for oil and vinegar on salads (or make some of the delicious salad dressing recipes you'll find in Chapter 11), drizzle it on steamed veggies, or even add it to fish or meat. You can learn how to make vinegar sodas called shrubs—they're delicious gut-healing tonics.

Add plenty of these 10 superfoods in Phase 2, and you'll give your gut microbiome that extra boost it needs to help you develop a lean metabolism, lose weight, and remain healthy for life. Don't forget, we've added lots of these foods to the recipes for this phase, and I definitely encourage you to try some of them out.

LOOKING AHEAD

You'll be done with Phase 2 when you've achieved your goal weight. For some of you, that may mean sticking with this part of the program for a month or two; for others, it may be longer. Whatever the case, Phase 2 is a healthy long-term eating plan designed to help you achieve optimal weight by rebalancing your gut microbiome. The superfoods you learned about in this chapter will help you do that.

Once you've achieved your weight-loss goals, it will be time to shift to Phase 3. The nutritional program in that phase is designed to help you sustain optimal weight for life while providing the flexibility to indulge in the occasional treat. At the heart of Phase 3 are the Mediterranean and Baltic Sea diets—arguably the two best-studied diets for long-term health and weight loss.

CHAPTER 8

Phase 3: Renew

KEEP YOUR FRIENDLY FLORA—
AND YOU—HEALTHY FOR LIFE

What is the best way to help a garden thrive? Does it take around-the-clock vigilance? Incessant watering? Aggressive fertilization with chemicals? Loads of herbicides and pesticides to kill weeds and pests?

None of the above! When it comes to gardens, sustainability is the name of the game. The ecological systems that succeed in the real world for the long term—whether it's a micro ecosystem like the vegetable garden in your backyard or a gigantic ecosystem like the Amazon rain forest—don't require massive work, chemical inputs, or constant vigilance to maintain. They thrive when nature's own strategies are used to sustain them— natural fertilizers, biodiversity to keep pests under control, periodic strategic watering, a little weeding, and some gentle nurturing are far more effective ways to sustain ecosystems.

The same is true of your gut microbiome and the larger ecosystem of your body. Trying to stick to an unsustainable dietary discipline won't keep you healthy and fit, just as massive doses of antibiotics and other medications won't cure the chronic illness epidemic we're facing in this country. These practices are unsustainable. We need a different approach to health and weight maintenance, one that's gentler, more realistic, and more applicable in our daily lives.

The Gut Balance Revolution isn't just about losing weight for swimsuit season and gaining it back around the holidays, it's about keeping it off for life while enjoying a diet that's sustainable for the long term. It's about seeking out a way of life that will help you achieve optimal health for good.

The problem with many popular diets is that they focus only on short-term weight loss—lose 7 pounds in 7 days. I know that sounds like an oxymoron—after all, why else would you go on a diet if you didn't want to lose a few pounds ASAP? But hear me out.

There are a million ways to drop a few pounds in the short term. You could restrict calories or carbs. You could fast. You could only drink liquids. You could try diet pills. You could even try one of the more bizarre fad diets like the grapefruit juice or cabbage soup diet that were popular in the 1980s. The cabbage soup diet limits food choices to veggies, fruits, and cabbage soup, so dieters lose water weight, then quickly rebound, creating a higher body weight set point, as discussed in Chapter 1. This means your body's metabolism is adjusted to maintain a higher weight than prior to dieting–a rebound phenomenon seen with yo-yo dieting. The grapefruit diet, which has been around since the Great Depression, also permits some nonstarchy veggies, emphasizes high protein intake with fish and some meats, and restricts sugars and carbs–it's a modified Atkins diet with grapefruit, eaten with every meal, as the main carbohydrate. The hypothesis–that grapefruit is fat-burning–has no science to support it. Instead, the low-calorie (800 kilocalories a day) and ketogenic aspects of the diet drive weight loss.[1] So barring the obviously ridiculous (the Twinkie diet or the beer and ice cream diet–yes, these are real), you can shed a few pounds using any number of popular diets. Dropping a few pounds for a couple weeks or even a couple of months is achievable for most people. You probably know this from experience.

The problem isn't weight loss. It's *weight maintenance.* That's precisely what this phase of the program is all about. By the time you come to Phase 3, you should be at your goal weight. So the big question is, how do you keep the weight off for the long term?

MOST DIETS DON'T WORK BECAUSE THEY *CAN'T* WORK

Most diets are unsustainable. That word gets bandied about a lot, so let's be clear about what it means. If something's unsustainable, it literally *cannot* be maintained forever. You cannot fast forever. You cannot drink grapefruit juice and exclude other wholesome foods that feed your good gut flora and expect to be healthy. You know from Chapter 4 that very low-carb diets (under 50 grams of carbs daily) tend not to work for most people in the long run, so you can't call them sustainable. And indefinitely keeping your caloric intake too low will cause your body to (1) respond with powerful hormonal and biochemical messages that make it nearly impossible to resist eating and (2) lower your metabolism so you burn *fewer* calories. Neither of these options keeps the weight off for good.

The approach of this book is different. It leverages the best data we have on what helps people lose weight and keep it off for life. I specifically designed it as a three-phase system to take advantage of this science, and I walk you through a sequence of steps that allow you to lose weight and recondition your gut microbiome in a healthy, achievable way. As you'll learn, this multiphasic approach is beginning to be tested and has shown excellent early success.

Now that you're in Phase 3, a brief recap will help you see my logic for building this program the way I did. Phase 1 was designed to be a 30-day low-carb, low-FODMAP, higher-protein ketogenic induction that would rapidly reduce inflammation, balance blood sugar, and till the soil of your inner garden while facilitating weight loss. I decided on this approach because ketogenic diets are an excellent way to jump-start weight loss, and reducing FODMAPs has been shown to facilitate a reduction in digestive symptoms (especially small intestinal bacterial overgrowth, or SIBO) and improve gut microbiome biodiversity. Unfortunately, this diet is difficult to maintain for long, and it may lower your intestine's bifidobacteria counts if you remain on it for extended periods. Phase 2 was developed to gradually enhance your healthy carb intake while diversifying your gut microbiome by focusing on pre- and probiotic foods packed with healthy bacteria. This critical step to weight loss is validated by the scientific literature, though it's been largely overlooked in popular diet books to date.

My mission with Phase 3 is to present you with a way of eating that allows you to maintain your weight loss for life. To do this, I dove into the scientific literature and found that such a diet is possible—and I discovered *tons* of scientific evidence proving its benefits, including weight loss and better health. In this chapter, you'll learn all about it. It's a traditional, flexible eating program filled with mouthwatering health-promoting foods to boot. First, I want to dig into this issue of weight maintenance a little more.

WEIGHT MAINTENANCE: THE NAME OF THE GAME

When you began the Gut Balance Revolution, you were probably more interested in weight loss than weight maintenance. That makes sense—you most likely had some pounds to lose. But by the time you start Phase 3, you will have achieved your goal weight. The next step is keeping the weight off, and that's where the real challenge begins.

How do we know if a diet works? Although there's no universally accepted definition of successful weight-loss maintenance, we all agree that the benchmark for a successful program isn't about short-term weight reduction. Losing a few pounds is nice, but keeping the weight off is the goal, and there are very little data about how successful popular diets are in the long run.

A Danish systematic review looked at 898 studies on weight-loss programs published between 1931 and 1999.[2] They defined successful dieters as those who kept all their weight off or maintained a minimum weight loss of 20 to 24 pounds for 3 years or more. One-third of the studies originally slated for review had to be thrown out because they didn't follow people this long. Of those that remained, few were designed well enough to provide meaningful data. At the end of the day, only 17 studies—a mere 2 percent of the total—held up to the Danish researchers' scrutiny and were included for analysis, although only 3 of these were well-designed randomized trials. What did these 17 studies show? Of the 3,030 participants, only about 15 percent—about 450 people—were considered successful dieters. Important indicators for success: Those who combined diet with group therapy had the best results for long-term weight maintenance, with a success rate of 27 percent. And those who were actively followed by their clinics experienced a higher success rate (19 percent) than those who weren't (10 percent). Behavior modification also appeared to have a positive effect on weight maintenance. (I'll explore this concept of connection, support, and behavior modification and more in Chapter 10.)

Another group of scientists from the University of Kentucky took a different approach to studying the efficacy of long-term weight-loss programs. Rather than identifying success or failure rates of dieters, they completed a meta-analysis of 29 studies done in the United States in which participants were guided through a structured weight-loss program for more than 2 years. Their objective was to determine the average weight loss a person might experience on one of these programs.[3]

They found that after 5 years, the average overweight or obese person would keep off an average of 6 pounds using the protocols studied. This may not seem like much, but, as the authors pointed out, people *not* on a diet program like this may gain weight. One of the control studies used showed that the average person gained 14 pounds over 5 years.

Think these criteria of long-term weight loss are too stringent? Some scientists would agree with you. A growing constituency of medical professionals believes that a good definition of successful weight loss/maintenance would be losing 5 to 10 percent of your body weight on purpose and *keeping the weight off for at least 1 year.*[4] Why 5 to 10 percent? Because in overweight or obese people, dropping 10 percent of body weight results in significant reductions in their risk for type 2 diabetes and cardiovascular disease.[5]

But this isn't as easy as it sounds. For example, if you're 165 pounds, dropping 10 percent of your body weight will mean losing 16.5 pounds. That's a lot of weight to lose. Keeping it off for a full year is no easy feat in the best of circumstances. To do it, you have to change your body weight set point as we discussed in Chapter 1. You have to reset the metabolic control mechanisms to be *balanced* at 148 pounds instead of 165. Your body at 148 pounds should leave you with an appetite to consume an amount of energy equal to your adjusted metabolic rate. When you try to do this with the latest unsustainable instant-weight-loss fad diet, it's all but impossible. You know what happens–you've probably experienced it. You lose a combination of muscle and water and perhaps some fat, but your percentage of body fat doesn't fall significantly–in fact, you look more flabby! Then you fall off the wagon, because these diets are impossible to maintain–your appetite is driving you to eat more so you weigh 165 pounds again. You yo-yo, moving your body weight set point and consequently your appetite even higher and making weight loss that much more difficult the next time around. And the cycle continues.

This may sound like grim news. On some level it is, but not in the ways you might think. What these studies really tell us is that we need more good research in the fields of nutrition and weight loss. The fact that only 1.8 percent of the 898 studies done over the course of 6 decades were of sufficient quality to be included by the Danish researchers in their systematic review is testament to a sad truth: Much of the research in the field of weight loss is suboptimal. Most of us working in this field would like to see a sequence of large randomized controlled trials comparing diets over long periods of time. Unfortunately, this is easier said than done. Studies like this are expensive and difficult to conduct; the compliance rate is often low and the dropout rate is high as people inevitably tire of the eating regimen they've been assigned.

We also need realistic expectations. Participant compliance has been a limiting factor in past studies. After all, if people who have agreed to be part of a scientific study won't stick to the diet, how likely is it that average Americans will? Probably not likely at all. To move the needle on the obesity epidemic, we must develop realistic eating programs that are *actually* sustainable, and we need to think about providing support through behavioral change, social intervention, and lifestyle alteration–factors repeatedly shown to influence weight and health outcomes.

We don't know what the perfect diet is for every person on the planet. (There probably isn't one.) We don't know, with 100 percent certainty, which of the thousands of diets work best for long-term weight loss. We don't know exactly how much weight the average person will lose on any given diet program. That may seem like a lot of uncertainty, but there are *many* things we do know.

We know that some diets don't work because they *can't* work. They can't work because they aren't sustainable. That's because (1) they don't provide your body and your gut microbiome the nutrients they need to maintain optimal health and weight, and/or (2) they don't provide the needed flexibility that allows you to follow the diet in your everyday life–and to enjoy the food you eat. And I believe that enjoyment is important in order to maintain a healthy diet.

We also know that the obesity epidemic is a relatively recent phenomenon, corresponding with the advent of highly processed foods packed with sugar, starch, inflammatory fats, and salt. Of course, correlation doesn't equal causation, but here the correlation is close enough to raise an eyebrow, which leads me to my next point.

For millennia, human beings thrived on a wide variety of diets, and obesity in most cultures across the world was rare or unknown. What can we learn from these traditional styles of eating that we can apply in our modern lives to mitigate our weight problems and the chronic illnesses associated with them? As it turns out, there is a lot we can learn. Some of the best-researched diets for long-term health and weight loss also happen to feature traditional patterns of eating that remained relatively stable until about the last 60 years. These are the diets we need to turn to in our quest to find a flexible way of eating–not a diet–that will allow us to keep weight off for the long term, reduce our risk of chronic illness, and provide the delicious foods we crave to keep body and soul together.

THE HERITAGE OF THE HUMAN DIET

The diets with the best data supporting long-term health and weight maintenance are what are sometimes called "heritage diets." The two that I'll focus on here (primarily because the data on them are excellent) are the Mediterranean and Baltic Sea diets, but there are many heritage diets in cultures from Africa to Asia to South America and beyond. These diets constitute centuries-old traditional ways of eating long associated with spectacular health and optimal weight. The beauty of heritage diets doesn't end there. These diets not only improve health but offer a way of eating that's delicious, enjoyable, socially connected, and relaxed. They bring pleasure to the experience of food.

A fascinating nonprofit organization called Oldways has been promoting heritage diets (and the Mediterranean diet, or MedDiet, in particular) as a healthy way of eating for more than 2 decades. Back in 1993, Oldways teamed up with the World Health Organization and the Center for Nutritional Epidemiology at the Harvard School of Public Health to review the implications of traditional diets for public health. (We'll look at some of the data they collected.) One of their objectives was to develop a series of food pyramids reflecting the dietary patterns of cultures around the world. The food pyramids you found in Phases 1 and 2 were inspired by these. For Phase 3, Oldways inspired

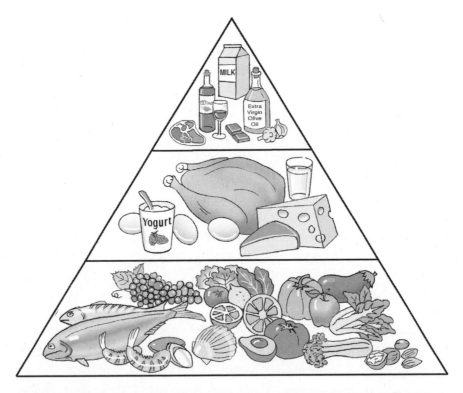

The Gut Balance Revolution Phase 3 Food Pyramid: This figure prioritizes foods in Phase 3, the renewal phase. Foods that are limited are at the top of the pyramid (i.e., alcoholic beverages—beer, wine—lean red meats (wild game preferred), coffee, dark chocolate, milk, and extra-virgin olive oil. Cheeses, yogurt, kefir, eggs, and poultry from the middle of the pyramid. Nuts, seeds, beans, green tea, herbs and spices, fruits, vegetables, seafood, wild fish, and vegetable poultry soups are at the base of the pyramid.

my adaptation shown opposite of their Mediterranean Diet Pyramid from that conference. It illustrates the basic principles of this healthy way of eating.

This is among the best graphic representations of a healthy human diet–far superior to the old US Food Pyramid or the new ChooseMyPlate initiative. For one thing, it's far simpler. For another, it organizes foods into meaningful groups and illustrates a reasonable way to eat–placing vegetables and whole grains at the bottom, fish and seafood right above them, chicken and dairy products (especially fermented dairy) in the next tier, and topping the pyramid with lean red meats (wild game preferred) and sweets–foods we should eat less of overall.

Oldways has published heritage diet pyramids for African, Asian, and Latino eating as well. Each is interesting in its own right, and I respect each of these traditional ways of eating. However, I wanted everything in the Gut Balance Revolution to have a strong foundation in science and clinical application, so I elected to build Phase 3 on two of the best-studied heritage diets around: the Mediterranean diet and the Baltic Sea diet. In the remainder of this chapter, we'll review the science supporting these diets and the similarities between them (and other traditional nutrition plans). Then I'll explain what foods you should forget, eat fewer of, and focus on in Phase 3.

Let's take a look at the most scientifically validated diet for long-term health and weight maintenance.

THE MEDDIET

The MedDiet isn't really a "diet" per se. Rather, it's a pattern of eating embraced by many people in olive-growing areas throughout the Mediterranean, including those in Greece, Crete, Italy, southern France, and Spain. Granted, these eating patterns have become less common in the last 60 years, thanks to the advent and worldwide influence of the modern, highly processed Western diet. And different studies focus more on the dietary patterns in specific geographical regions. But taking a broad overview of the area, we find the following are consistent, healthful trends.

- Abundant plant foods, including fruit, vegetables, bread, other forms of cereal grains, potatoes, beans, nuts, and seeds
- Fresh fruit as the typical daily dessert
- Olive oil as the principal source of fat
- Cheese and yogurt as the principal dairy products–these sources come from a wide array of animals including goats, sheep, and cows
- Fish in moderate to high amounts
- Poultry as the primary source of animal protein in moderate to small amounts
- Weekly consumption of eggs

- Low to moderate red wine intake
- Occasional inclusion of lean red meat (wild game preferred)
- Occasional sweet treats
- Overall, minimally processed, seasonally fresh, locally grown foods

Another factor important in the Mediterranean way of eating is the social and environmental context of meals. Delicious, artfully prepared meals are eaten slowly and enjoyed with friends and family, offering a relaxing respite from the workday and providing the social connections on which we thrive. Lunch is typically followed by a siesta, offering another opportunity for rest and relaxation and optimal digestion. These connections between lifestyle, diet, stress, and the overall health of the mind, body, and spirit are largely missing from today's world. We no longer connect the way we eat with the way we live. It's been my experience (and the data support this) that this disconnection between how we eat, interact, and live is a major contributing factor to the epidemic of weight gain and chronic illness in the Western world. We'll explore these connections more in Chapter 10, when we discuss how to live a healthy, gut-balancing lifestyle.

Exercise was also a key component of this traditional way of eating and living. Before the 1960s, those in this region were engaged in farm or kitchen work.[6] The exercise they received doing their daily chores was another contributing factor to the healthy Mediterranean way of life.

The data prove that the health outcomes of eating and living this way are spectacular. In fact, when Oldways in partnership with the Harvard School of Public Health developed the Mediterranean Diet Pyramid, they found that people in Crete, much of the rest of Greece, and southern Italy who ate this way had some of the highest adult life expectancies in the world, with relatively low rates of coronary heart disease, certain cancers, and a few other diet-related chronic illnesses. The MedDiet is clearly associated with big improvements in cardiovascular health. Notable studies, such as the PREDIMED (Prevención con Dieta Mediterránea) trial and the Lyon Diet Heart Study,[7-9] confirm that the MedDiet provides cardiovascular benefits and decreases all-cause mortality.

For example, in the PREDIMED trial, a randomized controlled 5-year study conducted in Spain, researchers assigned 7,447 people ages 55 to 80—more than half of them women—to one of three diets: a regular Western diet, the MedDiet supplemented with olive oil, or the MedDiet supplemented with nuts.[10] Originally scheduled for 10 years, the scientists elected to stop the study halfway through because their data were so powerfully in favor of the MedDiet that there were ethical concerns about keeping the control group on the regular Western diet. The groups on both versions of the MedDiet were 70 to 72 percent *less likely* to have a heart attack or stroke or to die from any other cause than the Western diet group.

A meta-analysis conducted by the Cochrane Collaboration reached similar conclusions.

Scientists reviewed 11 trials that included data on 52,044 participants and found that those eating a MedDiet saw reductions in total cholesterol, LDL, and blood pressure.[11]

While there are many reasons the MedDiet supports heart health, we know that one key component is olive oil–one of the Phase 3 superfoods you'll learn more about in the next chapter. Olive oil has been shown to enhance vascular endothelial function (cardiovascular disease oftentimes commences with dysfunction of the cells that line the vasculature, aka endothelium) and reduce blood lipids as well as the risk of atherosclerosis. Plus, the phytochemicals in olive oil have numerous anti-inflammatory, antioxidant, hypolipidemic properties.[12] You'll find more details in the next chapter, but for now suffice it to say extra-virgin olive oil (EVOO) is among the healthiest foods for your heart.

The MedDiet has also been shown to profoundly improve metabolic syndrome and type 2 diabetes. In another Spanish study, researchers randomly divided 3,541 people into three groups–they ate a MedDiet supplemented with EVOO, a MedDiet supplemented with nuts, or a standard low-fat diet.[13] The folks on the MedDiet did not alter their physical activity in any way. The conclusion? Both groups on the MedDiet had a reduced risk of developing type 2 diabetes. Another study from the Department of Nutritional Sciences at the University of Connecticut reviewed recent data on a wide variety of diets and their impact on metabolic syndrome–a cluster of symptoms including central obesity, hypertension, high fasting glucose, and increased inflammation that puts people at increased risk for heart disease, type 2 diabetes, and other chronic illnesses.[14] They concluded that the MedDiet, coupled with regular exercise, had the biggest impact on metabolic syndrome. Other studies have demonstrated that the MedDiet reduces inflammatory markers including those generated by fat cells (adipokines) in those with metabolic syndrome, even in the absence of weight loss.[15, 16] Of course, the effect is even greater in those who *do* lose weight. The MedDiet has been shown to improve nonalcoholic fatty liver disease; in a recent study, adherence to this diet was associated with lower abdominal fat gain.[17, 18]

There's mounting evidence that the MedDiet has a positive impact on the health of your gut microbiome. A small study working with nine overweight/obese men and women revealed that utilization of the MedDiet for 2 weeks decreased serum triglyceride levels by 14 percent and LDL by 12 percent while increasing the overall gut microbiome biodiversity and richness.[19] Little wonder–the MedDiet is rich in fermented milk products packed with probiotics and has tons of prebiotic foods and fiber that feed a healthy gut microbiome.

The MedDiet also has powerful anti-inflammatory benefits and is packed with prebiotics that enrich the diversity of the gut microbiome. It's not surprising that evidence suggests the MedDiet alleviates chronic diseases associated with inflammation and gut dysbiosis. It appears to provide protection against diseases associated with chronic inflammation, including metabolic syndrome, atherosclerosis, cancer, diabetes, obesity, pulmonary diseases, and even cognition disorders.[20] The gut microbiome has a strong influence on mood and behavior; dysbiosis has been linked to autism, mood and behavior disorders, and more.[21] The MedDiet has decreased depression in high-risk people with chronic lung disease.[22] Likewise, the PREDIMED study showed that the MedDiet supplemented with nuts could reduce risk of depression in patients with type 2 diabetes.[23] There is some preliminary evidence to suggest that the MedDiet may improve cognition and protect against senile dementia due to its anti-inflammatory properties and its biodiversifying influence on the gut microbiome.[24, 25]

But more to the point of this book, a number of studies indicate that the MedDiet helps facilitate weight loss and maintenance. Canadian researchers, for example, evaluated 77 women, who were randomly assigned to one of two diets (the MedDiet or a standard diet) for 12 weeks and attended seven individual sessions with a dietitian. Small but significant decreases in body weight and waist circumference were observed after the study's completion. Increased consumption of legumes, nuts, and seeds and decreased consumption of sweets were significantly associated with decreased waist circumference. As part of a MedDiet program, an increase in consumption of legumes, nuts, and seeds and a decrease in the consumption of sweets were associated with some beneficial changes across the board.[26]

In another study, 31 overweight-to-obese participants took part in the Spanish Ketogenic Mediterranean Diet (SKMD), which incorporated extra-virgin olive oil as the principal source of fat; moderate red wine, green vegetables, and salads as the main carbohydrate sources; and fish as the main protein source.[27] What made this study noteworthy? The SKMD was an *unlimited* calorie program. Participants were allowed to eat as much as they wanted; they were simply asked to follow the SKMD program. The result? An *extremely* significant reduction in body weight, body mass index, systolic blood pressure, diastolic blood pressure, total cholesterol, and glucose. There was a significant reduction in triglycerides and LDL cholesterol and a significant increase in HDL, the good cholesterol. The SKMD promoted weight loss, improved lipid profiles, lowered blood pressure, and decreased fasting blood glucose levels.

The bottom line: When it comes to sustainable diets that show improved health in the long run, few diets compete with the eating patterns long embraced by the people in the Mediterranean. There are similarities between these eating patterns and the diets of many traditional cultures. The historical evidence, scientific data, my clinical experience, and common sense all point to this way of eating—one that focuses on real, healthy whole foods—as the way human beings were meant to eat.

PROOF FOR THE GUT BALANCE REVOLUTION METHOD OF PERMANENT WEIGHT LOSS

Following the MedDiet in Phase 3 will not only help you cultivate a rich and biodiverse gut microflora but will also deliver a host of health benefits for a long, healthy life. Growing evidence confirms my weight-loss method of using the ketogenic diet (Phase 1) to induce weight loss, followed by gut microbiome restoration (Phase 2) and then a MedDiet (Phase 3) for maintenance and continued health promotion. This combination is the best approach for long-term weight loss and maintenance while providing numerous health benefits.[28] A recent study at the University of Padua saw magnificent long-term weight and health outcomes using a diet similar to the one found in this book. Though the study was small (only 89 subjects were followed over a period of 12 months), the results were extremely impressive. Over the course of 1 year, the average participant experienced:

- Significant decrease in weight—an average of 33 pounds
- 10 percent loss of body fat
- Reduction in blood pressure—systolic blood pressure was down 7 points, diastolic 4 points
- Decreased LDL and increased HDL—the good cholesterol
- Reduction in triglycerides
- Reduction in blood glucose

In addition, there was 90 percent compliance with the diet (unheard of with any diet program) and 88 percent of participants maintained for 1 year. The poststudy analysis found that those who didn't achieve successful weight loss hadn't complied with the program and went back to eating high-glycemic junk foods.

The magnitude of change, and the fact that people maintained their weight loss for a year after the study was completed, is compelling. Few studies have shown these kinds of results in as few as 12 months.

The science is beginning to prove what I've seen in my practice: A multiphasic approach to weight loss may be the way of the future. My only beef with the study? They didn't measure effects of their program based on gut microbiome health!

The Baltic Sea Diet

The other heritage diet we'll look at, the Baltic Sea diet, also has sound data to support it, and a validated tool called the Baltic Sea Diet Score (BSDS) has been developed by scientists to help judge adherence to the diet. The BSDS is based on the following nine dietary factors:

1. High intake of Nordic fruits like apples, pears, and berries
2. High intake of Nordic veggies like tomatoes, cucumbers, leafy vegetables, roots, cabbages, peas
3. Low-fat and fat-free milk
4. Nordic cereals like rye, oat, and barley

5. Nordic fish–salmon and other freshwater fish

6. Balanced ratio of polyunsaturated fats to saturated and trans fats

7. Low intake of red and processed meat

8. Moderate total fat percentage

9. Low to moderate alcohol intake

You may notice that this diet looks much like the MedDiet except for the use of low-fat and fat-free dairy products and an increased focus on specific groups of fruits and vegetables. Nevertheless, scientists have found that this diet, like the MedDiet, has a profound influence on health.

For example, in one study, researchers looked at food journal data from 4,579 people ages 25 to 74 and scored them based on their adherence to the Baltic Sea diet.[29] After adjusting for factors like age, socioeconomic status, length of education, and other lifestyle factors, they found that those who adhered to the diet most carefully had:

- Increased levels of adiponectin–more adiponectin in the blood is associated with reduced body fat percentage

- Reduced levels of inflammatory markers like interleukin 6 and C-reactive protein

These are the precise kinds of changes that lead to lower weight and lower risk for inflammatory and weight-related health concerns such as type 2 diabetes and heart disease. It appears that increased fruit, vegetable, and whole grain intake and reduced red meat intake associate most clearly with the reduction in inflammation. Moderate alcohol intake also seemed to be a primary dietary factor for reducing inflammation.[30] However, it's important to be aware that alcohol can cause gut dysbiosis and disrupt precious gut barrier function, so it's best to limit your moderate alcohol consumption to Phases 2 and 3 when your gut function is fully restored and you can benefit from some of the beneficial properties of alcoholic beverages.

A Finnish study showed that adherence to the Baltic Sea diet is associated with lower rates of abdominal obesity.[31] Researchers assessed the diet of 4,720 people between the ages of 25 and 74. Their findings were extremely straightforward: The closer participants adhered to the Baltic Sea diet, the less likely they were to be overweight and the less likely they were to carry belly fat. The effect seemed to be slightly stronger in younger age groups. The dietary factors that appeared to have the most effect were Baltic whole grain cereals and moderate alcohol consumption. How can carbs foster weight maintenance? It may be that low-carb dieting decreases your gut bifidobacteria and that whole grains are prebiotic and feed your good gut flora. These are the likely reasons that Baltic whole grain cereals help maintain weight, since they support the fertile soil of your gut's garden of life and promote a lean metabolism. As for alcohol, remember that "the dose is

What's the Real Story with Alcohol?

Alcohol has been villainized as a bad actor in society as abuse can lead to reckless behavior, lethal accidents, and numerous adverse health consequences. However, abundant data show that moderate alcohol consumption (150 milliliters of red wine a day) acts as a drug to improve blood lipid profiles, decrease chances of forming potentially lethal blood clots, increase coronary bloodflow, reduce blood pressure, improve insulin sensitivity and immunity, and decrease serum markers of inflammation.[32] But is it the alcohol itself that provides benefit or some other special properties in alcoholic beverages? Although the jury's still out, we do know that alcoholic beverages have identifiable plant-based nutrients (phytonutrients) that provide clear health benefits. Wine and beer contain many nutrients not related to alcohol, including soluble fiber that feeds your good gut bugs, minerals and vitamins, and polyphenols—which all help you combat disease. Specifically, red wine contains the polyphenol resveratrol, which improves immune function, prevents cancer, and cools down inflammation to help prevent disease. Likewise, beer has the polyphenol xanthohumol, an anti-inflammatory flavonoid regulating the immune system.[33] The more alcohol that a person drinks, the higher the risk of developing digestive tract cancers (mouth, pharynx, larynx, esophagus, colon-rectum, liver) but also female breast.[34] Moderate alcohol consumption may place women at higher risk for breast cancer (10 percent lifetime increased risk and may be related in part to alcohol's effects on estrogen metabolism or even subclinical folate insufficiency as folate requirements are higher in those who consume alcohol).[35]

the poison," but in certain cases, the poison can also be the remedy, depending on the dose. This yin-yang of alcohol reminds me of a process that I learned from Dr. Patrick Hanaway.* He brought to light the term "hormesis," which signifies how a stress to the body at low doses can cause a positive adaptive response but is harmful in higher doses.

The point isn't to determine whether the Baltic Sea diet or the MedDiet is superior. As we've discussed throughout this book, humans have thrived on a wide variety of diets for millennia. In fact, assessment tools like the Baltic Sea Diet Score[36] were developed because we've found that these diets don't always see the same success when they cross over into different cultures. The reasons for this are still obscure, but they likely include genetic predispositions and lifestyle and cultural factors that make adherence to these diets less likely when they are exported to other countries.

---

* Patrick Hanaway, MD, is the medical director, Cleveland Clinic Center for Functional Medicine (IFM)—an organization designed to promote the application of whole-systems practices to prevent and treat chronic disease by emphasizing nutrition and lifestyle-based interventions. Patrick, myself, Dr. Thomas Sult, and Dr. Elizabeth Lipski teach the GI Module at IFM-based symposia and elsewhere. To learn more about IFM, visit functionalmedicine.org.

Can You Stress Your Body to Health?

There's evidence that periodically indulging in low to moderate amounts of harmful substances (such as alcohol) may improve health in the long run. This idea is called hormesis. Gently stressing the body with these substances from time to time puts stress on your cells' power plants—the mitochondria—forcing them to adapt and making them stronger over time. We will discuss in Chapter 10 how interval training results in the division and expansion of fat-burning mitochondria in muscles. Since your mitochondria are your body's energy-producing factories, doing this may generate more energy in the long run. So periodic but limited indulgence can be a good thing. Substances such as curcumin (the curry in Indian food), even in low doses, have hormetic effects and are worthwhile in small amounts.[37] Homeopathy is another classical example of this concept. In homeopathy, "poisons" are given at infinitely low doses to stimulate a healing response.

Alcohol appears to operate according to hormesis as well.[38] Researchers explain it this way: One drink of red wine, beer, or stout provided equivalent increases in plasma antioxidant activity. Three drinks of red wine, beer, or stout provided equivalent increases in plasma prooxidant activity. This may explain, at least in part, the decreased risk of cataract and atherosclerosis from daily consumption of one drink of different types of alcoholic beverages, as well as the increased risk from daily consumption of three drinks of alcoholic beverages. The plasma prooxidant activity appears to be due to ethanol metabolism, whereas the antioxidant activity may be due to the absorption of polyphenols in the beverages. Hormesis may be one factor involved in this dichotomy of alcohol's effects—a true Jekyll and Hyde phenomenon.

In analyzing these data, it's more useful to come to consensus about what a healthy diet might look like for people in the long term.

Is There an Ideal Diet for Humans?

There's probably no one-size-fits-all diet perfect for every person on the planet. But by reviewing the data and comparing the heritage eating styles, we *can* come to a consensus about what dietary factors are involved in weight loss and health. I've identified 10 principles that should be the foundation for a healthy long-term eating program, and I've designed Phase 3 around these principles. Understand them and you'll be on your way toward creating a sustainable, lifelong, healthy eating plan to keep you at your optimal weight. (For more scientific details, refer to the article "Search for the Optimal Diet" that I wrote several years ago for *Nutrition in Clinical Practice*.[39] I was a guest editor for that issue, which discussed the holy grail of health diets and my no-spin-zone analysis and bottom line of what works and what to avoid.)

1. Nutritional Ketosis Works Short Term—Not Long Term

The data make it fairly clear that very low-carb, higher-protein diets that induce nutritional ketosis work as a short-term induction to weight loss. But these diets are difficult to sustain for long, and they may have a negative effect on the gut microbiome if maintained for too long.

Instead, a biphasic (or, as in this book, triphasic) approach seems to work best. By moving from a ketogenic diet in the short term to a Mediterranean/Baltic diet in the long term, you can lose weight and keep it off more effectively while improving many health outcomes. And if you start to backslide and regain weight, you can always go back to a 30-day ketogenic diet and work your way back through Phases 1 through 3.

2. Diets High in Sugar and Processed Carbs Don't Work

One of the problems with the low-fat dogma that has been dominant in our culture since the 1980s is that, in most cases, fat has been replaced with carbohydrates. Though I'm not a proponent of long-term, extremely low-carbohydrate plans, it's clear that carbohydrates–specifically, processed carbohydrates and processed, refined sugar–are the most prevalent dietary demons in the modern Western way of eating. Inflammatory fats run a close second.

While my reading of the data suggests that the inclusion of some low-glycemic-load whole grains in your diet can be part of a healthy way of eating for the long term, I want to be 100 percent clear that I *am not* encouraging you to overdo these foods, and I'm not condoning the overconsumption of carbohydrates.

Rather, it's been my experience clinically–and the data agree–that whole grains can be part of a long-term healthy diet for many. Healthy whole grains are a core part of both the Baltic Sea diet and the MedDiet, and they can be found in other healthy ways of eating the world over. Remember, when it comes to whole grains, portion control is important–the dose makes the poison or the remedy. However, whole grains are not typically the kinds of foods people binge on, so most of you will benefit from adding foods like oat bran, quinoa, and other healthy whole grains to your diet. They increase satiety, your gut bugs love to eat them, and, in moderation, they're a delicious addition to a well-rounded eating plan.

As we'll discuss later in the chapter, you can even "go off your plan" and indulge in an occasional dessert or pizza from time to time once your gut microbiome and metabolism have been rehabilitated and you've achieved your goal weight. I will give you all the details when we talk about taking a "rest" from the program and giving yourself permission to indulge in (but not binge on) your favorite foods from time to time.

The bottom line: Eating processed carbs can be a slippery slope. They can be addictive, and eating too much will upset gut microbioial biodiversity, lead to blood sugar and insulin imbalances, cause the fires of inflammation to burn once more, and set you up to regain weight and lose health. I don't like saying any food is bad, but of the many foods in the typical Western diet, processed carbs are among the most dangerous and insidious. Be wary of them.

3. Prebiotics and Probiotics Play an Important Role

Foods like live-culture yogurt and goat cheese are considered core components of the MedDiet. Little wonder why. These probiotic powerhouses are a wonderful way to balance the gut microbiome and keep your weight down, and good evidence suggests fermented milk products may reduce your risk of a wide variety of chronic illnesses. Vegetable ferments play a less prominent role in Mediterranean cuisine than in some other cultures (Korean and Japanese cuisine, for example), but they still exist. *Giardiniera* is a classic fermented Italian pickle that includes carrots, cauliflower, peppers, and other veggies. Cucumber pickles are known in both Greece and Italy. While probiotic-rich foods may not feature as prominently in the data on the Baltic Sea diet, many Nordic traditions were rich in fermented foods—including *surströmming,* a fermented Baltic herring that is a staple of traditional northern Swedish culture.

Plus, both diets are rich in vegetables and whole grains that have a prebiotic effect on the gut microbiome—and combining probiotic-rich foods with prebiotic vegetable foods is the one-two punch needed to maintain inner ecosystem balance for the long haul. Both these traditional dietary patterns include these types of foods.

4. Focus on Whole Foods

One of the most obvious and profound consistencies among traditional diets like the MedDiet and the Baltic Sea diet is the focus on real, whole, healing foods, not the processed junk food that dominates the modern Western diet. More than any of the other healthy elements of traditional eating, this may be the key differentiating factor.

Science has repeatedly shown the importance of whole foods. For example, a clinical study of 120,887 individuals who were nonobese and free of chronic disease were followed over 20 years to determine the dietary factors associated with weight maintenance and gain.[40] The findings, reported in the *New England Journal of Medicine,* showed that yogurt was the food best associated with maintaining a healthy weight.[41] The consumption of vegetables, whole grains, fruits, and nuts—all superfoods that feed our fat-burning friendly flora—was associated with maintaining healthy weight in ascending order of magnitude. In contrast, eating potato chips, potatoes, sugar-sweetened beverages, unprocessed red meats, and processed meats predicted long-term weight gain in descending order of magnitude.

A proper whole-foods-based diet rich in phytonutrients and pre- and probiotics, along with an active healthy lifestyle, is the best way to maintain a healthy weight. Other lifestyle factors independently associated with weight change in the study above included physical activity, moderate alcohol use (one 3-ounce glass of wine; one can, bottle, or glass of beer; or a 1-ounce shot or drink of hard liquor per day), quitting smoking, good sleep quality, and reduced television watching. The data on the influence of moderate alcohol consumption on weight change appear to vary in studies, perhaps because of technical measures, but I recommend that you wait until Phases 2 and 3 before enjoying an occasional alcoholic drink with your main meal and perhaps more on special occasions. There's little research on the potential benefits of distilled spirits.

The heritage diet of human beings is a whole-foods diet. After all, until about 60 years ago, there was nothing else. Remember that Oldways, the not-for-profit organization whose mission is "to guide people to good health through heritage," has developed food pyramids for traditional African, Asian, and Latino diets in addition to the MedDiet pyramid in this book.[42] While the data don't yet support these diets as a way to maintain health, it's easy to see the similarities between them when you compare these heritage-based diet pyramids. In fact, many of the key factors are the same across the board: lots of fruits and vegetables, moderate whole grains, seafood as a primary protein source, lots of probiotic-based foods like cheese and yogurt, little red meat, and few sweets.

What did these traditional cultures know that we don't? Good question, but it might actually be a matter of what they *didn't know*. Remember that these traditional ways of eating developed in the cradle of civilization, ages before food processing as we know it today existed. Ample evidence shows that when sugary, starchy, processed foods are introduced to these cultures, they begin to experience an explosion of weight gain and chronic illness similar to ours.

Modern food production has its advantages—it's fast, convenient, and accessible. We shouldn't sacrifice this entirely and go back to grinding our grain by hand with a stone mortar and pestle. But in our quest for convenience, we've lost our connection to fundamental truths about what it means to be a biological organism that consumes other biological organisms to live. We're no longer connected to the food we eat or the environment in which it is grown. Divorced from this outer ecology, it's no wonder we've lost contact with our inner ecology. The outcome: imbalance inside and out, driving an epidemic of weight gain and chronic illness.

Looking at traditional ways of eating offers us a connection back to our past that helps us understand and embrace real, whole foods once again. Whether you're in the Paleo crowd, love the MedDiet, or are interested in other traditional eating patterns, one thing is clear: Our ancestors didn't eat Doritos. Ever. Those comestibles were simply unknown. Our forebears wouldn't have recognized as food much of what fills the shelves of your local supermarket.

This transition from a cultural dietary paradigm of healthy whole foods to one built on highly processed foodlike substances has happened *extremely* quickly. Your grand-parents and great-grandparents wouldn't have known what Lunchables are, but I'd bet my life your kids do. Even if you never buy those processed-food lunch kits, their friends at school eat them, and your children see commercials for them during after-noon cartoons.

That transition from a world where processed food is unknown to one where it's one of the predominant sources of calories has correlated with the worldwide rise of over-weight, obesity, and chronic illnesses such as cardiovascular illness, type 2 diabetes, and more. A mere coincidence? I think not.

I'm not a food extremist. I won't tell you never to buy a can of soup again. But be aware that most of those cans contain your Recommended Dietary Allowance for sodium and then some, as well as a nice dose of sugar and/or HFCS to boot. The more you become aware of the foods you eat, and the more you choose to cook and eat real, whole, healing foods—organic and locally grown when possible—the healthier you'll be and the deeper the connections you will make between who you are, how you feel, and what you eat. This awareness supports your inner ecology as well as the broader ecological system of planet Earth.

Whether it's Mediterranean, Baltic, African, Asian, Latino, or some other traditional food culture, what you'll find at its base is the same: real food. That's the big difference between heritage ways of eating and the modern Western diet. Be aware of it.

5. Add More Fruits and Veggies

Increasing your intake of fruits and vegetables is an easy and delicious way to enhance your health. Studies have shown eating eight servings of veggies daily reduces your risk of heart attack and stroke by as much as 30 percent—and that's only the beginning of the health benefits these phytonutrient-packed plant foods provide. (Phytonutrients are plant-based natural products that provide disease-fighting health benefits.) Other studies have shown that increased fruit and vegetable consumption is associated with a reduction in all-cause mortality,[43] and health benefits directly correlate with an increased con-sumption of fruits and vegetables.[44] Those studies about the Baltic Sea diet and MedDiet corroborate this. The data are clear. Fruits and vegetables must be at the root of a healthy diet, so visit your produce section first on your next trip to the grocery store.

6. Try Lean Protein and Don't Overdo Red Meat

We've already reviewed why protein is an important part of your diet: It increases sati-ety, reduces fat production, has thermogenic effects, builds fat-burning lean muscle, and more. Recall that the type of protein you choose is essential. A little lean red meat from time to time is fine. I allow it on Phase 2, and you can keep it in your Phase 3 eating plan. But too much red meat, or too many fatty cuts, is unhealthy. It increases your risk of cardiovascular disease, upsets gut microbiome balance, and creates other problems, as we've discussed in earlier chapters. The Baltic Sea diet, the MedDiet, and *all* of the heritage diet pyramids created by Oldways to date keep red meat to a minimum.

But don't reduce your protein intake overall. In fact, many people should eat *more* protein. Remember that healthy protein sources like fish and chicken are just above fruit, vegetables, and whole grains in the Mediterranean Diet Pyramid. The point isn't to reduce protein, it's to focus on healthier protein options. Two standouts in terms of their satiating effects are whey protein and fish.[45] Fish is not only filled with high-quality, appetite-reducing protein but is also high in omega-3 fats, another critical component of a healthy diet. Whey protein has been used for millennia—Hippocrates, the father of Western medicine, prescribed it to help patients strengthen muscles and enhance their immune function,[46] purposes for which it's still used today.

7. Do Not Fear Fat

The amount of fat in the MedDiet is extraordinary by modern standards, ranging from 28 percent of total calories in southern Italy to as much as 40 percent in Greece. While the Baltic Sea diet may not contain quite as much fat, moderate amounts are still considered key. Those in the Baltic Sea region and those in the Mediterranean don't fear fat, and you shouldn't either.

Of course, the focus must be on healthy fats like olive oil, the main fat source of the MedDiet, not the trashy, inflammatory omega-6 fatty acid–rich fats of the modern Western diet. These inflammatory fats run a close second to processed sugary carbs in my list of dietary demons. The ratio of inflammatory to anti-inflammatory fats is way out of balance in America today, and it's not doing any good to the national waistline or our chronic illness epidemic.

So what fats can you eat? Extra-virgin olive oil (EVVO) is my number one choice. It's one of the key factors leading to the health outcomes we see from the MedDiet, and it's a veritable superfood. It should be your go-to oil for dressing salads and other veggies, sautéing, and other forms of medium-heat cooking. Other healthy fats include canola oil (for high-heat cooking) and coconut oil, avocado oil, and sesame oil (in limited quantities). Naturally, there are the fats in the fish you consume and in healthy plant foods like avocado, chia seeds, flaxseeds, and more. These types of fats should be the ones you focus on, and it's easy to do that by sticking to a whole-foods diet and avoiding overindulging in processed foods, which tend to be loaded with inflammatory fats.

8. Add Plenty of Fat-Burning Herbs and Spices

While herbs and spices aren't a focus in the research on the Mediterranean, Baltic Sea, or other heritage diets, I'm convinced they should be considered. These undervalued, phytonutrient-filled health helpers have nutraceutical properties that modern science is only now beginning to understand. You may remember that in earlier chapters I talked about superfood spices like cinnamon, ginger, cayenne pepper, and turmeric and the extraordinary health benefits they provide. I encourage you to add plenty of spices to your diet. They make food taste better and more enjoyable–and many of them support your fat-burning efforts and your overall health.

The Gut Balance Revolution recipes are packed with these and other healing spices. If you're not sure how to integrate them into your cooking, or if you're looking for delicious recipes that include these healing foods, try out the meal plans and recipes in Chapter 11.

9. For Many, A Little Alcohol Is Your Friend

In the studies we reviewed above on the Mediterranean and Baltic Sea diets, low to moderate intake of alcohol was not only healthy, it was among the most important factors correlating with reduced inflammation and increased health. Fermented beers and red wine have been part of the human heritage for millennia. In fact, in *Beer, Bread, and the Seeds of Change*, Thomas and Carol Sinclair argue that it was the production of beer, *not* bread, that led to the advent of agriculture.[47] We can never know whether or not this is true, but a little alcohol has been repeatedly correlated with a wide range of health benefits with the exception of breast cancer. This excess risk, though, may be reduced by consuming enough folate.[48-50]

So in Phases 2 and 3, enjoy a glass of wine or beer occasionally with your main meal. These fermented beverages nurture your body and your gut microbiome as they relax your spirit.

10. Enjoy Your Food—That's More Important Than You Think

This final point is critically important, yet it's tremendously undervalued by the medical community and, arguably, American society in general. Food is far more than a vehicle for energy and nutrients, though you'd never know this by reading scientific studies about diets that focus only on its nutrient composition and calories.

Food is one of the fundamental joys of life and a foundational element in human civilization. Richard Wrangham, the biological anthropologist from Harvard University, suggests that cooking food was not only critical to the development of human society as we know it but to the evolution of our species. Consuming calories is a necessary activity for all living things, but cooking and eating food are distinctly human. As with other human activities, there's a profound joy, a spiritually nutritive substance to food that goes beyond the vitamins it contains or the kilocalorie of energy it's worth.

Match this fundamental joy of eating with the vital social aspect of human existence, and what you have is the family meal–an institution unfortunately dying in the West. One of the essential features of the MedDiet (and many other heritage diets) is the slow, artfully prepared meal enjoyed with family and friends. Using meals as an opportunity to relax and connect adds another dimension to food's medicinal nature. Food is more than its constituent nutrients. Our way of eating is at the very heart of our species' development. So sit down and enjoy your food with friends and family. It's a wonderful way to deepen the connections between the community of microbes in your gut, the community of friends and family who surround you, and the nourishing food that feeds them both.

These 10 principles are what a healthy human diet is founded on. I'll share exactly what you should favor, what you should eat fewer of, and what you should forget in Phase 3. But all you really need to do is think through these 10 principles as you plan your meals day to day and week to week. There's great flexibility within these parameters. Some people might like to eat a little more animal protein; others may be vegetarians. For some, a higher dose of anti-inflammatory fat like olive oil may satiate hunger and satisfy a craving for rich foods; others may prefer a little less fat. Some may thrive on a few more servings of whole grains weekly than others. Just use these basic rules and tune in to what works for you and what doesn't.

How will you know? Your body will tell you. If you start regaining weight, that's a sign something has gone haywire and it's time to reevaluate your diet. If you begin to experience symptoms (such as digestive upset, joint pain, brain fog, mood imbalances, and others) that disappeared on previous phases, that's another sign. Medical tests like blood pressure, blood glucose levels, and C-reactive protein levels provide additional information. Together, these and other factors indicate how healthy or unhealthy you are and provide a benchmark for manipulating your diet to create optimal health. Pay attention to how the food you eat influences your weight and health and consciously make choices that help you thrive. Stay away from foods that diminish your health, lead to mood and energy imbalances, or cause you to gain weight. The particular foods will change, to some extent, day by day, but as long as you abide by these general criteria, you'll thrive and keep the weight off. There's truly no such thing as a "perfect diet"—any diet that helps you thrive is perfect for you. If you're honest and attentive to the signals your body provides, you'll find that the best diet for you fits somewhere inside these 10 principles through Phase 3 and beyond.

However, for those of you who want a little more detail, let's look more carefully at what you should favor, what you should eat fewer of, and what you should forget on Phase 3.

Don't Just Forget Foods

On Phase 3, you don't technically have to "forget" any foods. One key aspect of this phase is that you can eat off the program from time to time. Indulging in a dessert or having a little pizza once in a while shouldn't affect your weight or long-term health once you've rehabilitated your metabolism. In fact, the guilt some of us associate with "cheating" when eating foods like chocolate cake may actually cause us to gain weight. A fascinating study published in the journal *Appetite* appropriately titled "Chocolate Cake. Guilt or Celebration?" sought to determine if those who feel guilt about their eating behaviors (such as indulging in chocolate cake) actually lost weight and kept it off. The question these scientists asked: Do these guilty feelings have a positive or negative effect? After all, guilt has the potential to motivate behavior change, but it can also lead to feelings of helplessness and loss of control.

Researchers conducted an interesting experiment.[51] They examined whether feelings of guilt or celebration when eating chocolate cake were related to differences in attitudes, perceived control, and intentions to maintain a healthy lifestyle. Then they looked at weight-loss outcomes as they were associated with these feelings over a 3-month and an 18-month period. They found that guilt provided no motivation for healthy living– those who experienced guilt when eating chocolate cake felt they were less in control of their eating habits than their counterparts who felt eating chocolate cake was a celebration. At both the 3- and 18-month marks, people who felt guilt were less likely to achieve and maintain their weight-loss goals. Guilt had no positive benefits.

Our attitudes toward eating need a major overhaul. Food is a celebration, but that doesn't mean we should overindulge. We just need to keep things in perspective. That's why in Phase 3, I encourage you to "rest on the 7th day"–once a week, you can eat whatever you want–and you can take a break from this program on holidays, birthdays, and other special occasions. On these days, you aren't strictly forbidden from any foods. Taking a break and resting from your eating plan from time to time is essential to maintaining a healthy diet for life. After all, why bother to be fit and healthy if you can't periodically enjoy the good things in life, like a rich steak or a luscious piece of cheesecake? Our favorite foods are part of what makes life worth living.

First, remember that highly processed foods or those filled with substances toxic to the human body don't nourish you mentally, physically, or spiritually. If you tune in to your body and focus on what you truly enjoy, you'll find that you naturally shy away from foods such as:

- Overcooked, heavily breaded, creamed, or deep-fried foods
- Processed foods filled with hydrogenated oils and other unhealthy fats
- Highly processed meats and cheese–which are different from traditionally cured meats and cheese
- Highly processed soy and legume foods like "vegetarian cheese" or "chickpea chips"
- Foods filled with starch, like doughnuts, bagels, and muffins
- Soda and other sugary beverages
- Artificial sweeteners, high-fructose corn syrup, and other sugary substances made in labs but not found in nature

These are not food. We just don't have another appropriate word to define them. I referred to them as "ingestibles" in my book *The Inside Tract*,[52] and that seems fitting because they're products that can be ingested but they don't provide nutritional value. Even these foodlike substances aren't strictly forbidden in Phase 3, but I advise you to stay away from them. There are plenty of other options to satiate your cravings that don't poison your metabolism and decimate your gut microbiome.

Second, remember that periodic indulgences should be just that, periodic. Taking a break from healthy eating occasionally is fine. In fact, it can actually make you healthier! It's not the occasional treat that impacts health and causes weight gain. It's the daily assault of nutritionally vacant calories, sugary processed foods, inflammatory fats, stress, lack of exercise and sleep, and toxic exposure that deprives us of health. Enjoy a treat once in a while. Then get back to your healthy lifestyle the next day.

This leads me to my final point. Some foods may lead you down a slippery slope to overindulgence. You know who you are, and you know which foods do this for you. My recommendation: Stay away from these foods until you're confident they won't trigger bingeing or other unhealthy behaviors.

Foods You Should Eat Less Of

The foods you should eat fewer of in Phase 3 should be relatively clear. They include everything in the Forget section, as well as any that don't fit into the 10 principles mentioned above. However, there are a few "dishonorable mentions" to point out in this category, because though they're often considered healthy, they can be problematic unless consumed with caution–in moderation at best.

- **Store-bought fruit juices**. Juicing at home using whole fruits and vegetables is a great way to enhance your intake of healing plant foods. But store-bought juices are almost universally made of juice concentrate, high in sugar and stripped of the fiber and phytonutrients that make fruits and vegetables so healthy. They're basically sugar in disguise, so don't overdo them. For instance, while waiting in the checkout line at Baltimore's Mount Washington Whole Foods Market, I noticed some juice options in the refrigerator case. Naked Juice Company's Green Machine, with "no sugar added," caught my attention. An 8-ounce serving had 33 grams of carbs and 140 calories–and it came in a 16-ounce bottle. Most people will drink the entire bottle and pour 66 grams of carbs into their bloodstream, quickly setting off a strong insulin response. Even the Protein Zone smoothie, with 16 grams of protein, contains 220 calories per 8-ounce serving, due to the very high natural sugar content in the fruit juices used. I sampled it–one swig brought on an instant sugar rush. (Note that there was a class action settlement against Naked Juice Company for claiming their juice was "all natural." The suit also demands proof of the non-GMO status on the product label; see nakedjuiceclass.com.) And the organic, kosher, non-GMO Suja

Green Supreme drink, with kale, apples, and lemon, provides a whopping 110 calories per 8-ounce serving–plus a sugar rush. There are suitable choices available, if you go the purchased juice drink route. Some Suja products have as few as 35 calories per serving (Twelve Essentials, for example) and are rich in disease-fighting and fat-melting organic greens. The organic "Greens" drinks from BluePrintJuice have 110 calories and 24 grams of carbs–but contain more romaine lettuce and cucumber than any other greens with kale toward the bottom of the ingredient list. Another favorite brand is Evolution Fresh Organic Sweet Greens with either lemon or ginger (evolutionfresh.com/en-us/juice/organic-sweet-ginger). It contains 50 calories and 11 grams of carbs per 8 ounces–I highly recommend this product. The problem with some of these store-ready veggie juices is the lack of pasteurization, thus rendering them susceptible to contamination and foodborne illness. Otherwise, make your own fresh juice using greens that you hand-pick and wash thoroughly.

- **Dried fruit, applesauce, etc.** In moderation, dried fruit is a fine occasional snack, but be aware that drying fruit or making fruit sauces breaks down the fiber and concentrates the naturally occurring sugars–a little goes a long way in terms of total sugar intake.

- **Dairy.** Fermented dairy products like artisanal cheese, yogurt, kefir, and others are on the foods to favor list. But other forms of dairy such as cow's, goat's, and sheep's milk; custards; ice cream; and a few others should be kept to a minimum, mostly because they're higher in sugar than other forms of dairy and they cause adverse symptoms for many. Use them in moderation and watch to see how they affect you.

- **Gluten.** I am not 100 percent antigluten. Unless you're sensitive or allergic, a few servings of whole grains like barley, rye, spelt, and whole wheat are okay. Whole grains have some positive impacts on gut microbiome diversity. However, gluten-rich grains shouldn't be the predominant whole grains in your diet. Instead, focus on options with a lower glycemic load and higher protein content, such as amaranth, brown rice, quinoa, teff, chia, millet, and others. See the Phase 3 food charts on pages 251–256 for details.

- **Red meat and dark meat poultry.** These are associated with poor health outcomes and weight gain.

- **Sweeteners.** You can now reintroduce into your diet a few natural sweeteners, such as agave syrup, blackstrap molasses, stevia extract, and raw honey. However, these should be used as a condiment–a teaspoon in your coffee or morning shake is fine, but more really isn't healthy.

There are a few other foods to keep to a minimum, but we've covered most of them. For further detail, see the Phase 3 food charts on pages 251–256.

Foods to Favor

Once you've fine-tuned your Forget and Few lists, the foods you favor in Phase 3 will be everything else. Choose from the broad rainbow-colored array of fruits and vegetables in your produce section. Ask your butcher for lean cuts of red meat and chicken, and ask about available fish. Stock up on whole grains in the bulk section of your supermarket. Include a little goat's milk kefir or cow's milk yogurt (make it at home if you can) and a few delectable artisanal cheeses. Buy properly fermented vegetables or make your own ferments at home using the recipes in Chapter 11. The rich palette of healing whole foods is now open to you. Embrace them. Enjoy them with family and friends. And relish the foods that feed your inner ecology as well as your body, mind, and spirit.

I've included a Phase 3 meal plan and recipes in Chapter 11. These recipes represent quintessential Mediterranean dishes. They're exquisite, and I encourage you to try them. Use them as inspiration for your own creations. And as you dive deeper into this healthy way of eating and living, seek out more delicious recipes that fit the parameters of this program. The options are endless and include a broad array for cuisines from across the world. *Bon appétit!*

What You Can Expect During Phase 3

Phase 3 is a lifelong healthy eating plan built on heritage diets, especially the Mediterranean and Baltic Sea diets. It's a sustainable way of eating that will keep you trim and support optimal weight for life. Phase 3 never ends. It's not a diet—it's your lifelong eating plan, a way of eating and living in harmony with your inner ecology and the broader ecology around you.

What can you expect during this phase? Well, life is complicated, and it's hard to say what any individual will encounter. But my deepest hope is that this way of eating and living offers you a path toward reclaiming your human birthright: delicious food, slowly prepared meals enjoyed over a glass of wine with family and friends, optimal weight, excellent health, hope, happiness, and mental, physical, and spiritual nourishment.

LOOKING AHEAD

This chapter represents both an end and a beginning. You now understand what you need to know to create a healthy pattern of eating for yourself. The formal part of the program is complete. From here, it's up to you to decide which foods you'll favor, which you'll eat fewer of, and which you'll forget. I hope my guidelines offer you a road map to make nutrition decisions that will nourish you inside and out.

But there's always more to learn about healthy living. We're discovering more every day, adding nuance to what we already know. Now you have the tools you need to take control over your own health and become a full-fledged member of the Gut Balance Revolution club. That means you'll constantly be seeking new and innovative ways to support the garden of life inside and all around you.

The next step on your journey is to learn about the superfoods to include in Phase 3 for even more health benefits. After that, in Chapter 10, I'll explain how to take your progress toward healthy living to another level by creating a gut-balancing lifestyle. Then, in the Appendix, I'll give you the inside scoop on a highly controversial subject—the use of dietary supplements to support weight loss.

THE GUT BALANCE REVOLUTION SUCCESS STORIES

Monique Hendrix, 29

When your employer is the United States Army, keeping fit goes with the territory. Just ask Monique Hendrix. Her official job description may have been operating room technician at a base hospital, but, like all soldiers, she needed to stay in shape, too. "It was enforced that you exercise all the time," she explains. "I'd lift weights and run 3 or 4 miles, so you'd think I'd be pretty slim. But the problem was, I'd run right to McDonald's and grab a quarter-pounder. My diet wasn't healthy, and I really started to put on weight."

Even though her military career had come to an end, her unhealthy eating habits continued—but her exercise habits didn't. Little by little, she noticed that her clothes were getting tighter and she was having trouble catching her breath when she climbed up a flight of stairs. That's when she took the Gut Balance Revolution for a test drive.

"I've gone on lots of diets over the years," recalls Monique, a mother of four young children who's studying to become a registered nurse. "I tried everything from Weight Watchers to Jenny Craig. But nothing really worked until this program. In 8 weeks, I lost 12 pounds—and I felt so much better."

CHAPTER 9

Dr. Gerry's Top 10 Superfoods for Phase 3

The superfoods for Phase 3 are those you want to include in a healthy diet for life. Some were allowed in previous phases, as they constitute a healthy part of just about any nutritional program. I elected to feature them as superfoods in this phase for a few reasons. First, I want to highlight the types of foods to focus on as you move into this lifelong way of eating. They represent the broad range of choices now available to you. A few also feature prominently in the Mediterranean diet–another reason I feature them here. Finally, these foods are medicinal powerhouses that, when consumed regularly, can protect your health and waistline for years to come. So without further ado, here are my top 10 superfoods for Phase 3.

I. SALMON

The easiest way to increase your anti-inflammatory fats: Switch out red meat for salmon as much as possible. Try to consume this amazing superfood at least a couple times weekly. Salmon is chock-full of omega-3s–the healthy fats that reduce your risk of heart disease; enhance insulin sensitivity; support brain health, cognition, and mood; and help you burn fat. However, there are two important points to consider when adding this superfood to your diet.

Salmon has an outstanding ratio of omega-3 to omega-6 fats (5:1)–the opposite direction of the standard American diet ratio 1:14 to 1:25.[1] To maximize these anti-inflammatory omega-3 fats in your fish, go for wild, line-caught salmon–it's vastly healthier than farmed salmon, which has a higher content of the omega-6 inflammatory fats you're trying to avoid by adding fish to your diet. Why the difference between wild and farmed? For one thing, farmed salmon is fed genetically modified proinflammatory-rich soy and corn, given antibiotics, and contaminated with toxic chemicals such as dioxin and PCBs, which cause cancer and retard brain development *in utero* and in infants.[2]

Wild salmon, on the other hand, is extremely rich in health-promoting omega-3 fats while providing less toxic exposure.[3] These fats can even help protect you from Alzheimer's disease, the number three killer in America, according to Dr. David Perlmutter's bestseller *Grain Brain*![4]

Leading the pack for wild-caught salmon are Alaskan salmon—my favorite is king (sometimes called chinook) salmon, but I also enjoy sockeye, coho, pink, and Kodiak. Whichever species you prefer, I encourage you if possible to pay the premium for wild salmon to maximally support your health. You get what you pay for, so buy the good stuff.

Aside from the beneficial anti-inflammatory fatty acids, salmon contains bioactive peptides that regulate several hormones in the body that support cartilage and fight arthritis and may help prevent colorectal cancer.[5] Salmon is moderately high in purine, a food chemical that may flare gout in those who are susceptible, so if you have gout or are susceptible, beware.

But has salmon consumption been associated with weight loss? We've already discussed fish as one of the most satiating sources of protein—research shows that fatty fish can modulate hunger hormones and inflammation in overweight folks. During an 8-week intervention, salmon consumption modulated fasting insulin, as well as ghrelin and leptin, and lowered inflammatory markers.[6, 7] Varying the fish source has been demonstrated to improve compliance in those who favor fish as a protein source for weight loss.[8] Remember the Baltic Sea diet we discussed in Chapter 8? Rich in omega-3-fatty acid from fish, it's associated with weight loss and improved cardiometabolic markers.[9]

That's one reason I recommend that as you move into this lifelong journey toward health, you place fish on your menu often. Have fish as your main protein source two or three times weekly to cool inflammation. Use this high-quality protein source to regulate blood biochemistry and metabolic, satiety-controlling hormones. There are many varieties of fish to choose from and endless ways to prepare them. Some, like omega-3-rich Pesto Baked Cod (page 282), are included in your Gut Balance Revolution meal plans. In fact, a European study showed that consumption of cod increases weight loss in men and has other positive health effects.[10] A compelling study out of Iceland (which is in the Baltic region) reported a dose-response relationship between cod consumption and weight loss during an 8-week energy restriction diet.[11] Participants in the study ate diets consisting of one of these three seafood sources.

- Diet 1: 150 grams of cod five times per week

- Diet 2: 150 grams of cod three times per week

- Diet 3: No seafood

Those who consumed 150 grams (5.3 ounces) of cod five times weekly were found to have lost 1.7 kilograms (3.7 pounds) more than those who ate the same amount of calories without seafood.

Of course, other varieties of seafood may benefit weight loss by virtue of satiation and omega-3 content, or, like cod and salmon, they may have other properties that provide weight-loss benefits. However, not all fish of the same species are equally healthy—a wild salmon from the Pacific Ocean, for example, is different in many ways from a farm-raised salmon. The farm-raised salmon is much higher in cancer-causing organochemicals and lower in health-promoting omega-3 fatty acids and astaxanthin (a carotenoid pigment with powerful anti-inflammatory properties). In the Gut Balance Revolution recipe section, fishes high in astaxanthin, rich in omega-3 fatty acids, and low in mercury are favored.

Seafood Formerly Known as Healthy

Larger fish species like tuna (albacore, yellowfin, bigeye, ahi), swordfish, marlin, bluefish, grouper, halibut, orange roughy, skipjack, and shark were once among the healthiest foods on the planet but are no longer safe to eat in large quantities due to environmental mercury contamination.[12] That's because this toxic metal bioconcentrates up the food chain—small fish are exposed; medium fish eat the smaller, doubling their exposure; larger fish eat the medium fish—and they all end up with more mercury in their bodies, all the way up the food chain.

To reduce your mercury exposure, limit yourself to no more than one serving of albacore or yellowfin tuna weekly and avoid larger fish like shark, swordfish, king mackerel, or tilefish altogether. Limit fish with moderate mercury content to about one serving weekly. These include striped bass, carp, Alaskan cod, halibut, lobster, mahimahi, monkfish, perch (freshwater), sablefish, skate, snapper, tuna (canned chunk white, skipjack), and weakfish (sea trout).[13] The Crunchy Almond Tuna Salad in the recipe section (page 285) calls for chunk *light* tuna, which is lower in mercury.

I recommend consuming seafood that's low in mercury and organochemical pollutants, rich in omega-3 fatty acids content, and wild or fresh-caught in local waters. Examples include Atlantic or Pacific (US) cod, anchovy, butterfish, catfish, canned light tuna, flounder, haddock, herring, ocean perch, mussels, oysters, plaice, pollack, rainbow trout, rockfish, sardines, scallop, sea bass (black), shad (US), shrimp, sole, spiny lobster, striped bass, tilapia, trout (freshwater), wild eastern oyster, whitefish, and whiting. Pollack, rockfish, and black sea bass are threatened in certain waters; for more information, visit drweil.com/drw/u/ART02049/facts-about-fish.html. In general, farm-raised tilapia is loaded with antibiotics. The United States and Ecuador maintain the best practices for farming, and certain supermarket chains carry antibiotic- and hormone-free tilapia as an affordable whitefish option.[14]

A key superfood, seafood is underconsumed in the United States. The Dietary Guidelines for Americans suggest that everyone eat fish twice weekly,[15] but only about a third of Americans do. As you'll see in the meal plans, I recommend consuming safe seafood several times weekly during each phase. The health benefits are numerous—and you're worth it!

2. OLIVE OIL

I've highlighted the health benefits of olive oil throughout this book, but I decided to add it as a superfood in Phase 3 because it's the predominant source of fat in the MedDiet. Olive oil is, arguably, the healthiest oil on the planet, not only packed with monounsaturated fats but also containing high levels of phenols—antioxidants that play a role in heart health and fight chronic disease. The MedDiet features foods high in monounsaturated fatty acids (MUFAs), which may provide a nice perk to facilitate weight loss. Nuts, avocados, and olive oil, loaded with MUFAs, are anti-inflammatory superfoods. While many diet plans designed for short-term weight loss promote a low-fat approach, the Gut Balance Revolution favors foods that quench the fire of inflammation and improve satiation—that is what leads to a lean metabolism and weight loss. We need to move away from thinking that all fat-rich foods are evil and focus instead on eating fats that are anti-inflammatory. [16]

Another taboo is that energy-dense high-fat foods such as those high in MUFAs should be severely restricted. But this kind of thinking is based on the outdated calories in/calories out theory. While olive oil does contain 125 calories and 14 grams of fat per tablespoon, there's far more to health and weight than how many calories you consume. I'm not suggesting that you guzzle olive oil, but it has unquestionable therapeutic value and supports long-term weight maintenance.

A recent study published in the *European Journal of Clinical Nutrition* compared three diets: a low-fat diet against two slightly different MedDiets (nut rich versus olive oil rich as the prime source of fats). The MedDiets supplemented with virgin olive oil or nuts improved glucose metabolism as much as the typical low-fat diet. But unlike the low-fat diet group, both MedDiets groups lost significant body weight.[17]

What can explain these results? One reason: olive oil's effects on satiety. All fat enhances satiety to some extent, inducing gut hormones that make you feel full. However, there's a clever way that olive oil induces satiety: The scent of olive oil itself provokes a sense of fullness. A study published in the *American Journal of Nutrition* showed that spiking low-fat yogurt with the scent of a fat-free olive oil extract improved satiety and enhanced brain activity typically associated with fat consumption and reward.[18] Olive oil has special properties that profoundly impact satiety—its scent alone hits receptors in the brain promoting the sense of fullness.[19, 20] (There's even an ice creamery in Baltimore (Taharka Brothers, taharkabrothers.com) that developed an olive oil and sea salt flavor—a good way to feel more profoundly full with less ice cream!)

By now you know that fighting inflammation is a vital element of this program. Olive oil, especially extra-virgin olive oil (EVOO), is a strong anti-inflammatory compound with myriad health benefits.[21] EVOO has a very high polyphenol content and is considered a COX-1 and COX-2 inhibitor—the same class of anti-inflammatory as powerful medications like ibuprofen.[22]

These anti-inflammatory powers are important for cardiovascular health in particular. Anti-inflammatory fats are less likely to be involved in the oxidation of LDL that leads to coronary artery disease and atherosclerosis.[23, 24] Substituting carbohydrates for a calorically equivalent amount of olive oil has been shown in some studies to increase the good cholesterol—HDL—while having no effect on LDL. That's another excellent reason to incorporate more olive oil into your diet.[25] Olive oil is also high in oleic acid, which reduces the risk of blood clots, and it's a decent source of vitamin E–1 tablespoon contains 12.9 percent of the RDA.[26, 27]

Many people gain weight through a process called "emotional eating" in which they binge on food during periods of turmoil. Many factors can influence a binge eating disorder (BED), though good nutrition can help control this destructive impulsivity. A recent study showed that consumption of EVOO and nuts as part of the MedDiet decreased the risks of BED.[28] Compliance with the MedDiet was associated with a lower prevalence of BED, while the consumption of creams, butter, cakes, sweets, and baked desserts was a trigger for it.[29]

But what about weight loss? You guessed it. Olive oil probably helps you lose weight, too. A study on weight loss in 44 overweight breast cancer survivors used an olive oil–based diet, since studies have shown an association of olive oil consumption with a decreased risk of breast cancer development.[30] In the 44-week study, participants were randomly assigned to either an olive oil–enriched plant-based diet or a calorically equivalent diet from the National Cancer Institute (NCI). Their total fat intake was greater than 15 percent but less than 30 percent of the calories they consumed. Twenty-eight people completed the clinical trial. The olive oil–based diet proved to be more effective for weight loss, lowering serum triglycerides and raising high-density lipoproteins (good cholesterol), than a standard NCI low-fat diet. Significantly more women lost 5 percent or more of their body weight on the olive oil–based diet than on the NCI diet.

What other health benefits does olive oil confer on women aside from weight control and cancer protection? Olive oil has been shown in laboratory animals to protect female rats who have undergone surgically induced menopause against bone loss.[31]

Mediterranean people have used olive oil as their primary fat source for millennia, with no evidence of harm. In fact, it seems to be one of the key dietary factors in the long, relatively disease-free lives of those living in this region. So stick with EVOO as your main source of oil. It will keep the pounds off as it keeps your heart (and the rest of you!) healthy.

3. APPLES

According to researchers from the School of Food Science at Washington State University, an apple a day can literally keep the doctor away. These scientists evaluated the gut microbiome profiles of obese and lean laboratory rats before and after the consumption of apples and found that ingestion of apples normalized the maldistributed gut flora of the obese rats, making them similar to those of the lean ones. Several different varieties were tested, with all showing this benefit; however, the Granny Smith apple was found to provide the best protection against the development of obesity by promoting a healthy gut flora. The Granny Smith apple is highest in nondigestible fibers (gut flora food!) and anti-inflammatory natural products.[32]

These superfruits, cultivated in temperate zones the world over, have been around for nearly 3,000 years. Apple seeds are heterozygous—if you remove the seeds from the apples you buy in the store and plant them in the ground, four different types of apples will grow. This has several implications. One is that there's a virtually endless variety of apples. Unfortunately, few of them are the sweet, delicious fruit you're used to. Each of those store-bought varietals has been carefully cultivated by farmers, in some cases for centuries. Every apple in your local supermarket comes from a grafted tree. Some heirloom strains of apples have been passed down (and eaten!) by humans for hundreds of years. It's a good thing, too, as this superfruit comes with some real health benefits.

One reason we think apples are so healthy is their high levels of phytochemicals like flavonoids, carotenoids, and phenolics, plus powerful antioxidants like quercetin, catechin, phloridzin, and chlorogenic acid (the latter is also found in the weight-loss-promoting green coffee bean). This powerful combination of phytonutrients plus their soluble fiber—called pectin—and their relatively high amounts of vitamin C make apples a nutritional powerhouse that can reduce your risk of a wide variety of chronic illnesses. The anti-inflammatory activity, coupled with the feeding of the friendly flora by its pectin, makes apples a superfood for overall health and weight maintenance. For example, regular consumption of apples reduces your risk of heart disease. The Women's Health Study, which followed 40,000 women for nearly 7 years, showed that those with the highest consumption of flavonoids had the lowest risk of heart disease. Intake of apples and broccoli specifically further reduced the risk of cardiovascular events. Women who regularly consumed apples saw a 13 to 22 percent reduction in cardiovascular events[33]—a correlation that's been replicated in many studies.[34-37]

The antioxidant and anti-inflammatory chemicals in apples are one of the reasons they're so healthy for your heart. However, another factor is that apples seem to lower blood lipids. Remember that fiber has a powerful effect on blood lipids. While apples are reasonably high in fiber, the amount they contain doesn't seem to account for their overall effect on blood lipid levels. A group of French scientists designed a clever experiment to solve this mystery. They fed three groups of rats as follows:[38]

- Group 1 got apple pectin (the primary source of fiber in the fruit).

- Group 2 got a freeze-dried apple (in which the fiber was reduced) that was high in polyphenol content.

- Group 3 got both.

Guess which group had the lowest blood lipids? Group 3. It appears that apples (like many foods) are more than the sum of their parts. It's not just the pectin *or* the polyphenols that have this effect on blood lipids. It's the unique combination of these powerful phytochemicals and fiber that makes apples a superfruit.

These effects on heart health and blood lipid levels would be enough to recommend apples. But the benefits don't stop there. Apples have repeatedly been shown to have cancer-protective effects, especially against lung cancer. The Nurses' Health Study, involving 77,000 women and 47,000 men, showed that women who consumed one serving of apples or pears a day had a reduced risk of lung cancer.[39] In a study out of Hawaii, scientists sought to find out just how powerful this anti–lung cancer effect was. They took two groups of patients–582 with lung cancer and 582 without it–and compared their smoking history and food intake. Those with the highest consumption of apples, onions, and white grapefruit had a 40 to 50 percent reduced risk of developing lung cancer compared to those with the lowest intake of these foods.[40]

Apples appear to enhance pulmonary health in the absence of lung cancer. They seem to decrease the risk of asthma, reduce the severity of asthma attacks, and decrease bronchial hypersensitivity.[41] They also appear to enhance overall lung capacity. In a Welsh study, the lung capacity of 2,512 middle-aged men between ages 45 and 59 was assessed using a tool called forced expiratory volume (FEV), which measures how much air you can push out your lungs.[42] Scientists found that those who ate more apples weekly had better FEV scores, almost certainly due to high levels of flavonoids–especially quercetin–found in apples.

Not only do apples support heart and lung health, but they also seem to help people reverse type 2 diabetes and lose weight. In a Finnish study, the dietary history of more than 10,000 men and women was reviewed. Researchers found that increased apple consumption was associated with a reduced risk of type 2 diabetes.[43] Higher intake of quercetin, one of the major flavonoids in apples, was associated with a further reduced risk.

The bottom line for weight loss? The mighty apple helps you shed pounds and stay slim. A study conducted at the State University of Rio de Janeiro in Brazil randomly assigned 411 women to supplement their diet with one of three interventions: an apple, a pear, or an oat cookie snack three times daily. The women who ate one serving of apples three times daily lost 2.6 pounds in a 12-week period while lowering triglycerides and total cholesterol.[44]

Animal studies show similar results. An interesting controlled study in diet-induced obese rats demonstrated improved lipid profiles and loss of body fat and weight when these animals were fed either apple pomace (the residue after the juice extraction process) or apple juice concentrate (both having a high concentration of polyphenols and flavonoids as well as soluble fibers) *while consuming a Western diet high in saturated fat.* So what does this mean? Rats who become obese by consuming a diet high in saturated fats (aka diet-induced obesity) can reverse their obesity just with apple products.[45] The potential mechanisms of body-weight- and fat-loss-promoting benefits of apple products in this study include the soluble fiber blocking the absorption of cholesterol and bile acids, soluble fiber promoting healthy bacteria to improve metabolism, and the anti-inflammatory effects of the polyphenols in the apple products. A recent study confirmed that clear apple juice devoid of prebiotic pectin and lower in polyphenolics does not provide these benefits.[46]

These fascinating findings clearly demonstrate the healing power of this superfruit. But one other study brings home why superfood apples are especially suited to the Gut Balance Revolution. Scientists have recently shown in animal models that regular consumption of apples enhances the biodiversity of the gut microbiome.[47] Animals whose diet was supplemented with pectin (the primary fiber in apples) experienced a twofold increase of butyric acid—the primary fuel for cells in the large intestine, changes that didn't occur in controls or in animals fed apple puree, pomace, or juice. So go ahead and have an apple a day.

4. DARK CHOCOLATE

Chocolate is derived from tropical cocoa beans from the genus *Theobroma*, a word that translates as "food of the gods"–a name it deserves not only for its rich, luscious flavor but also for its health effects.

Chocolate contains two types of flavonoid: flavanols, made up of molecules called epicatechins and catechins, which are also found in tea; and procyanidins, longer flavanol molecules. Studies have shown that cocoa and some types of dark chocolate are higher in polyphenols, flavonoids, and antioxidant activity than many of the other superfoods highlighted here. Indeed, dark chocolate outscores acai, blueberries, cranberries, and pomegranates in each of these categories.[48] Fascinating information–but the real question remains: Do these increased levels of healthy phytochemicals in chocolate correlate with improved health outcomes? The data show that they do.

Much of the research on chocolate and health has revolved around its impact on cardiovascular disease, cholesterol oxidation, and hypertension. This superfood performs extremely well in each of these areas. Back in 2004, a coalition of scientists from the Netherlands, Belgium, and Australia joined together to identify dietary interventions to help people reduce their risk of heart disease.[49] To find out what this healthy meal would consist of, they reviewed data from the Framingham Heart Study and its Offspring Study (two of the largest studies ever conducted to determine the factors leading to heart health or disease). The scientists created the Polymeal–a diet that if eaten daily would decrease the risk of cardiovascular events by as much as 76 percent, a vastly better outcome than any existing medication, with no side effects. The meal consisted of fish, dark chocolate, fruits, vegetables, garlic, and almonds. Sound familiar? The researchers found that 100 grams of cocoa-rich chocolate alone could reduce risk of cardiovascular events by as much as 21 percent.

These are impressive findings and interesting dietary recommendations right in line with the Mediterranean Diet I recommend for Phase 3. But how does dark chocolate have such a profound effect on heart health? We don't have all the answers, but several mechanisms seem to be at play.

First, the high phenolic content of dark chocolate has both anti-inflammatory and antioxidant properties. In one study, an amino acid called clovamide and two phenolic extracts from roasted and unroasted cocoa beans were tested for their effects on proinflammatory cytokines and NF-κB gene activation (two primary markers for inflammation).[50] All three reduced these inflammation markers, and the clovamide also enhanced PPARy activation, which is a key factor in reducing systemic inflammation. As systemic inflammation plays a key role in heart disease, these effects suggest that consuming dark chocolate may mitigate your risk.

Another study showed that the antioxidant activity of dark chocolate may play an even more powerful role in cardiovascular health. Scientists at the University of Pennsylvania sought to determine how dark chocolate influenced heart health.[51] They divided 23 healthy subjects into two groups, giving one a standard Western diet and the other the same diet supplemented with 22 grams of cocoa and 16 grams of dark chocolate daily. The results? The dark-chocolate group experienced far less oxidation of LDL cholesterol—critically important because cholesterol oxidation is *the* leading factor in cardiovascular disease and heart attacks. It's also been shown that regular consumption of dark chocolate reduces blood pressure and enhances endothelial function, which seems to hold true both in healthy populations and in people with essential hypertension (high blood pressure with no known cause).[52, 53] We think that this effect on blood pressure has to do with the fact that the flavonoids in chocolate influence an important vasodilator called nitric oxide, important in regulating blood pressure. Dark chocolate is also high in oleic acid, the heart-healthy monounsaturated fat found in olive oil—perhaps another reason for its heart-protective effects.

Mounting evidence also suggests that dark chocolate may improve insulin sensitivity. A recent study in the *American Journal of Clinical Nutrition* revealed that healthy subjects who ate 100 grams of dark chocolate daily saw a significant increase in insulin sensitivity compared to those who ate a calorically equivalent amount of white chocolate. Plus, a decrease in systolic blood pressure was also observed.[54] British studies showed that higher consumption of flavones (found in berries and dark chocolate) was associated with a lower risk of diabetes, obesity, cardiovascular disease, and cancer. Higher flavone intake was also associated with improved insulin sensitivity.[55, 56]

This delectable superfood, rich in polyphenols that fight inflammation and improve insulin sensitivity, also turns out to be a prebiotic.[57] Investigators from Louisiana State University reported that fibers in dark chocolate are fermented by good obesity-fighting gut microbes, such as bifidobacteria and lactic-acid bacteria, which in turn make even more anti-inflammatory compounds, which benefits cardiovascular health and weight regulation.[58] So dark chocolate has prebiotic properties that make it a suitable Phase 2 or Phase 3 superfood.

Could something considered a sweet treat facilitate weight loss? Yes! Researchers from the University of Granada in Spain reported a European study involving 1,458 adolescents ages 12 to 17 showing that more chocolate consumption was associated with lower levels of total and central fat.[59] How can that be? A new study published in the *Journal of Agriculture and Food Chemistry* points to a possible answer.[60] It appears the flavanols in chocolate, especially the oligomeric proanthocyanidins (OPCs), are active obesity-preventing agents. Scientists fed mice a high-fat diet and then gave them a variety of flavanols found in chocolate. After 12 weeks, the mice receiving the OPCs were best protected against weight gain, fat mass accumulation, impaired glucose tolerance, and insulin resistance.

Please note that we're talking about *dark chocolate*, which is very different than the majority of chocolate you'll find in your local supermarket. When buying chocolate, look for products that are at least 70 percent cacao and not filled with sugar–that usually means paying a premium for specialty brands. Avoid milk chocolate and white chocolate (they're chock-full of sugar), and stick with the richest, darkest varieties.

Though I'm an advocate of dark chocolate, don't eat too much. Even dark chocolate has sugar in it. Enjoy a few servings–usually a couple of squares–three or four times weekly. More than this probably won't provide additional health benefits, and the sugar may indeed harm your health and your waistline if you overindulge. As long as you enjoy dark chocolate in moderation, you can (and should!) make this "food of the gods" part of your long-term eating plan.

5. GREENS (LEAFY GREENS, SALADS)

Leafy greens constitute a broad class of vegetables including but not limited to:

- Spinach
- Swiss chard
- Kale (this was a superfood for Phase 2, so I won't reiterate those points here)
- Mustard greens
- Collard greens
- Leaf lettuce

While these foods don't all possess the same health benefits or even come from the same plant family, it's useful to classify them together for one simple reason: Incorporating leafy green vegetables of *any* variety into your diet has a broad array of health benefits. Prepare them as salads, braised greens, or any of the other myriad ways–they're a relatively simple, low-cost, low-labor, delectable way to enhance your health. For ease, let's divide this immense group of veggies into salads and leafy greens. First, let's look at some of the data on leafy greens. Then we'll talk about the supermeal called salad.

Leafy Greens

One group of vegetables I haven't talked about at length is the Chenopodiaceae family, which includes spinach, Swiss chard, beets, and quinoa. The health effects of these foods are increasingly being celebrated because they contain a set of phytochemicals that confer cancer-protective effects. These protective plant chemicals are called carotenoids; a specific subset of these, called epoxy xanthophylls, seems to inhibit the proliferation of cancer cells. Spinach and Swiss chard both have high levels of these epoxy xanthophylls, which may be one reason these foods have been shown in repeated studies to protect against cancer.[61]

That's a big claim, so let's look at some of the studies backing it up. In animal models, it's been shown that the carotenoid neoxanthin stops the proliferation of prostate cancer cells.[62] A recent study published in the *International Journal of Cancer* analyzed the association between the intake of five common flavonoids and ovarian cancer incidences in the 66,940 women who took part in the Nurses' Health Study. They found that high intakes of the flavonoid apigenin—particularly high in spinach and parsley—was associated with lower rates of ovarian cancer. Kaempferol, an important flavonoid found not only in spinach but also in cruciferous vegetables, including leafy greens like collards and mustard, also seems to play a critical role.[63] Additionally, spinach consumption appears to reduce the risk of breast cancer. A study at the National Institute of Environmental Health Sciences reviewed health and food intake data from 3,543 women diagnosed with cancer and compared it to 9,406 controls. Their findings? Those who ate spinach and carrots twice weekly were 56 percent less likely to develop breast cancer than those who didn't eat these foods at all. Not only does spinach appear to mitigate cancer proliferation, but it also has antimutagenic properties (meaning it reduces the rate of cellular mutation). One study found that 13 chemical constituents of spinach acted as antimutagens in the human body.[64] And though the evidence isn't yet conclusive, it appears that increasing your spinach intake may decrease your risk of aggressive prostate cancer (stages III and IV).[65]

What about Swiss chard? Though fewer studies have been done on this vegetable, it stands to reason that Swiss chard has similar effects, since it contains many of the same specialized, cancer-fighting carotenoids as spinach.

Does this mean that you if you add a little spinach or chard to your diet you will be magically cured from cancer or remain cancer free for life? Certainly not—no one can promise that. Nevertheless, the growing research supporting the use of these foods in the fight against cancer is extremely compelling.

The health benefits of these leafy greens do not stop with their cancer-fighting properties. Spinach may reduce blood pressure. It's likely to have positive effects on eye health due to its relatively high levels of lutein and zeaxanthin, two carotenoids known to support eye health and mitigate macular degeneration.[66] Swiss chard, on the other hand, may help you fight high cholesterol levels and colon cancer and may protect liver function in type 2 diabetics.[67, 68]

No food is a magical cure-all. But taken together, the data suggest that a diet high in these leafy greens will protect your health on multiple fronts.

What about collards, mustard, kale, cabbage, and other leafy greens in the cruciferous vegetable family? Actually, this entire family of vegetables has medicinal properties and contains some of the healthiest foods you can consume. There are a few all-star players like kale (a Phase 2 superfood) and broccoli (part of the cruciferous family, with many of the same health benefits—and then some). You can't go wrong adding more crucifers to your diet—each is full of phytochemicals that can protect you from a wide variety of chronic illnesses. So let's take a few minutes to look at how cruciferous foods perform overall in terms of health outcomes.

Crucifers may have even more profound cancer-protective effects than those reviewed for spinach and Swiss chard. Though the evidence is mixed, over the last few decades epidemiological studies have shown an inverse correlation between cruciferous vegetable consumption and the risk of gastric, breast, lung, prostate, colorectal, bladder, and other cancers.[69-73] The correlation seems to be best illustrated for lung, gastric, and colorectal cancers,[74, 75] and most scientists now agree that eating more cruciferous veggies will help protect some of us from these three forms of cancer—and perhaps others as well. But which people are protected and why?

One reason these supergreens have cancer-protective effects is that they're a rich source of glucosinolates—unique phytonutrients metabolized in the body and turned into other chemicals called isothiocyanates (ITCs), which seem to have the powerful anticancer effect. They enhance elimination of potential carcinogens from the body, increase the transcription of proteins that suppress tumor formation, block enzymes used on carcinogen activation, and trigger cancer cell apoptosis (cell death).[76, 77] However, these effects appear to be somewhat dependent on individual predispositions. People with a gene called glutathione S-transferase M1 (GSTM1) don't seem to get the same protective effects from these greens. That's because this gene is involved in the urinary transport of ITCs, so those people pee out much of the goodness they get from cruciferous veggies. Thus, the cancer-protective effects you get from these veggies depend, to some extent, on your genetic makeup. How do you know if you have the GSTM1 gene? Well, you could get personalized gene testing to help determine if eating more greens may protect you from cancer, but it probably isn't worth the expense, as crucifers have plenty of other health benefits that justify their place in your diet.

Another area where these veggies shine is in their effect on blood lipids and cardio-vascular disease. In Chapter 7, I described the process by which eating kale enhances levels of bile acids that bind to cholesterol, allowing you to excrete it and lowering your overall blood levels of cholesterol. Kale isn't the only vegetable that accomplishes this. All crucifers can, and some are even better at it than kale–collards come in first place, and mustard isn't far behind. Cabbage is also a winner.[78] So if you want to lower choles-terol naturally, include plenty of cruciferous veggies in your diet. There's also some evi-dence that the same ITCs that may protect against cancer also have cardioprotective effects.[79] Again, the presence or absence of the GSTM1 gene appears to impact this effect.[80]

But how do cruciferous vegetables influence weight gain and type 2 diabetes? While there's little evidence that crucifers have a direct impact on type 2 diabetes and weight, increasing your overall intake of fruits and vegetables is inversely correlated with these con-ditions.[81] What's more, the phytochemicals in these leafy greens have anti-inflammatory and antioxidant effects, so they may indirectly influence type 2 diabetes and the complex of symptoms involved in metabolic syndrome. Of course, more research is needed to tease out all the relationships, but it's logical to conclude cruciferous vegetables don't have any nega-tive impact on these conditions–and they may improve them. So eat your greens–they're good for you.

Salads

It's difficult to ascertain the exact health benefits of salads for one main reason: They're all so different. A spinach salad is different from a mesclun mix, and both are different from a Cobb salad. But one thing's certain: As long as you avoid inflammatory fats (con-tained in many commercial salad dressings) and sugar (in candied nuts or in sweet dressings), you can't go wrong with a salad. It's not a superfood, it's a supermeal with health benefits more than the sum of its parts.

Since we're talking about greens, let's discuss the most common salad green of all: lettuce. There are hundreds of varieties of lettuce, and all of them are healthy except, perhaps, iceberg lettuce, which has zero nutritional value. Lettuce is universally low in calories, and most varieties are high in vitamins A and C as well as iron and calcium. Some lettuce varieties, like romaine, are also high in vitamin K (romaine contains 100 percent of the RDA for vitamin K) and folate. Research has shown that red and green leaf lettuces contain anthocyanins that are COX-1 and COX-2 inhibitors (the same class of chemicals as NSAID medications), and they mitigate lipid peroxidation–the process by which free radicals steal oxygen molecules from fat cells, causing oxidative stress that can contribute to cardiovascular damage and other conditions.[82]

There's also evidence that some types of lettuce have relatively high levels of the fla-vonoid quercetin[83]–the same antioxidant molecule contained in apples and onions. Both red and green lettuce have strong antioxidant and anti-inflammatory activities that vary by phenolic composition according to the type of lettuce. Higher amounts of phenolics, including anthocyanin, found in berries and present in red lettuce, may indicate that consumption of red lettuce provides better health benefits than green lettuce.[84] So it's logical to assume lettuce may have similar health effects to these foods, and increasing your intake of vegetables is one of the easiest ways to protect your overall health. And that's as easy as making a quick salad. Consider the overall potential health benefits of the following salad.

- Red leaf lettuce
- Spinach
- Baby chard
- Nuts
- Avocado
- Fresh feta cheese

Drizzle with olive oil and red wine or balsamic vinegar and you've got a supermeal if ever there was one. Every one of these ingredients is a superfood. The dish contains healthy protein, high-quality fat, a good amount of fiber, and probiotics all in a meal that takes you about 5 minutes to prepare. Want more protein? Add canned salmon or cooked chicken breast. Don't like feta? Shred fresh Parmesan instead. Not in love with the taste of chard? Replace it with baby kale. The variations are endless.

There's evidence that consuming salads as a preload facilitates weight loss.[85] "Preload" refers to a small meal eaten just before the main meal to curb appetite and ultimately lower caloric intake of the main meal so that the energy consumption of both meals combined is lower than from the main meal alone. A team of doctors demonstrated that salad preloading resulted in lower body weight, waist circumference, triglycerides, total cholesterol, and systolic blood pressure. The preload concept has been demonstrated to facilitate weight loss in a program called Volumetrics.[86] It involves eating low-energy-density foods as appetizers, which promote satiation and reduce appetite during the meal itself. Salads are popular preload appetizers shown to be effective, but others include soups[87] and even higher protein snacks.[88] That's why I view soup and salads as prime preload superfoods for weight control in Phase 3. As you'll see in the meal plans for recipes for this phase, I feature a Minestrone Soup (page 316) that has prebiotic and potent antioxidant properties to fight inflammation and add good bacteria to your inside tract.

One way preloading diminishes appetite is by slowing stomach emptying. The form and thickness (viscosity) of soup may alter the efficacy of the preload.[89] For example, pureed vegetable soup decreases gastric emptying time, slows down digestion, and gives a sense of fullness, but it also increases the insulin response (high glycemic response due to its predigested form and rapid absorption) and increases diet-induced thermogenesis (energy burning during digestion) compared to when the solid vegetables in soup are consumed with a glass of water. Eating soup can have gastrointestinal, endocrine, and metabolic consequences that may influence food intake and satiety, and the form of soup may influence these responses.

Eating soup regularly can reduce energy intake, enhance satiety, and promote weight loss.[90] A recent study reviewed epidemiological data from more than 10,500 adults who participated in the National Health and Nutrition Examination Survey.[91] Compared with non–soup eaters, those who ate soup had lower body weight and lower waist circumference. Soup consumption was associated with a lower dietary energy intake, independent of whether data on beverage or water consumption were included. Diet quality was significantly better in soup consumers as well–they ate less saturated fat and ate more protein and dietary fiber as well as several vitamins and minerals.

Soup appears to help you maintain a healthy weight in a number of ways, but the real key may ultimately be that it feeds your good gut bacteria to induce a lean metabolism and reduce your intake of energy-dense foods.[92] A word of caution: In this study, soup was also associated with a higher intake of sodium, which portends cardiovascular risks.

Epidemiological studies have revealed that soup consumption is associated with a lower risk of obesity. Moreover, intervention studies have reported that soup consumption aids in body-weight management. In 2013, researchers based in the University of Iowa looked at the US-based National Health and Nutrition Examination Survey (NHANES) that took place from 2003 to 2006[93] after reviewing health and dietary data on 4,158 participants. Their results were similar to a UK-based study: Non–soup consumers were at a higher risk of being overweight or obese and had a higher prevalence of reduced HDL cholesterol. The frequency of soup consumption was inversely associated with body mass index and waist circumference. Scientists concluded that "there is an inverse relationship between soup consumption and body weight status in US adults, which support laboratory studies showing a potential benefit of soup consumption for body weight management." A subsequent publication by these investigators using the NHANES database from 2003 to 2008 reported that soup consumers had a lower body weight, a lower waist circumference, and a trend toward a lower total energy intake.[94]

Several studies worldwide show that eating soup negatively correlates with body mass index, serum cholesterol and triacylglycerol levels, and blood pressure.[95, 96] So soups and salads are primo superfood appetizers for the Gut Balance Revolution weight-loss plan. Ultimately, the gut controls your figure, and just choosing the right foods that work with your gut physiology can help you lose fat in all the right places and keep your curves.

By now you should be aware that I have included many soups and salads in the recipes and meal plans in this book. Each is a supermeal in its own right. But don't stop with these. Use the recipes to inspire your own creations. The possibilities are endless when it comes to making supermeal salads.

6. FLAXSEED

Flaxseed has been with human beings a long time. It was known in the Stone Age, cultivated in Mesopotamia, has a long history of use in India, and was popular in Rome until the empire fell. Unfortunately, flax fell into obscurity until the modern era. In the 20th century, flaxseed was primarily used to produce linseed oil, a common ingredient in paints, varnishes, and other industrial chemicals.

It wasn't until the 1990s that flaxseed's health benefits became known to the public at large again. First off, it's one of the richest plant-based sources of omega-3 fats around, containing 132.5 percent of the DRI of these anti-inflammatory fats. Flaxseeds also contain extremely high levels of antioxidant polyphenols. Among 100 of the most common sources of polyphenols in the American diet, flaxseeds rank ninth, beating out such antioxidant powerhouses as blueberries and olives.[97] Researchers now consider flaxseeds to be *the* highest source of a unique type of fiber-related polyphenol called lignans, with seven times more of these important phytochemicals than their closest runner-up—sesame seed. These lignans are one of the key reasons flaxseeds are so good for us, and they only become bioactive when broken down by gut bacteria in a conversion process involving a wide mix of gut bacteria including those from the genera *Bacteroides*, *Bifidobacterium*, *Butyribacterium*, and *Eubacterium*. It's another glimpse into the important web of relationships between what you eat, the biodiversity of your gut microbiome, and your health.[98]

Another unique feature of flaxseeds is that when they're ground and mixed with water, they create a gel that seems to reduce appetite and overall food intake.[99]

This combination of factors—high omega-3 fat content, high polyphenol content, high lignan content, and a fiber that becomes gelatinous in water—is probably why their use produces such powerful, positive results in metabolic syndrome, insulin resistance, type 2 diabetes, and heart disease.[100]

The Importance of Lignans

Lignans are important fiber-related polyphenols. They:

- Are disease-fighting, plant-derived chemicals found in plants, seeds, whole grains, legumes, fruits, and vegetables.[101]

- Are precursors converted to other polyphenols by bacteria that normally colonize the human intestine, providing a weak estrogenic effect.

- May help prevent hormone-associated cancers, colon cancer, osteoporosis, and cardiovascular diseases.

- May improve menopausal symptoms and protect against breast cancer.[102]

Flaxseeds are the richest dietary source of lignan precursors. Sesame seeds are another rich source, followed by brassica vegetables, then grains (barley, oat, wheat, and rye).

For instance, a study at North Dakota State University randomized a group of obese, glucose-intolerant people, giving one group 40 grams of flaxseed and another group 40 grams of wheat bran baked bread. Each group took the prescribed supplemental fiber for 12 weeks. The group receiving the flaxseed saw reduced inflammatory markers, reduced blood glucose and insulin levels, and a 20 percent reduction in the prevalence of metabolic syndrome.[103]

Another study sought to determine whether or not flaxseed had an impact on cardiovascular disease risk in healthy menopausal women–a group whose number one risk of death is heart failure. The study investigators enrolled 199 women who were divided into two groups and assigned either 40 grams of flaxseed daily or 12 grams of a wheat germ placebo for 12 months.[104] After a year, those who took the flaxseed had increased levels of omega-3 fatty acids and reduced risk factors for cardiovascular illness including LDL, C-reactive protein, and blood glucose. This effect of flaxseed on LDL levels has been replicated several times. In one study, scientists found that LDL was reduced by as much as 12 to 15 percent with flaxseed supplementation, while fat excretion from the body was increased.[105] Another study showed that supplementation with flaxseed lignan for 12 weeks reduced cholesterol levels in men with moderately high cholesterol while decreasing liver disease factors.[106]

But can flaxseeds give you back your figure? Get this: Dietary flaxseed oil has been shown to reduce *fat cell size* and inflammatory mediators in obese insulin-resistant rats.[107, 108] In an interesting study, scientists induced obesity in rats by turning on inflammatory responses and appetite centers in their brains (the hypothalamus). They then showed that diet-, pharmacological-, and gene-based approaches could reverse this weight gain.[109] To do this, they used fire-quenching anti-inflammatory oils. They reported that either *partial substitution* of dietary omega-3–rich flaxseed-derived oil or omega-9–rich monounsaturated olive oil reversed hypothalamic inflammation and corrected the molecular mediator involved in inflammation in the first place. This intervention also helped rebalance hormones like insulin, leptin, and others. There are several important lessons from this study.

1. Bad diet can lead to inflammation in the brain, stimulating the appetite and leading to increased energy intake and insulin resistance.

2. This process is *reversible* with a healthy anti-inflammatory prebiotic diet.

In fact, researchers injected these anti-inflammatory oils directly into the hypothalamus and were able to emulate the dietary effects on appetite, metabolism, and body weight.

In a study of 115 women conducted by Laval University in Quebec, those with a higher consumption of lignans were healthier and thinner. They had a lower average body mass index (BMI), and those who ate the most flax had 8.5 kilograms (nearly 18 pounds) less body fat. Simply put, higher intake of lignans was associated with lower BMI and body fat mass and improved insulin sensitivity.[110]

So while I emphasize eating more olive oil through the Gut Balance Revolution, remember that ground flaxseed is a nice source of lignans that are prebiotic and whose oils are anti-inflammatory–a one-two punch to fight body fat.

You can grind flaxseeds and add them to baked goods, one of the typical methods they're administered in studies. But that's not the only way to enjoy them. Grind and add them to your morning shake, try them as a crust on broiled chicken, or add them to plain live-cultured yogurt with a little raw honey and blueberries for a superdessert. I love to stir a decadent blend of ground flaxseeds and chia seeds, cocoa, and coconut into a mixture of plain Greek and White Mountain yogurt (for a probiotic colony boost) and top it with berries and sliced almonds or walnuts. That's a superfood weight-loss-promoting healthy snack to be sure!

7. NUTS

Can a calorie-rich food packed with fat help you lose weight, lower your risk of type 2 diabetes and heart disease, and reduce your risk of mortality from all causes? That food does exist–it's the tree nut.

Nuts have basked in a lot of glowing press over the last decade, and for good reason. The data show that regular consumption of nuts has a wide array of health benefits, from the prebiotic effects of almonds to the cholesterol-improving, anti-inflammatory effects of pistachios. But that's only the beginning of the story about this superfood. Nuts in all forms–almonds, macadamias, pistachios, cashews, Brazil nuts, and others–have impressive effects on health and can help you lose and keep weight off. Let's go to the science that proves it.

A recent study published in the *New England Journal of Medicine* reviewed data from the Nurses' Health Study and the Health Professionals Follow-Up Study, which together included 118,962 people.[111, 112] Scientists found that nut consumption was inversely correlated with mortality from all causes–the more servings of nuts people ate per week, the less likely they were to die over the course of the studies. The researchers also noted that significant inverse associations were observed between nut consumption and risk of cancer, heart disease, and respiratory illness.

The long-studied correlation between nut consumption and reduced risk for cardiovascular disease has been replicated so many times that it's well accepted that nuts reduce your risk of cardiovascular disease and death from heart attacks for many reasons. We initially became aware of this correlation in 1992 with the completion of the Adventist Health Study, one of the first to show that nut consumption correlated with a reduced risk of cardiovascular illness.[113] This was quickly followed by another study published by the same group of scientists, revealing that eating walnuts reduced serum cholesterol levels and blood pressure in healthy men.[114] These two seminal studies kicked off what has now been more than 2 decades of research on the health effects of nuts.

A meta-analysis of four of the largest of these studies (Adventist Health Study, Iowa

Women's Health Study, Nurses' Health Study, and the Physicians' Health Study) showed that the risk of cardiovascular illness is 37 percent lower in people eating nuts four or more times per week.[115] Of the four studies reviewed, the Physicians' Health Study is of particular interest because the inverse correlation between nut consumption and cardiovascular illness was primarily due to a 47 percent reduction in sudden cardiac death and lowered total coronary heart disease mortality.[116] In each of these studies, there was a dose-response relationship between nuts and cardiovascular risk independent of gender, age, BMI, alcohol use, other nutritional characteristics, or other cardiovascular risk factors. That means simply eating more nuts—without changing anything else—may dramatically reduce your risk of heart disease.

Why do nuts have such a powerful influence on heart health? Most likely because they reduce cholesterol, inflammation, and oxidation, and they're also rich in fiber, which feeds your good gut bacteria, providing a wide array of benefits.

In a pooled analysis of 25 intervention trials in which nuts were given to participants, it was shown that on average 67 grams of nuts eaten daily reduced LDL cholesterol by 5 to 7 percent.[117] Again, nuts had this effect in a dose-response relationship independent of all other risk factors. Similar results were found in a meta-analysis of 13 studies done on walnuts.[118] When compared to control diets, walnut-enriched diets reduce LDL cholesterol by an average of 6.7 percent. In both these analyses, nuts had no influence on HDL. On the surface this sounds insignificant, but it's actually critically important. By reducing only LDL while having no effect on HDL, nuts improve the overall ratio of these different types of cholesterol in the body—very desirable for heart health.

Several studies have also revealed that eating nuts reduces systemic inflammation in the body—a primary risk factor for cardiovascular disease (as well as for weight gain, type 2 diabetes, and other chronic illnesses). One analyzed data from 6,000 participants in the Multi-Ethnic Study of Atherosclerosis in an attempt to uncover a relationship between nut consumption and inflammatory markers in the blood.[119] The results were astounding. People who ate nuts had reduced levels of C-reactive protein, interleukin 6, and fibrinogen—a powerful indication that nuts reduce inflammation. Other studies have come to similar conclusions.[120, 121] No doubt these effects are due to the fact that nuts are high in anti-inflammatory omega-3 fatty acids.

Growing evidence also shows that the tocopherols and polyphenols in nuts reduce lipid oxidation—another risk factor for heart disease. Studies in both animals and humans confirm this effect.[122]

The health benefits of nuts continue: They reduce your risk of metabolic syndrome, type 2 diabetes, and obesity. A recent study from the School of Public Health at Loma Linda University found that nut consumption had an inverse relationship to metabolic syndrome and obesity.[123] The data showed that people who ate the most nuts had a lower average BMI—they typically weighed less than their non-nut-eating counterparts.

How could it be that people who eat more calorie- and fat-rich nuts actually weigh less? It's likely because the protein, fiber, and fat in nuts reduce appetite and increase satiation.[124] A study from the School of Pharmacy and Medical Sciences at the University of South Australia showed that daily consumption of almonds reduced blood glucose, appetite, and the desire to eat.[125] This suggests that although nuts are a relatively energy-dense snack, they satiate hunger—when you eat them, you're likely to consume fewer calories over the course of your day. A number of studies have indicated that nuts induce satiation by eliciting the secretion of gut-slowing hormones that also act on the brain, such as cholecystokinin and peptide YY.[126, 127] Avoiding nuts because they're high in calories may be pennywise but pound foolish. The net result of eating nuts as a snack is overall daily caloric reduction that comes with a massive host of very well-documented health benefits.

Nut consumption has been firmly linked to a lean metabolism, a lower risk of obesity, and improved weight maintenance. Epidemiologic and clinical studies suggest that moderate consumption of nuts may provide people an enjoyable way to control their weight.[128-134] Most notable and widely cited throughout this book is the analysis performed by Harvard researchers led by Dr. Walter Willett,* who prospectively evaluated three separate cohorts,† including 120,877 US women and men who were free of chronic disease and who weren't obese at the beginning of the study.[135] Overall, those who increased the daily serving of nuts lost an average of 0.57 pound over a 4-year period of time, independent of many other dietary factors. In the Nurses' Health Study II, increasing nut consumption in women translated to a 1-pound weight loss per 4-year period, equaling yogurt as the two most prominent foods that help maintain body weight in women.

Although there are many choices for healthful and weight-loss-promoting nuts, there are interesting data about pistachios.[136] The pistachio is a nutrient-dense nut that promotes heart-healthy blood lipid profiles with potent antioxidant and anti-inflammatory activity. It enhances glycemic control while maintaining endothelial function.[137] When consumed in moderation, pistachios may help control body weight, because they signal satiety in the brain and have relatively few calories. In fact, those who eat nuts requiring removal of the shell actually consume fewer pistachio nuts compared to those who eat unshelled nuts—

---

* Dr. Willett is the Fredrick John Stare Professor of Epidemiology and Nutrition and the chair of the department of nutrition at Harvard School of Public Health. He is also a professor of medicine at Harvard Medical School and is the principal investigator of the second Nurses' Health Study, a compilation of studies regarding the health of older women and their risk factors for major chronic diseases—which was part of the analysis cited above. He has published more than 1,000 scientific articles regarding various aspects of diet and disease and is the second most cited author in clinical medicine. (hsph.harvard.edu/walter-willett/)

† The Nurses' Health Study (NHS) is a prospective study of a cohort of 121,701 female registered nurses from 11 US states who were enrolled in 1976. The Nurses' Health Study II (NHS II) is a prospective study of a cohort of 116,686 younger female registered nurses from 14 states who were enrolled in 1989. The Health Professionals Follow-Up Study (HPFS) is a prospective study of a cohort of 51,529 male health professionals from all 50 states, enrolled in 1986.

either from visual cuing and/or from the extra time and labor involved in eating more mindfully, which slows the process of eating.[138, 139] One study with subjects in a weight-loss program demonstrated lower BMI and triglyceride levels in individuals who consumed pistachios compared with those who consumed an isocaloric pretzel snack.[140] I strongly recommend that you incorporate pistachios into your diet–just beware that the pistachio is relatively rich in the FODMAP xylitol and may not be suitable for the Phase 1 diet plan.

Overall, nuts aid weight management by virtue of their strong effects upon satiation, the inefficiency of absorption of fats, and an elevation of energy expenditure and fat oxidation.[141] But given their high energy density, don't go totally nuts on nuts. It's easy to overeat them, and the effects can be deleterious. Two cups of nuts equals about 1,600 calories. I'm not a big calorie counter, but that's a lot of calories for not much food. My recommendation: Stick to a handful or two of nuts daily. Most of the studies have people consuming somewhere between 60 and 100 grams (around 30 to 50 nuts) daily–more than many of you will need to tide you over between meals. I strongly encourage you to include this crunchy, delicious snack in your daily diet–in moderation. There are few foods with such comprehensive data illustrating that they're truly medicine.

8. COFFEE

Almost everyone is surprised to find coffee on my list of superfoods, yet the data increasingly show that this ancient beverage, dating from 15th-century Ethiopia, has a plethora of health benefits, as long as you drink the right type of coffee in moderation and consider your personal health status while doing so. Let's address some of these issues.

The "right type of coffee" is most definitely *not* a grande frappucino from Starbucks. Coffee as a health food means the classic beverage brewed from ground coffee beans. It is the coffee, *not* the milk and sugar, that provides health benefits. If you prefer your coffee in the form of a milkshake, it won't benefit your health or your waistline. Plain old black coffee– possibly with a little cream (or almond milk if you're dairy sensitive) and a teaspoon of a stevia sweetener or raw honey, or a few sprinkles of cinnamon–is the way to go. Caffeinated or decaf are both fine, though caffeinated coffee may have slightly better health benefits. However, be careful about decaf, which is mainly processed using organochemical solvents (such as methylene chloride and ethyl acetate).[142] Decaf is also more acidic than regular coffee and can raise serum lipids levels, which raises cardiovascular risk.[143]

The key to coffee is moderation. Studies show that health benefits occur by consuming one to four 8-ounce cups daily. Less than this and you probably won't receive the same health benefits; more and you're liable to run into acid reflux, insomnia, and anxiety. Up to four cups may sound like a lot of coffee, but remember–that's a maximum of 32 ounces of coffee a day.

If you're anxious or have hypertension, minimize or eliminate your caffeine intake. Data show that drinking caffeinated coffee raises blood pressure–a primary risk factor for cardiovascular disease and heart attack—so if you have hypertension, I strongly encourage you to limit coffee or go for decaf and have your doctor monitor your blood pressure.[144] With these caveats in place, let's look at the research that supports the use of this superbeverage for supporting health and weight outcomes.

Perhaps the most profound evidence in favor of coffee as a superfood comes from a study published in the *New England Journal of Medicine*[145] that reviewed the data from 229,119 men and 173,141 women who participated in the NIH-AARP Diet and Health Study. Inverse associations between coffee consumption and deaths due to heart disease, respiratory disease, stroke, injuries and accidents, diabetes, and infections were observed. Put more simply: Coffee was correlated with a reduction in all-cause mortality.

As long as you don't have high blood pressure, there's strong evidence that regular coffee consumption *reduces* your risk of heart failure. Researchers at Harvard Medical School dug up studies on the relationship between cardiovascular disease and coffee consumption conducted from 1966 through 2011 and found five independent prospective studies including 140,220 participants. They performed a meta-analysis of this data and discovered that those who drank four cups a day had a significantly lower risk of heart failure than those who consumed no coffee. On the other hand, those who consumed more than four cups daily had a potentially higher risk of fatal heart attacks.

Coffee appears to have similarly powerful effects on type 2 diabetes. Researchers at the City University of New York conducted a meta-analysis of 20 epidemiological studies focusing on coffee consumption and type 2 diabetes risk. These studies include data on more than 300,000 people followed between 6 and 23 years. Seventeen of the 20 studies found evidence that coffee consumption can reduce the risk of type 2 diabetes. The other three showed no correlation; none of the studies showed that coffee had a negative effect. On the surface, this seems at odds with other data from the Netherlands that have shown a rapid intravenous infusion of caffeine over 15 minutes can raise blood glucose by reducing insulin sensitivity by 15 percent, at least in the short term.[146] Bear in mind this is likely because the caffeine shock induced by infusing the blood with so much at one time raised plasma stress hormones such as epinephrine and norepinephrine, which promote insulin resistance and inflammation. Still, how could drinking coffee reduce the risk of type 2 diabetes yet raise blood glucose in the short term? It doesn't seem to make sense. Well, one small study (this one had only 12 participants) may not completely emulate real life. Food eaten with the coffee and/or cream in the coffee would delay gastric emptying and the absorption of caffeine. Plus, noncaffeine compounds in coffee mitigate the blood sugar-raising effects over the long run, and research on such compounds is limited. However, there are three chemicals in coffee that show promising results in this area.

The first is chlorogenic acid, which is also a phytonutrient in apples. A study conducted at the University of Surrey in the United Kingdom showed that chlorogenic acid altered caffeine absorption rates and reduced blood glucose.[147] The researchers took three groups of people and gave them 25 grams of glucose in either water, regular coffee, or decaffeinated coffee. As expected, caffeinated coffee spiked blood glucose more than decaf or water. But here's where it gets interesting. Both coffee groups experienced a change in gut hormones directly responsible for insulin secretion and glucose absorption. This was not seen in the control. It appears that chlorogenic acid in coffee delays glucose absorption in the gut so that less ends up in the bloodstream. By the same token, less insulin is released, indicating enhanced insulin sensitivity. This is one mechanism scientists now feel is responsible for the relationship between regular coffee consumption and reduced risk of type 2 diabetes.

The second all-star player in coffee is quinidine. Animal models have shown that quinidine reduces liver glucose production, and we think the same thing may happen in humans.[148] Finally, there's the magnificent mineral magnesium. Coffee has relatively high amounts of magnesium (about 7 milligrams per cup, according to the USDA), and we know that magnesium enhances insulin sensitivity, reduces the risk of type 2 diabetes, and improves the metabolic profiles of those with metabolic obesity.[149, 150]

These effects on blood sugar, as well as caffeine's thermogenic effects and its positive impact on satiety, may be why coffee helps people keep weight off for the long term.[151] A prospective study of 18,417 men and 39,740 women who were followed for 12 years showed that those who drank more coffee gained less weight.[152] And a recent study out of the New York Obesity Research Center found that men who drank a beverage infused with mannooligosaccharides from coffee for 12 weeks lost more weight and visceral fat (that flab around the belly we all want less of) than did their counterparts who received a placebo.[153]

Since Phase 3 is all about weight maintenance, this makes coffee a particularly useful superfood for this phase. Coffee drinkers also seem to have lower rates of melanoma, depression, stroke, Parkinson's disease, cognitive decline/Alzheimer's disease, colorectal cancer, liver disease, gallstones, and vision loss.[154-161]

All that from a cup of coffee. Don't listen to the naysayers. Coffee's a superfood–no doubt about it. Just don't overdo it, avoid those sugar-laden coffee drinks, and choose lighter roasts–there's evidence that these retain more of the chemicals that help you burn fat.

9. BROCCOLI

The word *broccoli* comes from the Italian word for "cabbage sprout," and for good reason. Broccoli is a member of the cruciferous family of vegetables, and all these plants are derived from the same common, ancient ancestor. You'd never know it by looking at them in the produce department, but all crucifers–from bok choy to broccoli rabe–are a result of human selection occurring over the thousands of years these foods have been cultivated.

This makes it easier to understand why they have similar nutritional profiles and impacts on health. Like the other crucifers, broccoli is loaded with vitamins K and C and folate. It has the same power to bind to bile acids as its cousins, so it can reduce your cholesterol levels; it helps diversify your gut microbiome, as all the cruciferous veggies do; and studies have shown that eating crucifers may reduce your risk of cancer.[162]

Given all these similarities, why would I call out broccoli as a superfood?

Two reasons. The first is practical. Few people are aware that broccoli is in the same family as cabbage and kale. It's not intuitive, since they don't look much alike. So it made more sense organizationally to separate broccoli from the crowd. But the more important reason is that broccoli has special health benefits that other cruciferous vegetables don't.

Broccoli appears to have a powerful effect on prostate cancer. While all cruciferous vegetables seem to reduce the risk of cancer, few foods protect your prostate the way broccoli does, especially against more aggressive forms of prostate cancer. A study led by Dr. Victoria Kirsh and colleagues at Cancer Care Ontario's Division of Preventive Oncology in Ontario, Canada, reviewed data from 1,338 patients with prostate cancer and found that intake of cruciferous vegetables reduced the risk of aggressive stage III or stage IV prostate cancer.[163] Broccoli had the most powerful effect. People who ate more than one serving of broccoli per week were 55 percent less likely to develop aggressive prostate cancer than those who ate less than one serving monthly. A few servings of broccoli a week kept cancer at bay.

Why does broccoli, in particular, have such a powerful impact on prostate cancer? While more research needs to be done, scientists have tracked down a few of the biochemical properties that we think lead to these effects.

The first is that consuming broccoli appears to modulate the GSTM1 genotype—which is involved with inflammation and carcinogenesis in positive ways. Broccoli "tells" your genes to turn down inflammation and tumor production. Recent research showed that men who ate a broccoli-rich diet showed precisely these kinds of changes in gene expression.[164]

What is it in broccoli that produces these changes in gene expression? Broccoli, like all of those in the Brassica family, is particularly rich in the anti-inflammatory, antioxidant glucosinolates; in particular, it has high levels of glucoraphanin, gluconasturtiin, and glucobrassicin.[165] Scientists believe these chemicals may pull epigenetic triggers that mitigate the progression of prostate cancer. These three glucosinolates also happen to support various steps in the body's detoxification process, including activation, neutralization, and elimination of unwanted contaminants. So your detox system benefits from broccoli and the Brassica family of vegetables such as broccoli rabe.

As much as broccoli is an antioxidant-rich superfood, it's got plenty of soluble fiber to feed your good gut bacteria and induce a lean metabolism. Broccoli also has potent anti-inflammatory activities[166] and directly affects your fat cells, causing them to shrink into oblivion. For instance, the indole-3-carbinol (I3C) in broccoli and other cruciferous vegetables targets a specific receptor on fat cells to block their proliferation.[167] One study demonstrated that I3C—when given to mice with diet-induced obesity via a high-fat diet—improved blood lipid profile, reduced inflammatory markers, decreased the expression and levels of proinflammatory mediators, and modulated genes that control leptin and adipocyte protein 2 expression. This suggests that I3C has the potential to prevent obesity and metabolic disorders via multiple mechanisms, including decreased fat storage, reduced inflammation, and enhanced thermogenesis.

These phytonutrients appear to be most bioavailable when you lightly steam broccoli, though you can get them from raw broccoli as well. Don't overcook this vegetable, as some of its anticancer properties may be diminished if you do. I recommend preparing broccoli simply: Cut the florets into pieces and lightly steam for 3 to 5 minutes, or until just tender. Dress with olive oil, salt and pepper, and a splash of vinegar if you like. Broccoli rabe is a bold member of the Brassica family with a slight bitterness that is wonderful on the taste buds. Steam it and serve with olive oil, lemon juice, and a dash of salt–a Dr. Gerry favorite! Enjoy this delectable dish knowing you're fighting cancer, optimizing your fatty acid balance, and supporting excellent health all at the same time.

Honorable Mention: Broccoli Sprouts Powder

Broccoli sprouts are rich in antioxidants and have been tested for their ability to attenuate type 2 diabetes in humans in part by reducing oxidative stress and inflammation-induced insulin resistance.[168] Eighty-one patients were randomly assigned to receive either 10 grams daily of broccoli sprouts powder, 5 grams daily of broccoli sprouts powder, or a placebo for 4 weeks.[169] After 4 weeks, consumption of 10 grams daily of the powder resulted in a significant decrease in serum insulin concentration and improved insulin sensitivity. Broccoli sprouts may improve insulin resistance in type 2 diabetic patients.

Two marvelous scientists at Johns Hopkins put broccoli sprouts on the map: Dr. Paul Talay and Dr. Jed Fahey.[170] In fact, after their discoveries of the anticancer benefits of broccoli sprouts, the sales of these sprouts in the United States doubled. Thanks to these doctors, research has further elucidated the many health-promoting benefits of broccoli sprouts.

10. ARTICHOKES

We end the list of Phase 3 superfoods with a prebiotic edible thistle that has been with humanity for eons and was prized by Romans as a food of nobility. Artichokes are high in inulin–the prebiotic fiber that feeds your gut microbiome. These kingly foods share their name with two other foods they aren't related to: Jerusalem artichoke (also known as sunchoke) and Chinese artichoke. Don't get confused. The thistle with hard leaves that looks like a bulb is the one I'm referring to here.

Insulin is a natural oligomer of fructose that, following ingestion, is fermented by the bifidobacterial population of the colon, increasing its growth. Inulin added to food may prevent diabetes and obesity. Artichokes contain a special type of inulin called very-long-chain inulin (VLCI). In fact, artichokes have the longest chains of inulin of any vegetable,[171] and studies are showing that VLCI may have special effects on your gut microbiome.

A recent randomized, double-blind, placebo-controlled study (the gold standard in science) took two groups of people and gave them either 10 grams daily of VLCI derived from artichokes or maltodextrin.[172] The folks who took the VLCI supplement (remember, this is the same type of inulin found in artichokes) had significantly higher levels of bifidobacteria and lactobacilli and a reduction in pathogens such as species of *Prevotella* bacteria.[173] The health benefits of this superfood don't stop with its fertilizing effect on your gut microbiome. Artichokes may reduce LDL cholesterol, increase HDL cholesterol, and improve certain metabolic parameters in overweight people.[174, 175]

Most of the studies done in these areas have focused on the use of artichoke leaf extract, a supplement containing the phenolic compounds, flavonoids, and other protective compounds in the leaves of artichokes. While you'd have to eat a boatload of artichoke leaves to get the same amount in the supplements, it's logical to assume you'll still get some of the same positive effects by sticking with the whole-food version.

Artichokes may also balance blood sugar and improve other metabolic parameters associated with weight gain and type 2 diabetes. Research at the University of Paiva in Italy showed that supplementation with artichoke extract helped people reduce their fasting blood glucose, HA1c was reduced (meaning glycated hemoglobin in the blood was lowered), the patients' hyperlipidemic patterns improved, and patients saw improvements across several other metabolic pathways.[176]

To top it off, artichokes couldn't be easier to prepare. Just snip off the spiky ends of the leaves, drop the bulb in water, and simmer until tender. Then pull the leaves away and enjoy. Of course, don't skip the delectable heart.

LOOKING AHEAD

"Let medicine be thy food, and food be thy medicine." Hippocrates' words are more valuable today than ever. The superfoods I've highlighted in this book illustrate the profound healing power that food—real, whole food—can have. None of them individually will cure illness. But together they offer broad health-protective effects that may indeed shield you from chronic illness while keeping your waistline slim and trim.

So many people don't eat what I'd call food. The modern Western diet, filled with "ingestibles"—highly processed foodlike substances—is a poor excuse from both a health *and* a flavor perspective compared to the real, whole foods humanity evolved to eat.

The Gut Balance Revolution emphasizes superfoods found in your pantry to promote slimness by melting away your excess fat. Your pantry should be filled with items that can improve your metabolic fat-burning furnace. Remember that spiced foods and herbal drinks can lead to greater energy loss by thermogenesis, oxidizing fat and in some cases increasing satiety. These herbs have a wide range of effects that can upregulate the body's built-in weight-loss mechanisms. Capsaicin, black pepper, ginger, green tea, black tea, and caffeine have the potential to raise your metabolism and help you lose weight automatically just by incorporating these healthy functional foods into your repertoire.[177]

Adding the superfoods in this phase (and those from previous phases) back to your diet will provide not only a bevy of health benefits but also an opportunity to reconnect with the food that nourishes you and to experience a way of eating and living that's been part of the human experience for generations. When you do this, your gut microbiome will thank you, your health will thank you, and your waistline will thank you.

Another important step on the path to good health is learning how to reduce stress, exercise optimally, sleep better, and live a gut-balancing, health-promoting lifestyle. In the next chapter, I'll explain how to do that.

THE GUT BALANCE REVOLUTION SUCCESS STORIES
Stephanie Gittens, 37

Piling on the pounds might be easy, but as Stephanie Gittens knows, taking them off—well, that's another story. Over the years, she'd been on more diets than she could count. She'd quickly trim off a couple of pounds but gain them all back—and then some—even faster. Meanwhile, the number on the scale kept creeping up.

"When I reached my highest weight of 317," Stephanie recalls, "it definitely slowed me down, and I knew I had to try something else." When the Gut Balance Revolution came along, Stephanie realized she'd finally found a totally new eating plan that would work for the long haul. "I really liked learning about the connection between weight and the good and bad bugs in the gut," Stephanie says. "And I loved the ease of the plan—with the charts that showed us which foods to favor and which ones to forget, it was such a simple, effective diet."

Stephanie filled up her pantry and fridge with the Gut Balance Revolution foods and got started with the plan. And it worked—in 8 weeks, she'd lost 20 pounds. As it turns out, the other things she lost were even better. "I noticed that my moods were getting brighter," says Stephanie, who's a front desk receptionist at a surgeon's office. "I was so much happier, and I seemed so much more energized. And it was fantastic being able to go outside and play with my children. Everyone seems to notice that I've changed for the better!"

CHAPTER 10

Living a
Gut-Balancing Life

Creating a healthy, sustainable ecosystem inside and out is about more than how we eat. Certainly, what you feed your gut microbiome is at the foundation of good health–it's the first step you need to take to rebalance your inner garden, lose weight, and remain healthy for life. However, taking an ecosystems approach to weight loss means looking not only within our bodies but also at the broader picture of our lives and figuring out how to live in a way that supports our health, weight, and inner ecology. It's about learning how to live with the natural rhythms of life in a sustainable way that fits us for the long term.

Most of us don't live this way today. We're overworked and stressed out; we sleep too little and worry too much. We take our lunch at our desks because "we don't have time to eat," and we rarely make the time for activities that nourish us inside and out. We live in a world out of sync with the natural rhythms of day and night, work and rest.

We also have a bizarre relationship to exercise. We either exercise way too little or way too much. The most recent data from the Centers for Disease Control and Prevention reveal that 79 percent of Americans don't get the minimum recommended amount of exercise[1]–for adults, at least $2\frac{1}{2}$ hours of moderate-intensity aerobic exercise weekly or $1\frac{1}{4}$ hours of vigorous-intensity activity or a combination of both types. Those least likely to engage in physical activity were age 65 and older (nearly 16 percent of exercisers). Adults should also engage in muscle-strengthening activities like lifting weights or doing pushups at least twice per week. Research has shown approximately 25 to 35 percent of US adults are physically inactive,[2, 3] which translates to 40 million to 50 million Americans.

On the other side of the equation are those who overdo it at the gym, trudging for hours on the treadmill, hoping beyond hope (or reason) that if they exercise *a little more* they'll burn off the fat on their belly, butt, and hips. Those "weekend warriors" who are inactive all week, then overcompensate on weekends with high-intensity exercises, are exposing themselves to an increased risk of cardiovascular events.[4]

Put simply: Our lives are out of whack, and this impacts our health and our gut microbiome in surprising ways. Stress, sleep, exercise, the way you eat, when you eat, and other factors affect hormonal balance, metabolism, and the health of your inner garden.

That's why I want to provide you the tools you need to live a lifestyle that helps maintain balance inside and out. The Gut Balance Revolution is about more than changing your diet and reestablishing a relationship with the friendly gut symbiotes that keep you healthy and happy. It's about revolutionizing the way you live and relate to the world so that you can live in harmony with the broader ecology inside and around you.

Let's start by taking a close look at one of America's most unhealthy national pastimes–chronic stress–and review the ways it sends your life, your health, and your gut microbiome spiraling out of balance.

STRESS: THE UNHEALTHIEST PASTIME IN AMERICA

> *America is at a critical crossroads when it comes to stress and our health.*
>
> —Norman B. Anderson, PhD, CEO,
> American Psychological Association

Americans are a stressed-out people. A staggering 40 million of us over the age of 18– that's 18.1 percent of the adult population–have an anxiety disorder, costing the United States more than $42 billion per year.[5, 6] Forty-four percent of American adults report that their stress levels have increased over the last 5 years.[7] Unfortunately, it appears that the younger generations are getting hit the hardest. According to the American Psychological Association's report *Stress in America,* millennials (people who came of age during the 2000s) are the most stressed-out generation.[8] How come? Everything from money problems to work issues, from family troubles to personal challenges.[9] Stress is not just compromising our quality of life, it's also contributing to our chronic disease epidemic–and it's not doing any favors to our waistlines, either. Among the physical consequences of stress:

- It increases the amount of belly fat you have, makes it easier for you to store fat, and reduces your ability to burn fat.[10-12]

- It sets off a fire of inflammation in your body that can lead to metabolic syndrome, type 2 diabetes, weight gain, and other health problems.

- It increases your incidence of cardiovascular disease, especially among lower socioeconomic classes.[13, 14]

- It may lead to a 400 percent increase in the risk of developing hypertension.[15]

- It raises your blood sugar, makes it harder for sugar to get into your cells, and makes you less insulin sensitive, putting you at increased risk for type 2 diabetes.[16]

- It causes you to crave sugary foods and can set off emotional eating.[17]

- It leads to imbalance in your gut microbiome, causing a decrease in *Bacteroides* and an increase in *Clostridium* species. These imbalances may set off a downward spiral of continued stress and disrupt the harmony of the gut microbiome, since your intestinal flora has a significant impact on your mood and eating behavior, leading to a vicious cycle.[18, 19]

This is just the short list of detrimental effects of chronic stress, and it doesn't account for problems like lack of life satisfaction and relationship issues. For an in-depth look at the full host of health problems that can arise from chronic unrelenting stress and the underlying biochemistry that drives them, I recommend the book *Why Zebras Don't Get Ulcers* by Dr. Robert Sapolsky, one of the premier stress researchers in the country.[20]

Why does all this stress happen, and what can we do about it? Let's reach back to our caveman past to unearth the biochemical underpinnings of the stress response.

FIGHT OR FLIGHT: STAYING ALIVE IN CAVEMAN TIMES

Our stress response is an ancient survival mechanism easiest understood by considering why it likely evolved over time. Imagine you're a prehistoric man or woman out happily gathering and munching on berries. Behind you, in the brush, you hear a low growl, panting, and twigs snapping. What happens next is familiar to anyone who's been in a frightening or life-threatening situation: Your stress response–also known as the fight-or-flight response–is triggered, setting off a sequence of biochemical events that prepare you to either run like crazy or fight like a demon. Three primary chemicals are released into your bloodstream: epinephrine, norepinephrine, and cortisol. These chemicals trigger the physiological responses needed to prepare you for the imminent attack by the monster that wants to eat you. Your eyes dilate slightly so you can see more clearly, your blood is shunted toward your lower appendages so you can move more quickly, and your nonessential biological processes (digestion and the reproductive system, for example) are downregulated, conserving energy for the important work of staying alive.

This response is what gives you a fighting chance in life-threatening situations. Without it, humans very likely wouldn't be on the planet because most of them would have become dinner for stronger, faster predators. You can thank your stress response for saving you if you've ever been in a near-miss car accident or have accidentally stepped off the curb in the path of an oncoming bus only to quickly reel back onto the sidewalk before getting flattened. In fact, all these situations are examples how the stress response is *supposed* to work. An explosion of powerful biochemicals temporarily turns you into a superhuman so you can stay alive during trying circumstances. These chemicals are then rapidly ushered out of your bloodstream, your stress response cools down, and you go back to your regular, relatively relaxed way of life.

But there's one major problem in the modern world: The average life is not "relatively relaxed." Your body doesn't know the difference between perceived stressors and real, life-threatening stressors. It responds as though you're about to be eaten by a wild beast anytime something shakes you up. So if you're under heavy deadlines at work, your boss yells at you, you're stuck in traffic, you're having relationship problems, you don't sleep enough, your nutrition is poor, you don't exercise enough, or you exercise too much, your body will react to all these and the million other stressors you encounter daily as though you're in real, life-threatening danger. Physiologist Hans Selye, who coined the term "stress" in the 1950s, defined it as "the nonspecific response of the body to any demand made upon it." Decades of research since show that this definition is accurate. And it's this fact that has brought America to the "critical crossroads" Dr. Anderson was talking about in the quote earlier in this chapter.

Chronic, unremitting pathological stress is what most of us are facing today, and this form of stress is contributing to the chronic illness, weight gain, mental health problems, and general malaise so many people suffer from. Constant stress is like having the pedal to the metal all day, every day. Eventually, your engine begins to break down. The outcome? You gain weight, you're unhappy, you get sick—and your gut microbiome suffers.

So what's the solution? Most books will tell you to practice activating your relaxation response, and there's something to this. Your stress response is wired into your sympathetic nervous system, so you literally have no control over it—it's triggered by what stresses you out, period. However, we have a built-in antidote to this sympathetic stress response, known as the relaxation response. It's built into your parasympathetic nervous system—the part of your neurology you *do* have some control over. You activate a healing cascade when you make a conscious effort to deeply relax your body through activities like meditation, prayer, yoga, deep breathing, mindful eating, and progressive muscle relaxation.

Studies have shown that learning relaxation and stress-reduction strategies may be a key component of any effective long-term weight-loss program. Researchers at the University of Kentucky divided a group of 26 participants in half. They taught one group stress management techniques but provided no dietary intervention. Instead, they met with these participants for 75 minutes twice weekly for 7 weeks. They taught the other 13 participants an intuitive eating-based dietary intervention that encouraged them to tune in to hunger signals and only eat when hungry. At the end of 7 weeks, the group that learned stress management lost 17 pounds, a loss they sustained at their 14-week follow-up. Those who learned intuitive eating did not lose significant weight.[21]

There's been a recent explosion of research in this area. The Academy of Nutrition and Dietetics has published a position paper supporting the application of mindful eating and intuitive eating as part of nutrition interventions in those with eating disorders.[22] The organization has dedicated dozens of articles in its journal to this topic, demonstrating its efficacy for eating disorders and obesity management.[23-25] These and many other studies demonstrate the powerful tool of integrating mindful and intuitive eating practices into behavior and lifestyle modification plans.

Dr. Michelle May, who runs mindful eating workshops, notes in her programs that "many of the habits that drive overeating are unconscious behaviors that people have repeated for years, and they act them out without even realizing it. Mindfulness allows a person to wake up and be aware of what they're doing. Once you're aware, you can change your actions."[26]

Learning to relax is likely to improve your weight loss, and it's a central part of this program. Later in this chapter, I'll provide some relaxation exercises to integrate into your life. That's a good first step. However, recent research shows that to deal more effectively with stress, we need to do more than simply counter stress with relaxation. We need to develop resilience.

WHAT IS RESILIENCE—AND WHY IS IT IMPORTANT?

Dr. Mehmet Oz talked about resilience and reserve being vital elements to healthy aging at the Integrative Healthcare Symposium in 2013, which inspired me to research this topic and share its importance with you. Resilience is the ability to rebound from an illness, challenge, or life event without developing a maladaptive chronic stress response. Some people have that ineffable quality to be knocked down by life and come back stronger than ever. The more resilient you are, the less you become physically or emotionally compromised by life's stressors and more able to rebound when a setback occurs. After all, stress isn't going away anytime soon. You can reduce your life stressors and learn to relax more–important parts of becoming more resilient–but you won't eliminate all anxiety. In fact, as many as 90 percent of people will experience a traumatic event in their lifetime.[27] Even if you're one of the lucky ones who don't, you probably won't walk through life stress free–nor would you want to. We create deadlines, pressure ourselves to succeed at work, and have family responsibilities for good reasons. Though they can sometimes be stressful, they encourage us to engage with life in a meaningful and productive way. Other stressors—like exercise, which by definition puts stress on your body—are necessary for health and well-being.

Remember the concept of hormesis, which advocates that the human organism copes with a wide variety of harsh environmental conditions by acquiring physiological adaptive mechanisms that improve survival.[28] Exercise is the perfect example of a hormetic process that forces your body to adapt by acutely stressing the body, releasing catecholamines and other biochemicals that transiently alter cardiovascular and systemic physiology. When you overdo exercise or exercise in inappropriate ways, you unduly overstress your body and set off an alarm response with inflammation and other negative physiological reactions. However, when you exercise appropriately, inflammation is lessened. Some scientists think that hormesis is one of the ways by which inflammation is better managed when you exercise regularly.[29] Yet again—the dose makes the poison!

When it comes to stress, more is at stake than initially meets the eye. For example, it's not just the events in your life but the way you perceive and react to them that may make them stressors. In some cases, we may perceive something as a threat when it's really not. If these maladaptive thoughts are recurrent, then the stress response becomes chronic, eventually causing pathophysiological consequences. But if we perceive genuine stressors as a test of our tenacity and our ability to adapt and persevere, they may have a hormetic effect that only makes us stronger. Remember the old saying: What does not kill us makes us stronger.

As always, the key is balance and the ability to bounce back when adversity inevitably hits. That's what resilience is. How do we develop this useful trait? It's clear there are a few important factors that help. Here's what most experts in the field of resilience say you need to do to bounce back from adverse events more effectively.[30]

1. **Have a strong community and solid social support.** Friends, family, and loved ones provide the foundation we need to make it through the tough times.[31]

2. **Keep perspective and maintain a positive attitude.** Looking at the glass as half full instead of half empty seems to have a significant impact on our ability to manage stress.[32] Data from the Women's Health Initiative linked optimism to healthier eating.[33]

3. **Take care of yourself and maintain a positive self-image.** Developing self-confidence and trusting in your ability to overcome difficult challenges helps build resilience.[34] This is a key attribute to perseverance and success.

4. **Confront your fears.** The psychological literature increasingly shows us that avoidance isn't a successful strategy for managing adversity. Exposing yourself to what you fear helps you overcome it.[35]

5. **Accept that which you cannot change.** Change and trauma are a part of life. Ignoring this fact will not help you adjust to the difficulties you face. There is, perhaps, no better embodiment of this truth than the Serenity Prayer, which reads: God, grant me the serenity to accept the things I cannot change, the courage to change the things I can, and the wisdom to know the difference.[36]

6. **Rely on the spiritual.** Meditation and spiritual practices have been shown to help people cool off the stress response and recover more effectively.[37]

7. **Exercise regularly.** Those who exercise regularly tend to bounce back more effectively when confronted with acute stressors.[38]

How do we develop resilience? Some methods are fairly straightforward. Getting more exercise, for example, means setting a routine that makes sense for you—and then doing it. Later in this chapter, I'll outline several different routines based on your needs and fitness levels. Other attributes take time and personal exploration to develop. If you don't have a strong social support network, for instance, going out and meeting friends or reconnecting will take some effort and maybe even personal coaching or professional intervention. For some folks, creating a meditation or spiritual practice may seem difficult. For others, confronting their fears may feel impossible.

There's no one-size-fits-all prescription for resilience—you need to seek your own path, experimenting, testing, and keeping what works, rejecting what doesn't. Take the

Resilience and My Journey to Johns Hopkins: Ode to Dr. Tony Kalloo

If you've read my first book, *The Inside Tract*, you may remember that at one point I was sidelined by a bizarre series of medical mishaps resulting in disability. But as the old saying goes, "What doesn't kill you makes you stronger."

I returned to my roots of natural medicine and faith-based self-healing, and the rest is history. My family and close friends, old and new, rallied around me, and I defied another doctor to use the word *can't*. (After all, one of my favorite movie lines is from a Rocky movie, when Mickey, the trainer, tells Rocky, "Can't, there is no such thing as can't.") I fired my nay-saying doctors, and in due time, I grew stronger. Self-belief, motivation, and community are so important. They give people a reason to succeed, a reason to go on. Nature is smarter than people think.

time to tune in to your own needs and find ways to reduce the overall burden of stress in your life. Become more resilient so that when the inevitable stressors come your way, they won't take such a heavy toll on your weight, health, and life.

In the remainder of this chapter, I'll provide tips on how to build resilience. They include relaxation, mindful eating, improved sleep hygiene, exercise, and more. These techniques have been useful in my own life and with my patients, and the research supports them. This chapter is by no means a comprehensive program for reducing stress or building a more resilient character–it's a primer to introduce you to some valuable basics. If you integrate these steps into your life, I virtually guarantee the quality of your life and health will improve, you will lose weight more easily, and you'll be less likely to regain any weight you do shed. Consider what you're about to read as a beginning. Once you've added these steps into your life, then reach into the vast literature on stress reduction and resilience building on your own, tap into your personal resources, and seek out ways to better balance your life in a way that makes sense for you. You only live once. Enjoy the life you have and make the most of it. You deserve it!

Now let's learn how to relax and bounce back a little more effectively. It all starts with the breath.

LEARN TO BREATHE

Sometimes, all it takes to gain a new perspective on a stressful situation is to take a time out and a few deep breaths. Deep breathing is a simple, powerful, effective,

For me, this was a story of resilience, the ability to "take the hits in life and keep going." A year or so after starting my job at Johns Hopkins, my director, Dr. Anthony Kalloo, stopped by my office and looked at the poster of Rocky on my wall—a bit unusual for this academic workplace. Tony knew my story and was willing to gamble on hiring me—I was his first hire when he became chief of gastroenterology at The Johns Hopkins Hospital. When he looked at my poster, he said, "You need to see the movie *Rocky Balboa*.[39] There's a quote in it that will resonate with you." It was about resilience, which separates those who succeed from those who blame others for their failures. Here's the quote.[40]

> *You, me, or nobody is gonna hit as hard as life. But it ain't about how hard you hit. It's about how hard you can get hit and keep moving forward; how much you can take and keep moving forward. That's how winning is done!*

easy-to-learn relaxation activity you can take with you everywhere you go. It's been shown to reduce blood cortisol levels and improve heart rate variability–primary indicators of a more relaxed physiological state.[41, 42] You can do it anytime, anywhere, and it only takes a few moments. There are *many* deep breathing practices out there. Try this one and adapt it to your needs. Do this for 1 to 2 minutes to experience deep and immediate relaxation.

1. **Get comfortable.** Lie down on your back, sit comfortably in your chair, or just stand where you are with your arms loose and dangling at your sides. If you can, loosen any tight clothing.
2. **Inhale slowly through your nose for a count of 5.** As you slowly draw your breath down with your diaphragm, count 1-2-3-4-5. If you can't breathe through your nose, it's okay to breathe through your mouth.
3. **Exhale through your mouth to a count of 5.** Exhale as slowly as you inhale, counting 1-2-3-4-5.

Repeat the process five times anytime you're stressed, and you'll find the tension slowly fade away.

When you begin practicing deep breathing, I usually recommend doing it three to five times a day. Do this every day you're on this program. After you've integrated the practice into your life, you'll find yourself using it naturally when you're feeling tense or anxious.

Some people feel lightheaded or slightly dizzy when they begin this practice. For most, that fades away after a few times, but if it doesn't, discontinue the practice, use the relaxation techniques that follow, and check with a physician to see if you have an underlying medical problems causing this.

EAT MINDFULLY

It may be hard to believe that eating in a particular way can reduce stress and help you take life a little more lightly, but I assure you this technique will not only help you relax, it will revolutionize your relationship to what you put in your mouth.

Mindfulness is the state of simple, attentive awareness of what's going on around you moment by moment. In our fast-paced society, our mind races from one activity to the next with some seemingly simultaneous, chaotic, uncontrollable chatter. We think about the future ("What are we going to eat for dinner tonight?"), we think about the past ("Why did my boss say that to me?"), we tune in to our devices to check e-mail or work or play games at all hours of the day and night. During waking hours, life becomes a symphony of constant multitasking. Rarely do we take a step back, recenter ourselves, observe our own mind and surroundings, and connect with the inner peace and deep quiet within.

There are times when moving quickly to accomplish tasks is justified. In my job as a medical professional, for example, it's often absolutely necessary. Deadlines, benchmarks, and goals are all put in place as a way to encourage us to accomplish what we need to in a timely manner. But most of us are rushing from the moment we wake up until the moment we pass out at night, and this isn't healthy. It's stressful. It's exhausting. And perhaps most significantly, it diminishes the quality of our life.

So how do we beat the rush, step out of the rat race (at least for a moment), slow down, relax, and take the pause we need to reconnect with our inmost selves? There are lots of ways to do this, but one of my personal favorites is eating mindfully. This simply means putting aside other distractions, eating, and paying careful attention to food. It's about becoming attentive to your present experience and tuning in to what you're ingesting, how it tastes, and how it makes you feel. It's not difficult–it's actually very enjoyable–and doesn't take much time. Here's how.

1. **When you eat, just eat.** Don't take meals at your desk, in front of the TV, or while surfing the Internet. Just sit and eat, either alone or with family and friends. This allows you to be more attentive to the experience of eating. When I find myself finishing a fast-paced treadmill-like workday, rather than just running to the next task, I take a Stone Mill Bakery timeout to eat a simple meal (outdoors when possible).

2. **Acknowledge the food.** Before you begin eating, take a quiet moment to acknowledge the food and be grateful for the nourishment it brings.

3. **Pay attention as you eat.** Bring your full attention to the act of bringing the food to your lips, placing it in your mouth, and chewing. Pay attention to the flavors, consistency, taste, and smell of the food.

4. **Take your time.** Throughout the meal, take breaks. Just sit and breathe and enjoy your company (if you have any), the scenery, or the quiet time you're spending alone. Don't rush to gobble your food as quickly as you are otherwise programmed to do.

Eating this way not only allows you to relax and take a break, it also helps you draw the full nutritional value from the foods you eat. The first stages of digestion begin before you even put food in your mouth, so when you slow down and pay attention to what and how you eat, you take advantage of the full digestive process. And you're also likely to eat healthier, more nourishing foods and consume fewer calories overall.[43] When you bring your attention to the taste, feel, and flavor of what you eat, you will find that some foods you once thought delicious (like sugar) don't please you as they did, and others (like veggies) are actually more satisfying than you imagined. And by paying more attention to your hunger signals and feelings of fullness, you're likely to eat less.

Mindful eating has health benefits. Chewing food well helps regulate digestion and create a link between the digestive tract and the brain, improving satiety and tricking your brain into thinking you ate more food than you actually did. Plus, the simple act of enjoying food improves satiation. Mindful eating also helps keep digestion parasympathetic dominant by slowing the process down and providing adequate time for satiation signals to reach your brain. If you eat when you're stressed out, you don't digest as well since your body attenuates digestion in times of stress. When we gulp down our food, we don't give our body time to send signals to our brain telling us we're full. There is lag time between the moment food hits our stomach and when satiety signals are released. When we eat more slowly, we allow more time for those signals to travel to our brain and tell us we are full. So eating mindfully and slowly translates to eating less.

Mindful eating may positively impact type 2 diabetes. A 2012 study from Ohio State

Confucius Says: Eat Less, Weigh Less (or Digest Better)

Another principle worth discussing is one called *hara hachi bu*. Derived from the teaching of Confucius, this instructs a person to eat until he or she is about 80 percent full. Okinawans apply this principle rigorously. They have a typical BMI of around 20 (compared to the United States, where 67 percent of the population is overweight and/or obese with a BMI of 26 or greater) and are among the longest-living cultures in the world.[44] The practice of *hara hachi bu* trains the brain to sense satiety sooner and feel quite satisfied with less food. Similarly, Ayurveda and traditional Chinese practices espouse that a meal be eaten in a peaceful setting and until two-thirds full to promote healthy digestion—and never consumed late at night (a time of cleansing) lest small bowel overgrowth and gut dysbiosis ensue.[45, 46] All of these principles promote a relaxed parasympathetic-dominant state at the time of eating to maximize the enjoyment of the dining experience—and requiring less food to boot!

Are You an Emotional Eater?

The impulse to guzzle chocolate ice cream after a stressful day at work is understandable but unhealthy. We get trapped in this kind of impulsive eating because we're unconsciously seeking foods that satisfy reward centers in our brain. That's why the chocolate cake looks mighty tempting when you're feeling anxious or blue. This is called emotional eating, and some people engage in it to avoid or mitigate emotional stress, boredom, anger, fear, sadness, or anxiety.[47] The hunger emotional eaters experience isn't physical—your body doesn't need the calories or nutrients—it's emotional. So the question isn't "What are you eating?" but "What's eating you?"

While virtually all of us have experienced the psychological release that comfort foods bring from time to time, when emotional eating gets out of control it can become dangerous and lead to binge-eating disorders, bulimia nervosa, and more. If you're concerned that you may have an eating disorder, seek the help of a psychotherapist experienced in treating eating disorders. In such a case, dieting is unlikely to help you achieve your health and weight-loss goals without psychological support. Most eating disorder treatment programs have a nutritional component to them as well, and many clinics have you meet with both a psychotherapist and a nutritionist. You can ask whether or not this program would be a useful adjunct to your treatment.

Emotional eating can be related to food addictions. Growing evidence suggests that high-calorie junk foods may be as addictive as smoking or drugs of abuse. In a study published in *Nature Neuroscience,* researchers showed that rats that regularly consumed high-calorie, sugary, fatty foods like bacon, sausage, cake, and chocolate showed a pattern of blunted reward centers in the brain very similar to those in humans addicted to drugs.[48] These rats had decreased levels of the same dopamine receptors reported in drug-addicted humans. And this reward desensitization lasted for 2 weeks after the rats were taken off the diet.

To take these findings a step further, these scientists decided to see if the rats would continue to eat these junk foods even if they knew it was detrimental—a hallmark of addiction in any species. To do this, they trained the rats to expect a painful shock when eating these foods. They found that the addicted, obese rats kept right on eating despite the pain.

Although more evidence is needed to correlate these findings to human food addiction and weight gain, it's still extremely compelling and provides scientific support for something that many of us are aware of instinctually: The fatty, sugary, processed junk foods on the market today are flat-out addictive.

Eating mindfully and engaging in relaxation or exercise rituals may help you better manage your emotional states so that you don't engage in emotional eating as often.

University found that eating mindfully led to weight loss and blood glucose control results that were similar to adhering to nutrition-based dietary guidelines.[49]

Eating mindfully may also reduce our risk of turning to comfort foods for emotional upset.[50] Stressors and distractors can lead to emotional overeating, which in its most severe forms can turn into a binge-eating disorder (see "Are You an Emotional Eater?" on page 197). Becoming more mindful of the food we eat, and really tuning in to our hunger signals and our experience, can lessen this problem and return us to a more balanced relationship with food.

MEDITATE

Meditation is an ancient practice that includes a broad range of techniques from seated mindfulness meditation to moving forms of meditation such as yoga, tai chi, and qigong. Studies have shown that each of these techniques can help you feel more balanced and at peace and diminish your stress response; some have been directly shown to help you lose weight.

For example, a meta-analysis of 18,753 citations for mindfulness-based studies, which included 47 trials, was performed by my colleagues at Johns Hopkins. They found that regularly engaging in a mindfulness meditation program led to improvement for chronic conditions such as anxiety, depression, and pain.[51] Another study, which included 47 overweight or obese women, found that those engaging in mindfulness practices had reduced anxiety, better eating habits, and reduced abdominal body fat.[52] One study suggests that these effects may be increased when mindfulness is practiced in group settings.[53] A clinical trial under way now aims to identify how mindfulness-based stress reduction alters the gut microbiome in the context of irritable bowel syndrome.[54]

Yoga may have even more powerful results. Researchers at the Fred Hutchinson Cancer Research Center in Seattle reviewed data on 15,550 adults ages 53 to 57 who were recruited to the VITamins And Lifestyle (VITAL) Cohort Study. They found that practicing yoga lessened weight gain.[55] Those who were healthy and normal weight and practiced for 4 or more years were 3.1 pounds lighter than their nonpracticing counterparts. But here's what's really cool: Overweight participants who practiced yoga weighed 18.5 pounds less than those who didn't practice.

Indeed, the idea that yoga may lead to weight loss has been corroborated by a meta-analysis recently published in the *American Journal of Lifestyle Medicine*.[56] Scientists reviewed existing studies to find out if yoga could help you lose weight. Even though they found that the studies have some weaknesses such as small sample sizes, short durations, and lack of control groups, they still concluded that yoga likely leads to weight loss. According to these scientists the possible mechanisms were about more than the fact that you burn calories in yoga sessions. They include:

- Reducing joint and back pain, allowing for more exercise outside of yoga sessions
- Heightening mindfulness, improved mood, and stress reduction, all of which may reduce food intake
- Helping people feel more connected to their bodies, perhaps leading to an enhanced awareness of satiety and the discomfort that comes with overeating

While studies like these haven't been done on qigong or tai chi, we have every reason to believe they would work the same way, as these practices relax the mind and create balance in the mind, body, and spirit.

How to get started? You can look for local classes, which offers the additional benefit of putting you in a community of like-minded individuals where you're likely to make friendships. You might also try some of the many yoga, tai chi, and qigong resources online. And give my mindful eating exercise a chance. You can also experiment with the mindfulness meditation that follows.

I think that the institution of these practices may be helpful in your succeeding to control your weight and remain structurally sound. The figure on page 200 depicts the benefits of incorporating yoga as part of your weight-loss plan. I practiced tai chi for my first 2 years at Johns Hopkins and found it useful in my recovery. For others, qigong may be quite useful and effective. The key is to move, balance the healing life force, or chi, and improve health in mind, body, and spirit.

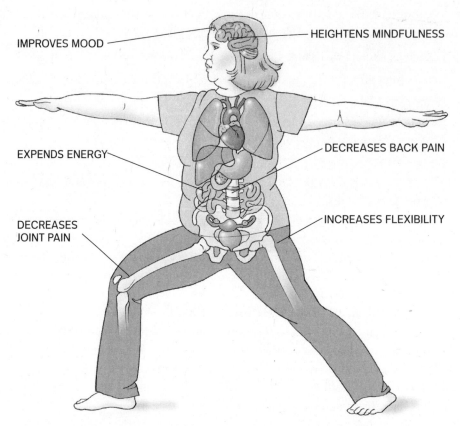

IMPROVES MOOD

HEIGHTENS MINDFULNESS

EXPENDS ENERGY

DECREASES BACK PAIN

DECREASES
JOINT PAIN

INCREASES FLEXIBILITY

How Yoga Reverses Obesity: Yoga may improve flexibility, decrease joint pain, and enhance mobility, which facilitates energy expenditure. Yoga also helps attenuate stress, depression, anxiety, insulin resistance, hypertension, and dyslipidemia.[57] By improving mindfulness, yoga is felt to diminish emotional eating behaviors, improve satiety, and make one more immune to the influence of external stimuli to the ear.[58] Studies have shown that yoga as a lifestyle intervention decreased body fat, body mass index, and body weight while improving lean body mass by building muscle.[59, 60] Regular yoga (1 to 2 times per week, 45-minute sessions weekly) has been associated with lower cortisol levels, a stress hormone that promotes obesity. Yoga practice has been associated with a decrease in inflammation, which improves cardiovascular function and insulin resistance.[61] Bernstein et al recommend 3 months of instructor-led yoga (45- to 60-minute sessions one to two times per week), with 25 minutes of independent practice where there are no formal sessions (5 minutes of meditation, 15 minutes of poses, 5 minutes of rest).[62] Those with cardiopulmonary disease should consult a physician before engaging in yoga. Musculoskeletal pain is the most common adverse event, which should be reported to the instructor.

THE GUT BALANCE REVOLUTION SUCCESS STORIES

Terri Meekins, 58

Arthritis, tummy troubles, weight gain—just a couple of years ago, Terri Meekins chalked it all up to aging. When her hands were too stiff to knit, she figured that arthritis went with the territory. When she started to pile on pounds and suffer from anxiety and depression, she figured it was menopause. And when the digestive issues from IBS—which had plagued her for years—started to worsen, she figured that now that she was in her fifties, this was just a normal way of life.

"I always tried to eat healthy foods," Terri recalls, "and I made it a point to choose small portions. But nothing seemed to help, and I just kept gaining weight. I hated going to the beach—no bathing suits for me! And with arthritis in my hands and knees, it was tough to do any physical activities." That is, until she met Dr. Gerry Mullin and learned about the Gut Balance Revolution.

About to undergo a series of serious surgeries, her doctor sent her to Dr. Gerry for a checkup in June 2013. That's when she learned that the root of all her health concerns was small intestinal bacterial overgrowth—SIBO—and that, with Dr. Gerry's help, she could feel better once and for all.

Terri was a willing patient, and she followed the doctor's orders to a T. "When Dr. Gerry told me that what I was suffering from was abnormal, and that it could be improved," she says, "I was willing to do anything to feel better." So she went on the low-FODMAP eating plan, and in a matter of weeks, her life began to change. "It was like a fog lifted," she recalls. "Many of my symptoms got better or just went away."

Now, a year and a half later, she's 40 pounds lighter and feeling better than ever. She's outside every day, going for her "run-walk," and she's been knitting sweaters for her grandchildren—and for herself. The headaches she experienced daily? Now that she's eliminated processed foods from her diet, they're a distant memory. "My skin looks better, and I have so much more energy," Terri says. "People tell me that I look younger. This new way of eating has changed my life."

YOGA POSES IN THE MANAGEMENT OF OVERWEIGHT AND OBESITY

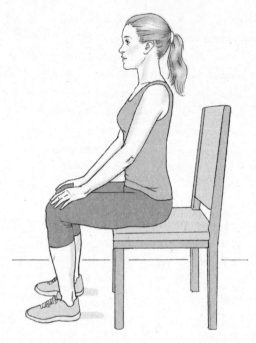

1 **SEATED POSITION:** Sit at the edge of your chair and keep your feet flat, under the knees; lightly rest your palms on your upper legs and keep your spine straight. (This is the alignment for all seated postures.)

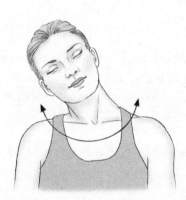

2 **NECK ROLL:** Sit straight and with your eyes closed. On an inhalation, drop your chin to your chest; on the exhalation, roll your right ear to your right shoulder. Return your head to center, then switch sides.

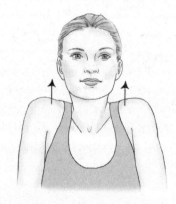

3 **SHOULDER ROLLS:** Sit straight and, on the inhalation, gently lift your shoulders to your ears and gently roll your shoulders around and back, squeezing your shoulder blades together and dropping them away from your ears.

4 **EASY SPINAL TWIST:** Sitting at the center of your seat, with your spine straight, place your right hand on your left knee and lightly rest your left hand on the edge of the seat or the back of the chair for support, keeping your shoulders parallel to ground. Inhale and twist, looking over the left shoulder. Return to center, then switch sides.

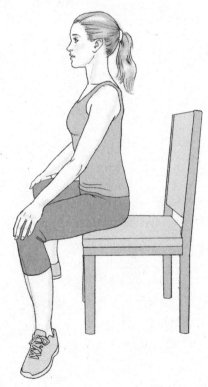

5 **GROIN STRETCH:** Sitting at the center of your seat, with your spine straight, gently open your legs as far apart as possible, keeping your feet flat on the ground and pointing in the same direction as the knees. Lightly rest your palms on the upper legs and ensure the knees are directly above the ankles.

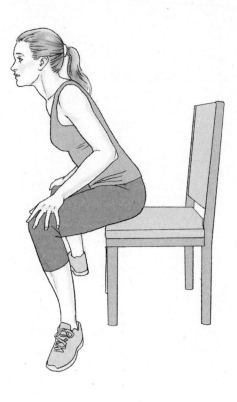

6 **LEANING GROIN STRETCH:** Keeping your spine straight, with your hands on the upper legs, inhale and lean forward with your chin and chest pointing forward.

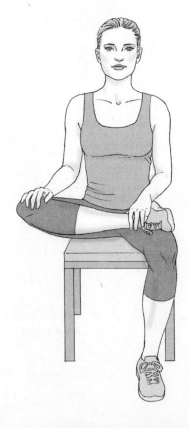

7 **NUMBER 4 STRETCH:** Keeping your spine straight and your left leg at a 90-degree angle, bring the outside of your right ankle above the left knee. Lightly place your right hand on the inside of the right upper leg and your left hand on your right ankle. Inhale and lean slightly forward. Repeat on the other side.

8 **LIFTED HAMSTRING STRETCH WITH DEEP FOOT FLEX:** Return to the center of your seat, with your knees at a 90-degree angle and your spine straight. Holding a yoga strap with both hands, loop it over the arch of the left foot and, on inhalation, lift and straighten the left leg, using the yoga strap for support. Exhale and slowly lower your leg. Repeat on the other side.

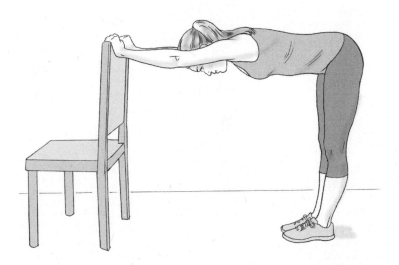

9 **TABLE POSE:** Stand up and walk around the chair; put your hands on the back of the chair and walk backward. With your spine straight, lean forward until your body forms a table position and your arms are straight; keep the hips over the feet and the feet slightly apart. On exhalation, tuck your chin to your chest and slowly roll up and walk back toward the chair.

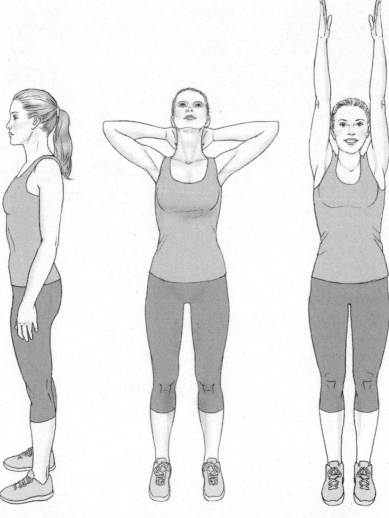

10 MOUNTAIN POSE: Stand with your feet slightly apart, your hips over the feet, your shoulders over the hips, your chin parallel to the ground, and your weight evenly distributed.

11 EASY BACK BEND: In Mountain pose, clasp your hands behind your head and pull your elbows back. Inhale and pull your abdomen in, gently look up, and slowly bend back.

12 RULER POSE: From Mountain pose, inhale as you gently lift your arms toward the ceiling (your arms should be perpendicular to the floor and parallel to each other) and tuck your shoulder blades under. Exhale and, slowly lowering your arms, return to the center position.

13 PRESS-UPS: From Mountain pose, focus your eyes straight ahead. Pressing your toes into the ground, lift your heels up and down three times and, on the fourth, hold, then come down.

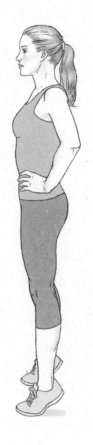

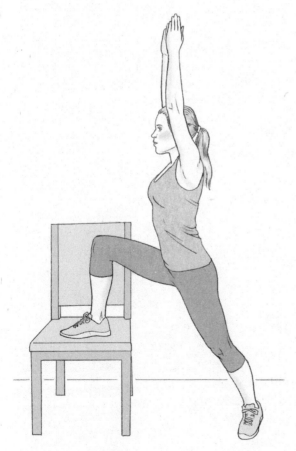

14 WARRIOR 1: Face the side of the chair with the seat back on your right side. Start in Mountain pose with parallel feet, then gently lift and place your right foot on the chair seat, your knee in a 90-degree angle. Lean slightly forward, keeping your left leg straight, and press your left heel down, taking care to keep the foot at a 45-angle from your spine. Gently lift your arms toward the ceiling (your arms should be perpendicular to the floor and parallel to each other). Step slowly back into Mountain and switch sides.

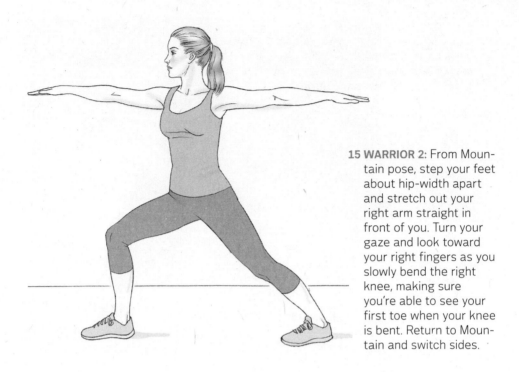

15 WARRIOR 2: From Mountain pose, step your feet about hip-width apart and stretch out your right arm straight in front of you. Turn your gaze and look toward your right fingers as you slowly bend the right knee, making sure you're able to see your first toe when your knee is bent. Return to Mountain and switch sides.

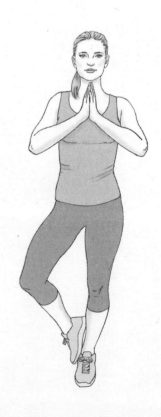

16 TREE POSE: From Mountain pose, focus your eyes straight ahead. Slowly shift your weight slightly onto the left foot and bend your right knee. Draw your right foot up and place the heel against the inner left shin, keeping your left leg as straight as possible. Put your hands together, close to your chest, and hold. On an exhalation, lower the right foot. Repeat on the other side.

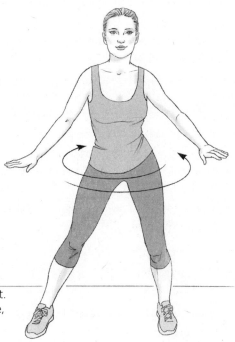

17 HIP CIRCLES: From Mountain pose, move your feet about hip-width apart. Keeping your knees and ankles loose, gently move your hips in a circular motion using the balls of your feet.

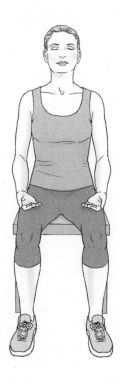

18 RELAXATION POSE: Lightly rest your palms, facing up, on your upper legs. Keeping your spine straight, close your eyes and rest, concentrating on breathing.

Meditation: Watching Your Thoughts

One of the hallmarks of mindfulness meditation is becoming aware of your thoughts, feelings, and bodily sensations *without doing anything to change them.* The objective isn't to change your world or your experience but to become more deeply aware of and attentive to that experience. By a lucky, but tricky, set of cognitive, behavioral, and emotional human tendencies, when you become more aware of your own internal experience, that experience tends to shift on its own. You become less stressed and more at peace simply by paying attention to what's happening in your mind, body, and spirit. But be careful! Becoming mindful and meditating *because* you want to feel more peace may not work so well. If you sit down to meditate and think, "Don't stress out. Don't stress out," all that's likely to happen is that you'll become even more stressed. Instead, gently begin to notice what comes up for you emotionally, intellectually, and physically by following these guidelines.

1. Find a quiet, comfortable, distraction-free place to sit. Sit cross-legged on the floor with a pillow underneath you (a more traditional style of meditation) if that suits you, or simply sit in a chair with your back straight.

2. Take a few deep breaths using the deep breathing exercise on page 194 to enter a state of relaxation.

3. Just sit and breathe. As you do so, many thoughts, feelings, and bodily sensations are likely to arise. When they do, gently bring your attention to them and acknowledge them without trying to change them.

4. To help with this, you may want to label your experiences. For example, if you become aware of a slight pain in your ankle, you might label it "pain in the ankle." Or if you find yourself becoming anxious or angry, you could label these emotional experiences as such. The same with thoughts–you may find yourself getting distracted by the thought "I need to get to work." Just notice it. Label it. And let it be.

5. Float your experiences down the river of life. Thoughts, feelings, and bodily sensations tend to have an ebb and flow to them. Imagine standing next to a beautiful river, and as experiences come up, you write them on a leaf and watch them float away. For example, if you begin to feel tense, imagine yourself writing the word *tense* on a leaf. Then place the leaf on your river of personal experience and watch it float away.

Try this exercise two or three times a week for 10 to 20 minutes at time. As you grow more accustomed to meditating, explore it more often, for longer stretches of time. This simple exercise will put you in deeper touch with your personal experience and the array of thoughts, feelings, and sensations humans experience. It may affect you in unexpected ways. Answers to questions you've long struggled with may suddenly arise, no longer as challenging as they once seemed. When you tap into the deep inner wisdom of your own mind, body, and spirit, you'll be pleasantly surprised at what you find.

VISUALIZATION, GUIDED IMAGERY, AND HYPNOSIS

Take a moment to imagine you're relaxed. Close your eyes. Imagine yourself completely at peace. You might see yourself sitting on a quiet beach where the crystal blue water gently laps against long stretches of white sand. Or maybe you envision yourself walking slowly, meditatively, through an ancient redwood forest. Perhaps you find yourself in a cozy cottage where the delicious fragrances of home-cooked foods permeate the air. Simply visualize yourself at peace in your most cherished personal place. Go ahead: Close your eyes and do it now. Then come back to this book. How do you feel? I'd bet you feel more relaxed. Don't you? You just completed a very simple visualization exercise.

Our bodies respond to our thoughts. When you use your imagination, enter a state of absorbed and focused attention, and intentionally concentrate on specific images and ideas, you can help yourself relax, change mental and physiological processes, and enhance your belief in yourself and your goals. Hypnosis, visualization, and guided imagery are different techniques with this state of focused attention in common. Each has a broad range of ways to influence your mood, your weight, and your overall health. For example, they can help you:[63]

- Feel more relaxed, more positive, and less anxious, angry, or depressed

- Make better food choices

- Get motivated to exercise

- Uncover unconscious psychological barriers that may stand in the way of your health and weight-loss goals

- Increase your self-esteem and self-confidence

- Believe in your ability to stick to your health and weight-loss goals

Hypnosis can work as an adjunct for weight loss. In a recent study, 32 females and 5 males were recruited and divided into groups.[64] One-third were placed on a weight-loss plan with no other interventions. One-third were on a weight-loss plan and received cognitive-behavioral therapy (CBT) from a certified CBT therapist. The final group was on a weight-loss plan and got both CBT and hypnosis intervention. The group receiving hypnosis outperformed both other groups in total weight lost. This is just one study with a small sample size, but it's an important finding that lends credence to the long-held belief those of us in the complementary and alternative medicine (CAM) community have embraced—mind-body medicine is an important piece of the weight-loss and antiobesity puzzle.

Give these techniques a try. You can get hypnosis, visualization, and guided imagery CDs or download electronic versions. One resource I like is healingwithhypnosis.com.

ACUPUNCTURE AND OTHER ALTERNATIVE TECHNIQUES

A growing base of research supports traditional medicine (such as traditional Chinese medicine and Ayurvedic medicine) for assisting with weight loss. Manual acupuncture (needling by hand), electroacupuncture (with an electronic device), and auricular acupuncture[65] (acupuncture delivered through the earlobe) all have evidence to support their use in the treatment of weight problems and obesity.

For example, a meta-analysis of 44 trials on acupuncture and 3 trials of combined therapy (Chinese herbs and acupuncture) that included 4,861 participants found that both acupuncture and the combined therapies were more effective than placebo or lifestyle modification for helping people lose weight.[66] The analysis stated that these methods work similarly to Western antiobesity drugs but with fewer adverse side effects. A similar study on auricular electroacupuncture that included 56 obese women randomly selected to receive electric stimulation or placebo found that the treatment group had a significant reduction in weight and BMI. Scientists think that acupuncture has these effects because it's known to:[67]

- Affect appetite
- Regulate intestinal motility–contractions that move food through your gut. This is important for reasons we will discuss later in this chapter.
- Speed up metabolism
- Increase neural activity in the hypothalamus (the command center of the brain that governs appetite and more)
- Increase serotonin levels and enhance mood
- Reduce stress

Preliminary evidence suggests that Ayurvedic medicine may also be a useful adjunct for long-term weight loss. Twenty-two women in a 3-month Ayurvedic treatment program for weight problems were encouraged to change their eating habits and activity patterns; improve self-efficacy, quality of life, well-being, vitality, and self-awareness around food choice; and manage stress more effectively. The results were positive–12 women completed the intervention as well as the 6-month and 9-month follow-ups. At the end of 9 months, each of these women had lost more than 10 pounds.

GET SUPPORT

Humans are social creatures–we need other people to survive and thrive. It could be argued that we depend on one another more today than we ever have, but we're ironically more isolated than we've ever been before. We rely on others for virtually everything in our lives, in ways we don't always realize. The water in your tap comes into your home because other people have built and managed an infrastructure of pipes to deliver that water to you. It's very likely that your home, your furniture, your car, your clothes, your computer, even your food was made by another person. And that only scratches the surface. Our cities, governments, and nations are the outcome of the interdependence of human beings. As I said in Chapter 1, our industrialized society has evolved to a highly sophisticated synchrony of symbiosis, so it's such a tragic irony that so many suffer in isolation today. Between 1985 and 2004, the number of people who said they had no one with whom they could discuss important matters tripled to 25 percent.[68] Computers, cell phones, instant messaging, e-mail, and social media allow us to connect in ways never before imagined, yet we feel more disconnected, more isolated than ever.

This isolation impacts our health and weight in distinct and disturbing ways. When scientists reviewed a sample of the women included in the Community-based, Heart and Weight Management Trial, they found that those with stronger social support groups and less perceived stress were more likely to engage in healthy behaviors and less likely to be obese.[69] And a systematic review that sought to determine the factors that worked in weight loss for men found that interventions delivered in social settings were far more likely to work and that group-based programs providing support for men with similar health problems were far more effective than interventions delivered in the clinical-care setting.[70]

Research also indicates that isolation leads to health problems and early death.[71] A 2014 University of Chicago study suggested that feeling lonely impairs executive function, sleep, and mental and physical well-being, all of which may lead to higher rates of morbidity and mortality, especially in older adults.

We humans need one another, and I encourage you to connect with others. It will improve your health, your weight-loss outcomes, and the quality of your life. Here are some ideas on how to do that.

- Ask a coworker or friend to do this program with you. This has many advantages, one of which is having an "accountability partner" to help you stick to the plan.
- Call an old friend you haven't talked to in a long time or, better yet, meet for lunch.
- Invite a coworker out to lunch.
- Join a support group, club, or gym.
- Go to a sporting event.
- Go on a date with your spouse or friend.
- Join a reading club.
- Create a game night with friends.
- Go for a walk or a hike with a buddy.
- Try team sports with a group of friends: baseball, softball, Ultimate Frisbee. Or go back to your childhood and try kickball or invite a friend to play catch.

When You Need Professional Guidance

In some cases, underlying psychological problems, mood disorders, eating disorders, and other issues can lead to weight problems. If you try everything in this program and it doesn't work, or if you know that your issues with eating and weight have a psychological underpinning, it may be time to consider seeking professional help. I recommend you look for someone trained and certified in cognitive-behavioral therapy (CBT) or acceptance and commitment therapy (ACT). Both treatment approaches have been validated as effective interventions for weight loss and a wide variety of psychological issues.

Don't lose hope. Don't be afraid. And don't be embarrassed. Many people could use some help at times, but precious few are brave enough to reach out for it and do the hard work it sometimes takes to heal. You deserve to be a whole, healthy, happy person. Seek the help you need to get you to that place.

The possibilities are endless. Get out and connect with real people in real life, away from electronic devices when possible. Facebook makes it seem like you have a thousand friends (and maybe you do!), but you'll get a lot more out of meeting people face-to-face. When it comes to human social interaction, there's nothing like seeing a real person in real life and giving them a handshake or a hug.

LIVING IN HARMONY WITH YOUR GUT CLOCK

It's not only what you eat and how you eat that can either stress out your body or relax it. *When* you eat is important, too. We're a culture that often eats until right before we go to bed. This can cause unnecessary physiological stress, weight gain, gastrointestinal distress, and an unhealthy, fat-forming gut microbiome. Here's why.

Your body operates on its own set of circadian rhythms—a kind of biological clock that helps you know, for example, when to sleep, when to eat, and when to release certain biochemicals. All animals have these internal clocks, but humans are the only ones who can consciously choose to ignore them. We stay awake after dark, eat whenever we want, and generally ignore our natural biological impulses.

But living this way can adversely impact our health if behaviors become too extreme. Sleep deprivation is a health epidemic, but many of us wear it as a badge of pride. We'll talk more about sleep and why getting too little can lead to weight gain and chronic health problems shortly. For now, let's focus on the circadian rhythms of your gut—your gut clock and the cleansing waves it sets in motion.[72]

Your gut clock determines when and how your gut contracts, a movement called gut motility—an extremely important part of your digestive health. These contractions occur with a certain regularity and become pronounced when your stomach is supposed to be empty (in between meals and during sleep). This is what I call the cleansing wave. It not only helps you digest food but helps keep bad bugs from getting a foothold in the wrong places in your gut, especially your small intestine. Remember when we talked about small intestinal bacterial overgrowth, or SIBO? Well, this cleansing wave is a critical part of preventing that condition.

These contractions happen outside your conscious control, but how and when you eat can affect them. Imagine you have a clock in your gut. If you eat a certain way, it sets an alarm that, when triggered, releases powerful cleansing waves that wipe away bad bugs and debris from your stomach and small intestine. But when you eat in a different way, the alarm is delayed and the waves become smaller and weaker. The technical name for the cleansing waves is the migrating motor complex (MMC), and it's strongest when you're asleep and fasting. In this state, the waves occur frequently and are quite vigorous. But when you eat late in the evening, the waves become weaker and less frequent. The later you eat, the less you'll clean out the small bowel, setting the stage for SIBO and all the problems that come along with it, including dysbiosis and weight gain as we mentioned on page 196 when discussing the practice of *hara hachi bu*, Ayurveda, and traditional Chinese eating principles.

Studies have shown that changes in gastrointestinal motility force your body to pack on the pounds.[73] I illustrated the connections between SIBO, GI distress, and weight gain more fully in Chapter 4. So remember that *when* you eat is nearly as important as how you eat. Here are some recommendations to help you live in harmony with your gut clock.

- **Eat your last meal earlier in the evening**. Stop eating at least 3 or 4 hours before bed; eating your last meal by 6:00 is ideal.

- **Drink water or herbal tea**. Instead of eating late into the evening, try drinking more water or a relaxing herbal tea like chamomile or peppermint.

- **If you're hungry, have a light snack**. Try to eat dinner by 6:00 p.m. If you're hungry later in the evening, have a light snack like a few nuts or plain Greek yogurt with a little raw honey–just enough to satiate your hunger.

You don't want bad bugs building up in the wrong part of your GI tract. To keep your inner garden healthy and radiant, keep the bugs out of your small bowel. Luckily, you have a built-in mechanism for doing this. So eat earlier and let the cleansing wave do the weeding for you.

Sleep Like a Baby

Americans seem to hate sleep. Unlike our Mediterranean counterparts, we don't have siestas, we don't take naps, and the less we sleep, the prouder we seem to be of ourselves, regarding our sleeplessness as proof of just how industrious we Americans are. The result? Forty million men and women in this country are chronically sleep deprived.[74] Think this doesn't affect your health and your waistline? Think again.

Disruptions in sleep, getting too little sleep, and having your circadian rhythms interrupted have all been implicated as contributing factors to type 2 diabetes and obesity.[75] This is likely due to the fact that not sleeping enough, even for one night, has negative impacts on your neuroendocrine system that cause you to feel hungrier and eat more as hunger hormones become altered–increasing ghrelin and decreasing leptin.[76] Restricting sleep to as little as 5 hours nightly reduces insulin sensitivity, sets off systemic inflammation, and puts you at increased risk of mortality by all causes.[77-79]

Scientists have learned that kids who stay up late to play video games are at an additional risk for obesity from the sleep deprivation itself.[80] A recent study concluded that compared with decreased sleep, increased sleep *duration* in school-age children resulted in lower reported food intake, lower fasting leptin levels, and lower weight. And other researchers recently observed that chronic sleep curtailment from infancy to school age was associated with higher overall and belly fat in mid-childhood–a fact further confirmed by yet another study.[81, 82] The potential role of sleep duration in pediatric obesity prevention and treatment warrants further study.[83, 84]

A 2010 study published in the *Annals of Internal Medicine* put all these data in perspective. Investigators at the University of Chicago demonstrated that insufficient sleep undermines dietary efforts to reduce overall body fat.[85] They conducted clinical trials in 10 overweight, nonsmoking adults who underwent 14 days of moderate calorie restriction with either 8.5 or 5.5 hours of nighttime sleep. Sleep curtailment decreased the portion that lost weight as fat and increased the loss of lean muscle mass. The scientists also found those who were sleep deprived experienced body weight set point adaptations that shifted them toward a state mimicking caloric deprivation: increased hunger and a relative decrease in fat oxidation. In fact, those who slept 8.5 hours burned twice as much fat as the 5.5-hour group. And over a year, the 8.5-hour group lost an average of 10 more pounds than the 5.5-hour group and preserved twice as much lean body mass.

There are no questions about it: Sleep deprivation compromises your efforts to lose weight. Your goal should be to get 7 to 9 hours of deep, restful sleep nightly. If you think you don't have the time to sleep that much, I suggest you rethink that position and make sleep a priority over other activities. Sacrificing sleep for the sake of productivity is seriously overrated. It's great to want to be more productive. But how much do you think you'll get done if your health suffers? Sleep deprivation has been linked to a number of adverse health conditions. Even evening shift workers have increased inflammatory markers portending adverse health outcomes,[86] and health-care shift workers aren't immune to these adverse effects of circadian rhythm disruption.[87] Whatever it is you're working on can wait a few hours.

On the other hand, if you have trouble getting or staying asleep at night, don't despair. Some simple interventions can improve the quality of your sleep and make it

The Adverse Health Effects of Sleep Deprivation

- Accidents
- All-cause mortality
- Alzheimer's disease
- Cardiovascular events
- Cognitive impairments
- Decreased quality of life
- Diabetes
- Gastrointestinal disorders
- Hypertension

- Impaired athletic performance
- Impaired work performance
- Increased colorectal cancer risk
- Memory loss
- Metabolic syndrome
- Osteoporosis
- Stroke
- Weight gain
- Worsening of mood disorders[88-95]

easier to fall asleep and stay that way. Most people with sleep problems are engaged in negative lifestyle or behavior habits prohibiting them from getting enough good sleep. You can change this by improving your sleep hygiene, and it isn't hard to do. Here are some tips to help you improve your sleep hygiene starting tonight.

- **Create a sleep ritual.** Doing the same thing before bed every night helps remind your body that it's time to go to sleep. You might change into pajamas, brush your teeth, turn out the lights, spread back the covers, or any other number of things. Just keep it consistent.

- **Relax before bed.** Try doing something relaxing every night 30 to 60 minutes before bed. You could try some deep breathing, mindfulness meditation, visualization, or even a little light, relaxing stretching.

- **Go to bed earlier.** If you need more sleep, it's probably best to go to bed earlier. Try climbing into bed 10 or 15 minutes earlier each week until you're enjoying 7 to 9 hours of shut-eye.

- **Don't stress before bed.** Getting stressed before you go to bed won't help you sleep better. Think of how many ways we amp up our stress hormones right before bedtime: watching the evening news or violent TV shows, surfing the Net, even checking e-mail. Try to make rational decisions about using electronic devices, and stay away from alcohol as well as caffeine and other stimulants.

- **Sleep in a completely dark room.** Light alters your circadian rhythms and may make it difficult to get or stay asleep—not just the lamps in your bedroom but also those little lights from phones, computers, TVs, DVD players, clocks, streetlamps, and more. Get blackout blinds for your windows if you need them. Turn your phone off and point your alarm away from the bed. If you have a computer, TV, or DVD player in your room, plug it into a power strip you can shut off easily before you go to bed. For millennia, humans went to sleep when it was dark. That ancient way of living is stenciled into our DNA. Respect your circadian rhythms and provide them the dark they need.

- **Experiment with naps (if you can).** For some, naps can actually improve nighttime sleep. For example, if you've learned to rely on a coffee at 2:00 p.m. to get through your day, you may find that a 20-minute nap does a better job of rejuvenating you without that jolt of caffeine. On the other hand, if you have a hard time sleeping already, napping during the day may not be the ticket. Try naps if you can and see if they work for you.

- **Drink a cup of tart cherry juice.** A small randomized clinical trial recently found that insomniacs who drank a cup of tart cherry juice twice daily (in the morning and evening) increased their sleep time by nearly 90 minutes.[96] The scientists hypothesize it's because the juice inhibits an enzyme that degrades tryptophan–an essential amino acid in your body's production of melatonin, the master circadian rhythm hormone. Speaking of which . . .

- **Try melatonin.** Supplemental melatonin can help put your sleep rhythms back on track and may provide support for people who either don't make enough or need to replete their levels. Try 1 to 3 milligrams 60 to 90 minutes before bedtime.

If you still have sleep problems, seek out the help of a sleep specialist. You may have undiagnosed sleep disturbances, such as sleep apnea, that can adversely impact your health and your weight. Don't take this lightly. Sleep apnea, in its worst forms, is a life-threatening condition. Even less severe forms of sleep apnea or other sleep disorders can compromise your health. Sleep is one of your most precious commodities. Don't short-change yourself by ignoring it.

EXERCISE MORE EFFECTIVELY IN LESS TIME

I cannot overstate the importance of exercise. It's a magnificent stress reducer that even enhances resilience. Movement reduces inflammation, makes you more insulin sensitive, improves your mood (exercise releases "happy" neurochemicals like serotonin), and builds lean muscle mass that enhances your fat-burning machinery by increasing the number of mitochondria (your body's fat-melting organelles).

It's too early to say whether or not exercise has a direct impact on your gut microbiome. A few studies, like one recently published in *Environmental Health Perspectives*, suggest that exercise may mitigate the damage done to your gut microbiome by environmental toxins and other factors.[97] However, even if exercise doesn't directly impact your inner garden, it indirectly impacts your flora by reducing inflammation. Exercise is one of the healthiest things you can engage in, and I would be remiss not to address it in a book about weight loss.

Our bodies were built to move. When we don't exercise enough, or when we live a sedentary life, our health breaks down. An Australian study looked at data from more than 220,000 people age 45 or older and found that those who sat more than 11 hours a day had a 40 percent increased chance of death from all causes.[98] Findings like these have been replicated by the American Cancer Society, the American College of Sports and Medicine, and other organizations.

Does that mean more is better when it comes to exercise? Well, yes and no. Certainly, most of us could afford to exercise more. But it doesn't necessarily follow that because an activity is healthy we should do it nonstop. Exercising too much or in the wrong way can lead to inflammation, injury, and metabolic adjustments that make it difficult to burn fat. This point is particularly important to keep in mind in light of our cultural addiction to the calories in/calories out theory of weight loss. We used to believe that if we burned more calories by exercising more and ate less, we'd lose weight. We used to believe this was the equation for weight loss. But we were wrong. The human body simply doesn't work this way. You gain or lose fat based on a wide variety of factors, including the health of your gut microbiome, your metabolic rate, hormonal balance, and more. All that plays a part in figuring how much—and how—to exercise.

The good news: You no longer have to spend long hours plodding on a treadmill to receive the many metabolic, neurochemical, and other advantages of moving your body.

The Health Benefits of Exercise

Exercise has so many health benefits, it's hard to catalog them all. These include but are not limited to:[99]

- Decreased risk of cardiovascular (heart) disease, high blood pressure, and stroke
- Decreased risk of colon and breast cancers
- Decreased risk of diabetes
- Decreased risk of osteoporosis
- Decreased risk of depression and dementia
- Decreased body fat

- Improved metabolic processes—the way the body breaks down and builds necessary substances
- Improved movement of joints and muscles
- Improved oxygen delivery throughout the body
- Improved sense of well-being
- Improved strength and endurance

Novel approaches to exercise have been developed in recent years, allowing us to exercise better and in less time and still achieve the results we want.

I'd like to share some of what I know about these breakthroughs. As you'll see, I've divided my exercise program into beginner, intermediate, and advanced options. Select the program that's right for you, and get moving!

Beginner: Walk

Walking may not be the most novel approach to exercise, but if you've been sedentary for a long time, it's the perfect place to start. There are dozens of studies that show walking as little as 15 to 45 minutes daily can reduce your risk of heart disease, stroke, type 2 diabetes, and more.[100-102]

If you don't exercise at all, you're out of shape, or you're injured, start with light walking. I recommend 15 to 45 minutes three to five times weekly, depending on your health status and conditioning. Why such a broad range? Because I want you to do what you're comfortable with. As the old saying goes, "The best kind of exercise is the kind you will do." If you set the benchmark too high, you'll resent and avoid your exercise routine, especially if you haven't been moving around much for a long time. Start where you can. If that means 15 minutes three times a week, great! If it means 30 minutes three times a week, great! If it means varying your routine based on what your lifestyle will allow, great! Just get moving–around the block, to the market, in the hills, on a trail, in the mall. I like getting outside in the fresh air and sunlight when I can, but for some folks, that's not possible. Bad weather, dangerous neighborhoods, and other factors may prohibit this. In that case, you can walk on a treadmill, use an elliptical machine, or climb stairs in your building.

Over time, you'll naturally feel yourself become accustomed to walking. When this happens, increase the amount of time you walk. You can also vary your routine by walking up stairs, walking up hills–or trying intervals. Here's how.

Intermediate: Walk with Intervals and Add Some Weight

Interval training allows you to get an excellent cardiovascular workout in less time, and some studies have shown it's a more effective way to burn fat and balance insulin than traditional cardio routines.[103-105] When doing interval training, you push as hard as you can for a set period of time, then you go at a more moderate pace, then you push again. One cycle of pushing and going slower is called an interval.

How long do you push, how long do you back off, and how many intervals are involved? That depends on the program or routine–there are many options available. Probably the most common interval sequence comes from the world of running. In this routine, runners sprint as fast as they can for 1 minute and run slower for 2 minutes. Six intervals are typically completed for a total workout time of about 18 minutes. That may not sound like very much exercise, but I can assure you the routine is extremely challenging (in fact, I don't recommend you do it for the intermediate routine). It also provides the same or better cardiovascular and metabolic benefits as a 60-minute jog, with less wear and tear on the joints. I encourage you to give intervals a try. They can give you a better workout in less time, and they make exercise more fun.

Intervals: Where to Begin?

If you're at an intermediate level of exercise, or if you've worked through the beginner's program and you're ready to try intervals, here's what I recommend.

Plan to exercise five times a week for 20 to 30 minutes. You may do a little less on some days, a little more on others. Two days a week, you'll walk with intervals. The other 3 days, you'll do body-weight training (more on this in a moment). To integrate intervals into your walking, start with something manageable. Here is what I recommend.

TIME IN MINUTES	INTENSITY
0:00–5:00	Warm up with some slow, relaxed walking.
5:00–7:00	Walk at a moderate pace—quick enough to be a little difficult, but not to make you breathless. You'd be able to talk to a friend during this time.
7:00–8:00	Walk as quickly as you can without running. This should make you breathless, and you may feeling burning in your legs and arms.
8:00–10:00	Resume a moderate pace of walking for about 2 minutes, or until you're recovered.
10:00–25:00	Repeat minutes 5:00 through 10:00 for five intervals.
25:00–30:00	Cool down by walking at a slow, relaxing pace.

When you're ready to enhance the intensity of the routine, do more intervals–up to 8 or 10–and/or shorten your rest period. Here's an example.

TIME IN MINUTES	INTENSITY
0:00–5:00	Warm up with some slow, relaxed walking.
5:00–6:00	Walk at a moderate pace—quick enough to be a little difficult, but not to make you breathless. You'd be able to talk to a friend during this time.
6:00–7:00	Walk as quickly as you can without running. This should make you breathless, and you may feeling burning in your legs and arms.
7:00–8:00	Resume a moderate pace of walking for about 1 minute, or until you're recovered.
8:00–21:00	Repeat minutes 5:00 through 8:00 for seven intervals.
21:00–26:00	Cool down by walking at a slow, relaxing pace.

There are plenty of other options, so you can customize the routine to fit your personal preferences. Another possibility, for example, is to walk as fast as you can for as long as you can, rest when you need to, and walk fast again. Hills and stairs will further increase the intensity.

Integrate a routine like this into your schedule twice a week, and you'll be getting all the cardio you need. The other 3 days of the week, I want you to integrate body-weight exercises. Here's why.

Weight Training Using Your Own Body

Resistance training is an important part of any exercise program–possibly more important than cardio. It builds up your lean muscle mass, increasing your mitochondria, and is good for your skeletal structure as well. In fact, cardio and resistance training aren't actually different things. You can get a good cardio and resistance routine all in one go if it's structured correctly. The traditional wisdom that you need to exercise your aerobic and anaerobic systems separately is no longer considered valid. The systems are interrelated, and you can get far more benefits for far less work by weight training quickly a few times weekly.

So why do I suggest you divide the routines in the intermediate program? Mainly because working out this way is hard–too hard for a lot of folks. When you're building back up to your optimal fitness level, it's still useful to do weight training and interval walking on different days.

There are almost endless options for weight training, and I encourage you to seek a program that works best for you. I like body-weight training, possibly with light hand weights if needed. Most everyone can get a solid resistance workout with body weight alone, and you can do it anywhere. Here are two training routines I recommend.

WEIGHT-TRAINING ROUTINES

For the routines that follow, do all your 5 to 10 reps for each exercise in a row. This is one set. Take a 2-minute rest between sets, then repeat. The entire routine won't take more than 20 to 30 minutes, and if you do it correctly with good form, you'll feel like you spent an hour in the gym. When you're done, cool down with a walk and/or some full-body stretching.

WORKOUT I

Hinge and Row

A. Stand with your feet about shoulder-width apart. Hold a dumbbell in each hand in front of your legs, palms facing thighs.

B. Keeping your abs tight, bend forward from your hips, sliding the weights down your thighs. Slowly lower (about 4 counts) until your torso is almost parallel to the floor. If you notice that your back is rounding before that point, stop there. The dumbbells should be below your shoulders.

C. Bend your elbows toward the ceiling and pull the dumbbells up until your arms are bent at 90 degrees.

D. Straighten your arms. Do one more row, then slowly stand.

EASIER (OR IF YOU HAVE BACK PROBLEMS): Hold on to the back of a chair with one hand and do one-arm rows.

HARDER: Do one-legged hinges. Lift one leg behind you as you bend forward.

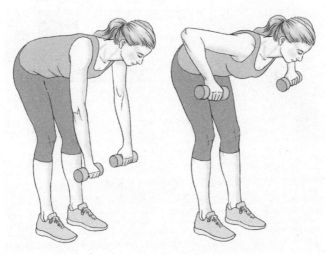

Plié Squat and Curl

A. Stand with your feet wider than shoulder-width apart, toes pointing out. Hold a dumbbell in each hand with your arms bent so your hands are by your shoulders, palms facing you.

B. Keeping your abs tight, bend your knees and lower yourself until your thighs are almost parallel to the floor. At the same time, straighten your arms and lower the dumbbells between your legs, palms facing forward.

C. Straighten your legs, squeeze your buttocks, and stand back up. Simultaneously, curl the dumbbells up toward your shoulders without moving your upper arms. Repeat.

EASIER: Don't bend your knees as far.

HARDER: As you stand up, raise one foot off the floor to do a side knee lift.

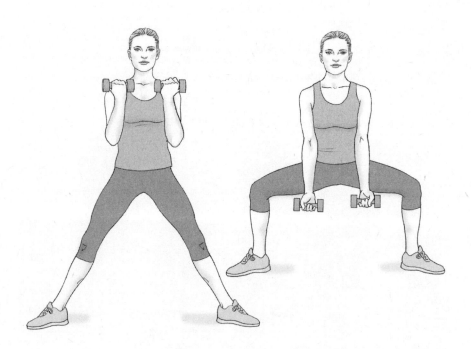

Lunge and Twist

A. Stand with your feet together. Hold a dumbbell with both hands and with your arms bent so the dumbbell is in front of your chest.

B. Keeping your abs tight, step back with your left foot about 2 to 3 feet and bend your knees. Lower yourself until your right thigh is parallel to the floor, keeping your right knee above your ankle. Your back heel will be off the floor. At the same time, rotate your torso to the right, bringing the dumbbell down by your right hip.

C. Press off your back foot to stand up as you rotate back to the starting position. Repeat for the recommended number of reps, then switch sides.

EASIER: Do stationary lunges, beginning with your feet apart and keeping them in that position the entire time.

HARDER: As you stand up, raise your back leg up in front of you to a knee lift.

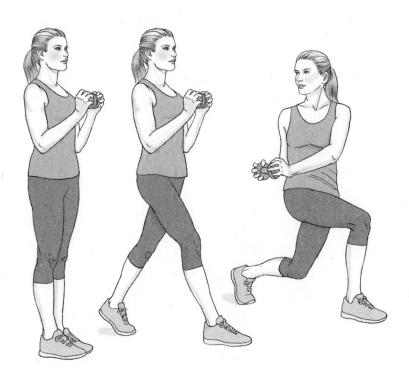

Bridge with Flies

A. Lie on your back with your legs bent and your feet flat on the floor. Hold a dumbbell in each hand with your arms extended out to your sides, elbows slightly bent and palms facing up.

B. Squeeze your glutes and abs and lift your lower and middle back off the floor. At the same time, raise the dumbbells over your chest as if you were hugging a ball.

C. Lower your back and arms to the floor. Repeat.

EASIER: Lift into the bridge first, then raise your arms. Lower your arms and back separately or at the same time, whichever is easier for you.

HARDER: Hold in the up position and raise one foot off the floor. Hold for a second, then lower your foot to the floor. Then lower your arms and back to the floor at the same time. Alternate legs with each rep.

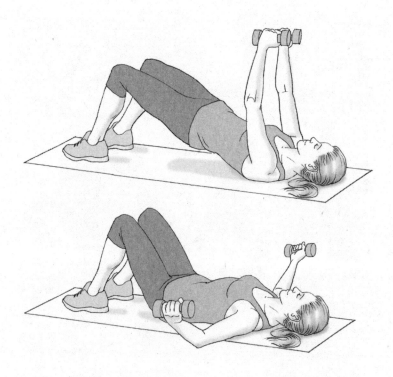

Kneeling Arm Raise

A. Get down on the floor on all fours. Hold a dumbbell in your right hand with your arm bent 90 degrees, your elbow by your hip, and your palm facing your thigh. Extend your left leg behind you and off the floor so you're balancing on your left hand and right knee. If your left wrist bothers you, hold a dumbbell so your wrist isn't bent.

B. Slowly straighten your right arm and raise the dumbbell behind you. Keep your abs tight and look at the floor a few feet in front of you to keep your head in line with your spine.

C. Slowly bend your arm back to the starting position. Your upper arm should remain still throughout the move. Repeat for the recommended number of reps, then switch sides.

EASIER: Keep both knees on the floor.

HARDER: Bend and straighten your leg as you bend and straighten your arm.

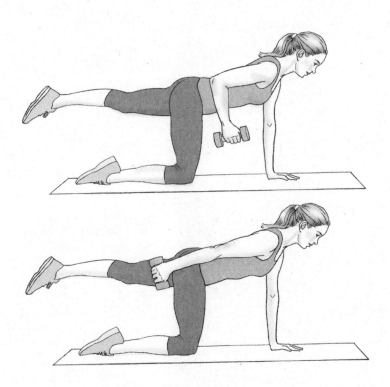

WORKOUT 2

Step and Extend

A. Holding the dumbbells at your shoulders, with your palms facing in, stand facing a staircase. Plant your right foot on the first step. (You can use the second or third step, depending on the height of the stairs and your fitness level.)

B. Press into your right foot and straighten the right leg while lifting the weights overhead. Tap your left toes on the step, then lower both feet back to the starting position. Complete a full set. Switch legs for your second set.

EASIER: Perform the move without the overhead press.

HARDER: Keep the foot you're stepping up with planted on the step throughout the exercise (lowering just the other foot to the floor).

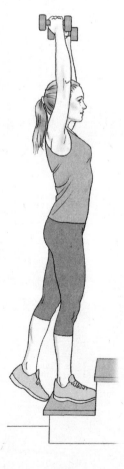

Split Squat, Biceps Curl

A. Stand with your right leg 2 to 3 feet in front of your left leg. Hold a pair of dumbbells down at your sides.

B. Bend your right leg until your right thigh is parallel to the floor and the left leg is extended, with the knee bent and almost touching the floor. Be sure to keep your back straight, and don't allow your right knee to jut beyond your right toes. As you lower, bend your arms and curl the weights to your chest. Pause, then push back up to the starting position, lowering the weights as you stand. Complete a full set. Switch leg positions for your second set.

EASIER: Place one hand on a chair back for balance, and curl with only one arm at a time.

HARDER: Place the top of your back foot on a step.

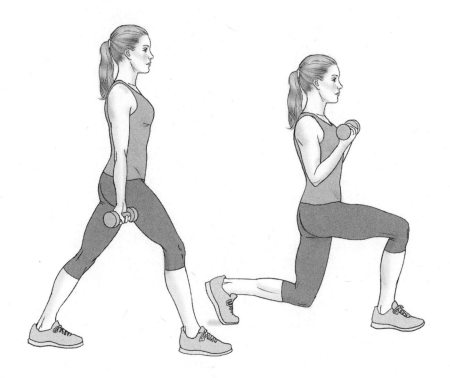

Single-Leg Row

A. Stand with your feet about hip-width apart, holding the dumbbells down at your sides, with your palms facing in.

B. Bend forward toward the floor while extending your right leg straight behind you until your body forms a T (or as close to it as possible). Allow your arms to hang straight down toward the floor, with your palms facing each other.

C. Squeeze your shoulder blades together and raise the weights to either side of your chest. Repeat for half a set, then switch sides.

EASIER: Hold on to a chair back with one hand, and perform the rows one arm at a time.

HARDER: After rowing the weights to your chest, extend your arms straight back to add a triceps kickback.

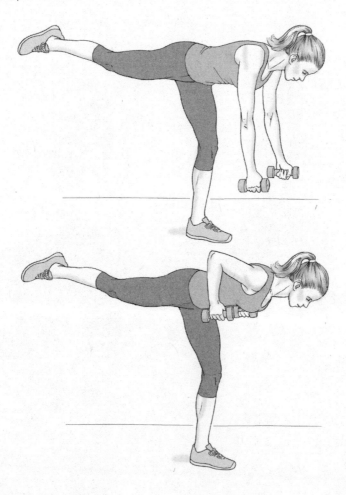

Flamingo Lateral Lift

A. Stand with your feet about hip-width apart. Hold the dumbbells down at your sides, with your palms facing in.

B. Bend your right leg and lift your right foot off the floor as high as comfortably possible while maintaining your balance. Tighten your glutes and abs for support, then slowly lift the weights straight out to the sides until your arms are parallel to the floor. Lower your arms back to the starting position and repeat for a full set. Switch legs for the second set.

EASIER: Lightly place one foot on a step instead of suspending it in the air.

HARDER: Extend the lifted leg, holding it as high as possible while maintaining good form.

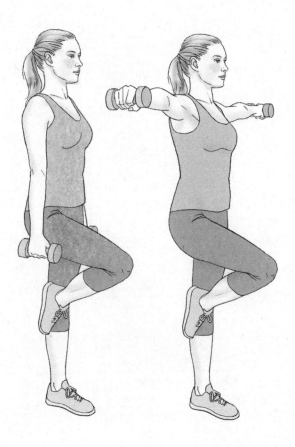

Dip and Crunch

A. Sit on the edge of a chair with your feet flat on the floor and your knees bent 90 degrees. Grasp the chair seat on either side of your butt. Walk your feet out slightly and inch yourself off the seat. Extend your right leg and plant the heel on the ground, keeping your foot flexed.

B. Bend your elbows straight back and dip your butt toward the ground while simultaneously contracting your abs and pulling your right knee toward your chest. Don't dip your elbows past 90 degrees. Return to the starting position. Complete a set (you may not be able to do 10 the first few times). Switch legs for the second set.

EASIER: Keep both legs bent while performing the move.

HARDER: Extend both legs while performing the move, bending the leg you bring to your chest.

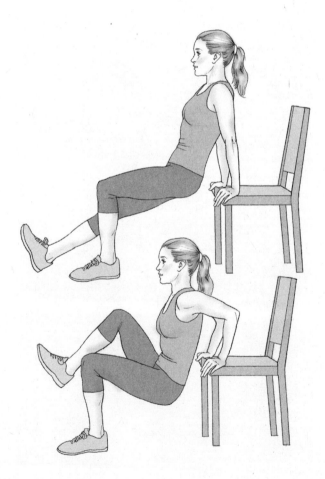

Chest-Press Punch

A. Lie on your back on a mat or carpeted floor and bend your knees. Hold two dumbbells at either side of your chest, with the ends facing each other.

B. Contract your abs and curl your head, shoulders, and torso off the floor. As you come up, extend your left arm across your body to the right as though throwing a light punch in that direction. Return to the starting position. Repeat on the opposite side. Alternate for a full set.

EASIER: Perform the move without weights.

HARDER: Punch to each side before lowering back to the starting position.

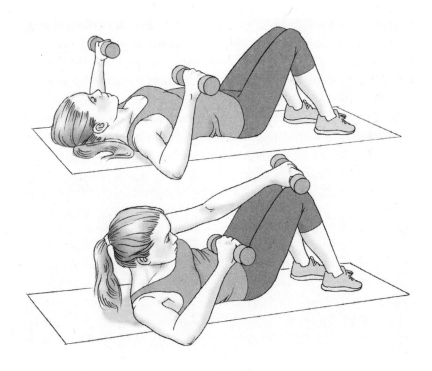

Advanced: High-Intensity Intervals

Most of you will get extremely fit just doing the intermediate program. But if you want to take it to the next level, or you're already in super shape, I definitely have some options for you.

First, forget about splitting your cardio and weight-training days. Instead, just do the weight-resistance program on pages 223–233 three to five times a week, but do it *as fast as you possibly can while maintaining good form*. This will help you achieve failure. Yes, that's an oxymoron, but it's precisely accurate. Lifting to the point where you cannot lift anymore–which in weight-lifting circles is called "lifting to failure"–has a number of metabolic benefits to help you burn more fat and shape muscle. There are many ways to do this: You can go heavy and slow or fast and light. It doesn't matter for our purposes. You just want to get to the place where lifting more is very, very hard.

To do this with your own body weight, select three to five exercises (such as the routines on pages 223–233) that will hit all your major muscle groups and do three to five sets of 10 to 12 reps, moving as quickly as you can while still maintaining good form. If you hit failure before that point, you can either try a simplified version of the exercise, reduce the amount of reps and sets you do, or try fewer exercises at a time.

For most of you, that will be enough. Pumping through 30 to 50 Hinge and Rows, Pilé Squat and Curls, Lunge and Twists, Bridge with Flies, and Kneeling Arm Raises in 10 to 15 minutes is enough to keep you in amazing shape. And there's no question it will get your heart pumping. If you want to take it to the next level, reduce the amount of time you rest and/or add more weight.

If you really enjoy cardio and can't wait to get out for a run, try doing the classic high-intensity interval training (HIIT) running sequence, in which you sprint as fast as you can for 1 minute and rest for 2 minutes. Here's how to do that.

TIME IN MINUTES	INTENSITY
0:00–3:00	Warm up with a light jog.
3:00–5:00	Increase your pace. This should be quick enough to be a little difficult but not enough to make you breathless. You'd be able to talk to a friend during this time.
5:00–6:00	Sprint as fast as you can—you should be completely out of breath after your sprint.
6:00–8:00	Resume a moderate jog for about 2 minutes, or until you are recovered.
8:00–18:00	Repeat minutes 3:00 through 8:00 for two intervals.
18:00–20:00	Cool down by walking at a slow, relaxing pace.

As you improve, you can shorten your rest periods and increase your intervals as desired. Figure out what works for you.

Once you've mastered this, you'll probably be in the best shape of your life. This is an intense program, and no one needs more exercise than this to get fit and remain healthy. But if you love a challenge, there are always ways to take your performance to the next level. Just remember not to overdo it—too much exercise doesn't serve you any better than too little.

LOOKING AHEAD

You now have all the tools you need to optimize your nutrition, reduce stress, enhance resilience, and exercise optimally. If you do everything you've learned so far, you'll go a long way toward enhancing the health of your microbiome, losing weight, and getting healthy.

That said, there's one more subject I want to address—supplements to help you lose weight and diversify your gut microbiome. There's a lot of nonsense out there when it comes to this topic. A few supplements work to support weight-loss attempts. But most of them are bunk with little or no good scientific evidence behind them. In the Appendix I'll separate the wheat from the chaff and tell you the real truth about which supplements work, which don't, and how to integrate them properly into this program.

CHAPTER 11

THE GUT BALANCE REVOLUTION

FOOD CHARTS, MEAL PLANS, SHOPPING LISTS, RECIPES, AND OTHER TIPS ON HOW TO EAT ON THE PROGRAM

F ood is medicine, and there's no better way to improve your health, lose weight, and rebalance your gut microbiome than to optimize your nutrition using the three-phase plan outlined in this book. This chapter gives you all the tools you need to do that.

I'll share more than 50 delicious anti-inflammatory, blood-glucose-balancing, fat-burning, gut-microbiome-diversifying recipes that I developed especially for this program. These recipes are something special. I worked extensively with a chef to create spectacular gourmet meals you can prepare on a budget and that follow the nutritional criteria for each phase of the program. They're easy to make–most take less than 30 minutes of prep and cook time–and they're tasty, and each and every one has the Dr. Gerry seal of approval. In fact, most of the recipes contain at least one (and in many cases more than one) of the superfoods in this book. I like to call these my WFMDs–weapons of fat mass destruction–because they'll blow the fat right off your body.

But I didn't stop there. For each phase, you'll also find a 2-week rotational meal plan to guide you on your way. I'll tell you more about how to use these in a moment. We also developed shopping lists to make your shopping experience a breeze.

If you don't want to make the recipes in this book every night, just use the Gut Balance Revolution food charts. These include the foods you should favor, eat fewer of, and forget altogether. Use these lists to create your own gut-microbiome-enhancing meals.

You'll also find tips on how to prepare foods ahead of time. You'll even find guidelines for eating out at restaurants, tips on how to prepare your pantry for the program, and more.

In short, you have all the information you need to lose weight, improve your lifestyle, and integrate the best-researched supplements for fat-burning into your daily routine.

Now it's time to put it all together, to get going with the program. And it all starts with preparing your pantry.

PREPARING A GUT-BALANCING PANTRY

The idea that the kitchen is the heart of our homes is an ancient concept that in modern times is often forgotten–it's disappearing from our culture so fast that some people see cooking as a lost art and wonder whether generations to come will have the skill set–let alone the interest–to cook. And that's something we should stand against. According to Michael Pollan in his recent book *Cooked*, each day the average American spends only 23 minutes preparing food in the kitchen and another 4 in the kitchen cleaning up. The USDA reports that the average American spends 78 minutes eating outside the home.[1] That's a real concern.

More to the point, evidence has begun to show that the amount of time you cook at home is inversely proportional to your risk of weight gain and obesity. In a study published in the *Journal of Economic Perspectives*, researchers looked at data on the correlation between obesity and home cooking across several cultures. Their findings? Cultures in which cooking at home was prominent had dramatically reduced rates of obesity.[2]

A big part of the Gut Balance Revolution is preparing your own meals. And that means reclaiming the kitchen and making it the center of family life once more. Doing this starts with setting up your kitchen and pantry with the foods you'll need to prepare (and eat!) the meals in this book. It also means cleaning out the junk food that may take up an enormous portion of the real estate in your cupboards, refrigerator, or freezer.

To prepare for the Gut Balance Revolution, here's what to do: Before Phase 1, go through your pantry (and your refrigerator) and throw out anything not allowed on the program. You can donate it if you'd like, but get it out of your house. That's because you're far more likely to eat junk food if it's around. When cravings strike, you can't give in if the food isn't there waiting for you.

Next, stock your pantry with weapons of fat mass destruction (WFMDs)–the ingredients to make the healing, gut-balancing recipes in this book. To do this, you can shop weekly for the items on the relevant shopping lists on pages 270–275. Make sure you have plenty of the superfoods for each phase on hand. And stock your spice shelf with the delicious, medicinal spices outlined in this book. Don't forget the extra-virgin olive oil (EVOO)! Consuming this good fat will help you feel satiated and actually burn fat.

Once you bring these foods into your home, organize them so they're easily accessible. Cooking in your kitchen should be an enjoyable experience. If you're scrambling around trying to buy ingredients at the last minute, or digging through the dark recesses of a disorganized dry goods cabinet, you're more likely to give up, go out, and eat off the program.

So take the time and prepare your pantry. I know it sounds like a chore, but do it. Don't underestimate this step. It will make sticking with the plan far easier, and it will set you up for long-term success.

DO-AHEAD GUIDELINES

Here are quick tips for preparing foods ahead of time to make cooking at home more convenient. The more preparation you do in advance, the more time you'll save, the easier your cooking experience will be, and the more likely you are to cook and eat at home. So strive to integrate these tips into your weekly routine.

Breakfast

Make a double batch of smoothies to freeze in airtight containers for a fast on-the-go breakfast that thaws in transit. Freezing yogurt or kefir doesn't kill their probiotics, but warming or heating in the microwave does. So let them thaw naturally.

Power Breakfast Bars (page 279) freeze well, too. Purchase a box of snack-size resealable bags–the perfect packing for individual servings–pop the bars in the bags, and toss in the freezer or fridge. Grab and go, or tuck one into your gym bag for an afterworkout meal.

You can also freeze the fully cooked Muffin-Size Frittatas (page 295) in sandwich bags. Use a permanent marker to jot down the freeze date. For a portable breakfast or a relaxing brunch entrée that's ready in minutes, thaw the frittata, unwrapped, in a 300°F oven for 10 minutes.

Lunch

Prep your greens up to 3 days in advance for fast cooking. Bok choy or Swiss chard, kale, romaine, and other mature greens can be trimmed, prewashed, and stored in large resealable plastic bags lined with paper towels to prevent wilting. Avoid washing baby greens that can easily rot, or opt for "prewashed" baby greens and tuck in a dry paper towel to keep them fresher long.

Prechop nuts and store them in the freezer to keep them from going rancid. No need to thaw them before use–just toss into salads and smoothies.

Soups freeze well and don't lose their nutrients. For Phase 1, make a double batch of the Spiced Pumpkin Soup (page 283) and Chicken Vegetable Soup (page 288). For Phase 2, prepare and freeze Cool Cucumber-Avocado Soup (page 296), Miso Soup (page 300), and Creamy Asparagus Soup (page 303). For Phase 3, rely on Wild Rice and Turkey Soup (page 314), Minestrone Soup (page 316), Turkey Chili (page 319), and Curried Red Lentil Soup (page 320), or mix and match the soups from other phases.

The Massaged Kale Salad (page 286) minus the toppings stores well in your fridge for up to 3 days. Use it as a base for any phase-appropriate protein from chicken to fish, beef, or turkey.

Prep salad dressings ahead and store in airtight containers in your fridge, like this tasty Greek Dressing for Phase 1 that you can use throughout the program.

Greek Dressing

MAKES 4 SERVINGS (2 TABLESPOONS EACH)

¼ cup extra-virgin olive oil

¼ cup lemon juice

2 teaspoons dried oregano

1 teaspoon Dijon mustard

⅛ teaspoon freshly ground black pepper

In a blender, combine the olive oil, lemon juice, oregano, mustard, and pepper and process until smooth. Transfer to an airtight container to store. Serve over the Greek Village Salad (page 280) or your own favorite medley of greens.

Dinner

Stock your freezer with frozen shrimp and place under cold running water to thaw in minutes. Similarly, if you don't have time to cook fresh shrimp, opt for cooked frozen shrimp (that's more economical) and thaw under cold running water.

Shop for a wide array of frozen berries as fast snacks to store in your freezer for up to 6 months.

Stock your pantry with low-sodium canned beans, such as chickpeas or black beans, and add this nutrient-dense prebiotic food to meals and snacks.

Both the Massaged Kale Salad (page 286) and the Greek Village Salad (page 280) will store in your fridge for up to 3 days and make perfect snacks or fast no-cook meals. Feel free to make them ahead or during the weekend.

Slow-cook your proteins to use for a quick-to-assemble supper. Cook boneless, skinless chicken breasts on low for 2 to 2½ hours with flavorings appropriate for each phase. Or cook salmon fillets (skin on) or raw shrimp on low for 1½ to 2 hours with flavorings appropriate for each phase.

Cook chicken breasts in batches. Cool and cube them, then store for up to 3 days in the fridge or freeze in 1-cup portions for fast weekday meals. See the recipe on page 240.

Buy items in bulk or family-pack sizes to save cash and trips to the store. For all phases, shop for low-sodium chicken or vegetable broth, tomato paste, kale, spinach, salad greens, frozen berries, eggs, and olive oil. Use baby or spinach greens within 5 days, but heartier greens will last up to 10, and so will eggs. For Phases 2 and 3, yogurt, kefir, lemons, avocado, and fresh ginger will store in your fridge for up to 2 weeks.

Have leftover tomato paste from a recipe? Freeze it in tablespoon-size portions in snack bags for future recipes.

Prechop celery, carrots, and garlic in a food processor for fast soup-batch cooking or for stew and salad prep.

Short on herbs for a particular recipe? Parsley and basil are all-purpose herbs that can make a tasty substitution.

Bulk Cooking Chicken

MAKES ABOUT 12 CHICKEN BREASTS

Cook chicken in bulk for fast mealtime salads.

4 pounds boneless, skinless chicken breasts

1 teaspoon salt (omit for low-sodium diets)

1 teaspoon salt-free garlic powder

1 teaspoon chili powder or mild paprika

½ teaspoon freshly ground black pepper

1. Preheat the oven to 400°F. Cover a baking sheet with foil and set aside.

2. Sprinkle the chicken with the salt (if using), garlic powder, chili powder or paprika, and pepper. Coat 2 large skillets with cooking spray and place over high heat for about 5 seconds. Place 3 or 4 breasts in each skillet without crowding them. Reduce the heat to medium and cook for 2 to 3 minutes, or until the chicken begins to brown. Turn the breasts and cook for 3 minutes. Transfer the chicken to the prepared baking sheet and repeat with the remaining breasts until the sheet is full.

3. Bake for 8 to 10 minutes, or until a thermometer inserted in the thickest part registers 165°F and the juices run clear. Let stand for 5 minutes before slicing. To store, allow the chicken to cool completely, then place in resealable bags. Store in the fridge for up to 5 days or in the freezer for up to 3 months.

Note: Cooking for just one or two? Cut the ingredient amounts in half and cook in a small skillet or use a loaf pan to bake in your toaster oven.

THE GUT BALANCE REVOLUTION FOOD CHARTS

Here are the food charts for each phase. Use these as a guideline for creating your own meals.

FOOD CHART   PHASE I

Baking Ingredients/Condiments

FAVOR

Baking powder (aluminum free)
Baking soda
Coconut, shredded
Flavor extracts, 100% (almond, orange,
    maple extract, etc.)
Mustard powder
Vinegars, clear
Wasabi powder (no colorings)

FEW

Arrowroot powder
Cocoa powder
Miso (gluten free)

Sea salt
Soy sauce (gluten free)
Tamari (gluten free)

FORGET

Condiments with unacceptable
    ingredients:
Chutney
Ketchup
Mayonnaise
Pesto
Sun-dried tomato paste

Beverages

FAVOR

Coffee
Teas: Emphasize green tea; black, white,
    and herbal teas
Water

FORGET

Apple cider
Chicory-based coffee
Fruit beverages and juice drinks or -ades
Sodas, regular and diet

PROTEIN/FAT SOURCES

Dairy

FAVOR

Butter
Cheese (Colby, Edam, feta, Gouda,
    Parmesan, Swiss)
Cheese, ripened (blue vein, Brie, Cheddar)
Fromage fraise

FORGET

Cheese, soft (cottage, ricotta, cream
    cheese, mascarpone, crème fraîche)

Cow's milk
Custard
Dairy desserts
Evaporated milk
Goat's milk
Ice cream
Milk powder
Sheep's milk
Sweetened condensed milk
Yogurt (cow's, sheep's, goat's)

Dairy-Free Alternatives

FAVOR

None

FEW

Almond, hemp, coconut, or rice nondairy
  beverages, plain and unsweetened

Coconut water

FORGET

See Dairy above

Fats and Oils

FAVOR

Canola oil (baking only)

Extra-virgin olive oil

FEW

Almond, canola, flaxseed, grapeseed,
  olive, palm, pumpkin, safflower, sesame,
  sunflower, walnut oil, etc.

Canola oil

Coconut oil, 100% palm oil (dairy-free,
  nonhydrogenated shortening)

Peanut oil

FORGET

Corn oil

Cottonseed oil

Lard

Shortening

Fish

FAVOR

Wild-caught favored over sustainably
  farmed seafood. Salmon, tilapia, Atlantic
  or Pacific (US) cod, anchovy, butterfish,
  catfish, canned light tuna, flounder,
  haddock, herring, ocean perch, mussels,
  oysters, plaice, pollock, rainbow trout,
  rockfish, sardines, scallops, sea bass
  (black), shad (US), shrimp, sole, spiny
  lobster, striped bass, trout (freshwater),
  wild eastern oyster, whitefish, and
  whiting.

FEW

Striped bass, carp, Alaskan cod, halibut,
  lobster, mahi-mahi, monkfish, perch
  (freshwater), sablefish, skate, snapper,
  tuna (canned chunk white, skipjack),
  and weakfish (sea trout), albacore or
  Yellowfin tuna (1 time weekly)

FORGET

Shark, swordfish, king mackerel, or tilefish

Meat (Organic, Pasture Fed and Raised)

FAVOR

Poultry (chicken, turkey, duck) without skin

Whole eggs, egg whites

Wild game

FEW

Lean cuts of meat (beef, lamb, pork);
  grass-fed, organic favored

FORGET

Fatty cuts of meat (beef, pork, lamb)

Poultry with skin

Processed or aged meat and poultry
  products (hot dogs, deli meats, canned
  meat products, etc.)

FOOD CHART PHASE I

Fruits

FAVOR

Banana (green)
Blueberry
Cantaloupe
Cherries (sour)
Cranberries (whole)
Honeydew melon
Kiwifruit
Lemon
Lime
Passionfruit
Plums
Raspberries

FEW

Avocado
Grape
Grapefruit
Orange
Papaya
Pomegranate
Rhubarb
Starfruit
Strawberry

Tangelo
Tangerine
Tomato

FORGET

Apples
Applesauce and apple cider
Apricots
Blackberries
Boysenberries
Dried fruits (dates, figs, prunes, etc.)
Fruit beverages
Fruit juices or fruit concentrates (100%)
Fruits, canned in syrups
Mango
Nashi fruit
Nectarines
Peaches
Pears
Persimmon
Pineapple
Plantains
Tamarillo
Watermelon

Herbs and Spices

FAVOR

Fresh and/or dried herbs and spices:
  Cardamom
  Cayenne (ground red) pepper
  Cinnamon
  Cumin
  Ginger

FORGET

Herb or spice mixes or seasonings with
  unacceptable food ingredients

(continued)

Legumes (Vegetable Protein), Nuts, and Seeds

FEW

Almonds

Cashews

Chia seeds

Flaxseeds (linseed)

Hazelnuts

Natural nut butters made from almonds,
  Brazil nuts, pecans, walnuts

Natural seed butters made from chia,
  flaxseeds, hempseeds, pumpkin, sesame,
  sunflower

Nut and seed beverages

Pistachios

Poppy seeds

Pumpkin seeds (pepitas)

Sesame seeds

Sunflower seeds

FORGET

Baked beans, bean sprouts, black-eyed
  beans, borlotti beans, broad beans (fava
  beans), chickpeas (garbanzo beans),
  kidney beans, lentils, navy beans, peas,
  split peas

Highly processed soy foods or legume
  products (tofu hot dogs, soy chips,
  garbanzo bean chips, etc.)

Highly processed vegetable protein
  alternatives (Quorn, seitan)

Nut and seed butters made with
  hydrogenated or peanut oils

Nut and seed products with unacceptable
  toxic ingredients

Soybeans (edamame, tofu, miso, tempeh)

Tahini

Other

FAVOR

Garlic-infused olive oil

Ginger

Stevia

FORGET

Agave syrup

Brown rice syrup

Chocolate, cocoa products

Evaporated cane juice

Fruit sweeteners

Glucose

High-fructose corn syrup–containing
  foods and beverages

Honey

Mannitol

Maple syrup, artificial

Maple syrup, 100%

Molasses, blackstrap

Sorbitol

Sucrose (table sugar)

Xylitol

Vegetables

FAVOR

Alfalfa sprouts

Bamboo shoots

Beans (green)

Bean sprouts

Bok choy

Butternut squash

Capsicum

Celery

Chard (Swiss)

Chives

Choy sum

Cucumber

Eggplant

Endive

Escarole

Greens (mustard, collard)
Kabocha squash (Japanese pumpkin)
Kale
Lettuce
Olives
Parsnip
Pumpkin
Radish
Silverbeet
Spaghetti squash (baked)
Spinach
Spring onion (green part only)
Squash (yellow, zucchini, butternut)
Turnips

FEW
Artichokes (globe and Jerusalem)
Asparagus
Beetroot
Broccoli
Brussels sprouts
Button mushrooms

Cabbage
Carrot
Cauliflower
Fennel
Garlic
Green peas
Leek
Okra
Onions (mature, cooking)
Shallots
Snap peas
Snow peas
Sweet corn
Sweet potato
Tomato juice (100%)
Vegetable juice (100%)

FORGET
All vegetables breaded, creamed, and fried
Overcooked tempura
Vegetable juices made with vegetables on
   Forget list
White potato

Whole Grains and Flours

FEW
Buckwheat
Corn
Gluten-free bread, cracker (plain,
   unseasoned), and cereal products*
Millet
Oat bran
Oats

Polenta
Quinoa
Rice
Sweet biscuit

FORGET
Barley-, rye-, and wheat-based bread,
   crackers, pasta, cereal, couscous, gnocchi,
   noodles, croissants, muffins, crumpets

*All grain and flour-based products must be labeled gluten free.

Beverages

FAVOR

Black tea
Ginger-herbal teas
Green tea
Water
Whey
White tea

FEW

Coconut water
Coffee
Fermented beers*

Limit to 1 serving (glass) per day.

Kefir (variety of animal, seed, and nut milk sources)
Milk: 2% organic animal milk; nondairy (soy, almond, hemp), plain and unsweetened
Red wine*

FORGET

Fruit juices
Rice milk
Sodas
Sugar-sweetened beverages

Condiments

FAVOR

Arrowroot powder
Baking powder (aluminum free)
Baking soda
Cocoa powder
Flavor extracts, 100% (almond, orange, maple extract, etc.)
Mustard powder
Vinegars (clear)
Wasabi powder (no colorings)

FEW

Fruit-based condiments:*
  Chutney
  Ketchup
  Sun-dried tomato paste
Miso (gluten free)
Sea salt†
Soy sauce (gluten free)
Tamari (gluten free)

FORGET

Condiments with unacceptable ingredients:
  Mayonnaise
  Pesto

High FODMAP
†High sodium

Fruits

FAVOR

Apples
Apricots
Avocado
Banana**
Berries (blue, black, etc.)
Cantaloupe

Carambola (star fruit)
Cherries (sour)
Cranberries
Figs
Grapefruit
Grapes (concord)
Honeydew melon

**Bananas are high in resistant starch and feed beneficial bacteria; it's best to eat a firm greenish banana.*

Kiwifruit
Lemon
Lime
Oranges (tangelo)
Papaya
Passionfruit
Peaches
Pear (Asian)
Persimmon
Plums
Rhubarb

FEW
Grapes (green, red)

Mango
Oranges (navel, Florida)
Pears (Anjou, Bartlett)
Pineapple
Plantains
Watermelon

FORGET
Apple cider
Applesauce
Dried fruits (dates, prunes, etc.)
Fruit beverages
Fruit juices or fruit concentrates (100%)
Fruits, canned in syrups

Grains

FEW
Amaranth
Brown rice
Buckwheat
Oat bran
Popcorn
Quinoa
Teff

FORGET
Barley
Millet
Rye
Spelt
Wheat products

Oils

FAVOR
Canola (baking only)
Extra-virgin olive

FEW
Almond
Butter (from grass-fed cows)
Canola (baking preferred)
Coconut
Flaxseed
Grapeseed
Palm
Pumpkin

Safflower
Sesame
Sunflower
Walnut

FORGET
Corn
Lard
Margarine
Palm, hydrogenated
Safflower
Shortening

FOOD CHART   PHASE 2

Soups

FAVOR

Vegetable, bean, chicken (white meat, no
  noodles)

FORGET

Cream-based

Spices

FAVOR

Black pepper

Cardamon

Cayenne (ground red) pepper

Cinnamon

Cumin

Garlic

Garlic-infused olive oil

Ginger, fresh or ground

Herbs

Mustard

Turmeric

Sweet Additions

FAVOR

Stevia

FEW

Brown rice syrup

Chocolate (dark)

Cocoa products

Evaporated cane juice

Glucose

Honey, raw

Maple syrup (pure)

Molasses, blackstrap

Sucrose (table sugar)

FORGET

Agave syrup

Artificial sweeteners

Fruit sweeteners

High-fructose corn syrup (foods and
  beverages)

Honey, refined

Mannitol

Sorbitol

Xylitol

Vegetables

FAVOR

Alfalfa

Artichokes (globe and Jerusalem)

Asparagus

Bamboo shoots

Beans (green)

Bean sprouts

Bok choy

Brussels sprouts

Butternut squash

Cabbage

Carrots

Cauliflower

Chard (Swiss)

Chicory root, raw

Chives

Choy sum

Cruciferous vegetables

Cucumber

Dandelion

Eggplant

Endive

Escarole

Fennel

Garlic
Green peas
Greens (collard, mustard, turnip)
Kabocha (Japanese pumpkin)
Kale
Leek
Lettuce
Mesclun greens
Mushrooms
Okra
Olives
Onion
Parsnips
Pumpkin
Radish
Shallots
Silverbeet
Snap peas
Snow peas
Spaghetti squash (baked)
Spinach
Spring onion (green part only)
Squash (yellow, zucchini, butternut)
Tomato

Pickled foods:
Fermented tofu
Korean kimchi
Miso
Natto
Pickled beets
Pickled cabbage
Pickled corn relish
Pickled cucumbers
Pickled garlic
Pickled radish
Sauerkraut
Soy sauce
Tempeh

FEW
Beets (nonpickled)
Sweet corn
Sweet potato*

FORGET
All vegetables breaded, creamed, and
   fried
Overcooked tempura
Vegetable juices made with vegetables on
   forget list
White potato products

Baked with skin—highly satiogenic, high fiber, anti-inflammatory.

PROTEIN/FAT SOURCES

Dairy

FAVOR
Butter
Cheese (Colby, Edam, feta, Gouda,
   mozzarella, Parmesan, Swiss)
Cheese, ripened (blue vein, Brie, Cheddar)
Cheese, soft (cottage, ricotta, cream
   cheese, mascarpone, crème fraîche)
Fromage fraise
Greek yogurt
Yogurt (cow's, sheep's, goat's), home-
   made preferred
Yogurt, nondairy (almond, soy, coconut)

FEW
Lactose-free frozen yogurt
Sour cream

FORGET
Cow's milk
Custard
Dairy desserts
Evaporated milk
Goat's milk
Ice cream

(continued)

Fish

FAVOR

Wild-caught favored over sustainably farmed seafood. Salmon, tilapia, Atlantic or Pacific (US) cod, anchovy, butterfish, catfish, canned light tuna, flounder, haddock, herring, ocean perch, mussels, oysters, plaice, pollock, rainbow trout, rockfish, sardines, scallops, sea bass (black), shad (US), shrimp, sole, spiny lobster, striped bass, trout (freshwater), wild eastern oyster, whitefish, and whiting.

FEW

Striped bass, carp, Alaskan cod, halibut, lobster, mahi-mahi, monkfish, perch (freshwater), sablefish, skate, snapper, tuna (canned chunk white, skipjack), and weakfish (sea trout), albacore or Yellowfin tuna (1 time weekly)

FORGET

Shark, swordfish, king mackerel, or tilefish

Legumes

FAVOR

Chickpeas and other white beans (i.e., cannellini)
Kidney beans

Lentils
Mung beans
Soybeans

Meat

FAVOR

White meat poultry
Wild game (deer, buffalo, bison)

FEW

Lean meats (beef, lamb, pork), grass-fed, organic favored

FORGET

Dark meat poultry

Fatty cuts of meat (rib eye, lamb, duck)
Hamburger
Milk powder
Poultry with skin
Processed cheeses
Processed meats (hot dogs, deli meats, canned meats like Spam)
Sheep's milk
Sweetened condensed milk

Nuts

FAVOR

Almonds
Brazil nuts
Hazelnuts
Peanuts
Pecans
Pine nuts
Pistachios
Walnuts

FEW

Cashews
Macadamia nuts

FORGET

Processed nut and seed butters with hydrogenated oils and sweeteners

FOOD CHART — PHASE 2

Other

FAVOR
Soy
Eggs (whole, whites)

Seeds

FAVOR
Chia seeds
Flaxseeds (ground)
Hemp seeds
Poppy seeds
Pumpkin seeds (pepitas)
Sesame seeds (tahini)
Sunflower seeds

FOOD CHART — PHASE 3

Beverages

FAVOR
Black tea
Ginger-herbal teas
Green tea
Kefir (variety of animal, seed, and nut milk sources)
Water
Whey
White tea

Coffee*
Fermented beers*
Fruit juices
Milk: low-fat organic animal milk; nondairy (soy, almond, hemp), plain and unsweetened
Red wine*
Rice milk

FORGET
Any except for sodas, sugar-sweetened beverages, which are consumed rarely

FEW
Coconut water (without added sugar)

*Limit to 1 serving (glass) per day.

Condiments

FAVOR
Arrowroot powder
Baking powder (aluminum free)
Baking soda
Cocoa powder
Flavor extracts, 100% (almond, orange, maple, etc.)
Mustard powder
Vinegars (clear)
Wasabi powder (no colorings)

FEW
Mayonnaise
Miso (gluten free)
Pesto
Sea salt†
Soy sauce (gluten free)
Tamari (gluten free)
Fruit-based condiments:††
  Chutney
  Ketchup
  Sun-dried tomato paste

†High sodium
††High FODMAP

Fruits

FAVOR

Apples
Apricots
Avocado
Banana*
Berries (blue, black etc.)
Cantaloupe
Carambola (star fruit)
Cherries (sour)
Cranberries
Figs
Grapefruit
Grapes (concord)
Grapes (green, red)
Honeydew melon
Kiwifruit
Lemon
Lime
Mango
Oranges (navel, Florida)
Oranges (tangelo)
Papaya
Passionfruit
Peaches
Pears (Anjou, Asian, Bartlett)
Persimmon
Pineapple
Plantains
Plums
Rhubarb
Watermelon

FEW

Apple cider
Applesauce
Dried fruits (dates, prunes, etc.)
Fruit juices or fruit concentrates (100%)
Fruits, canned in syrups

FORGET

None

*Bananas are high in resistant starch and feed beneficial bacteria—best to eat a firm-greenish banana.

Grains

FAVOR

Amaranth
Brown rice
Buckwheat
Oat bran
Popcorn
Quinoa
Teff

FEW

Barley*
Millet*
Rye*
Spelt*
Wheat products (whole grain)*

FORGET

None except for white-flour-based
    products, which should be limited: noodles,
    croissants, muffins, crumpets, etc.

*Those with celiac disease, nonceliac gluten sensitivity, and/or wheat allergy should avoid these grains.

FOOD CHART   PHASE 3

Oils

FAVOR
Almond
Canola
Coconut
Extra-virgin olive
Flaxseed
Grapeseed
Palm
Pumpkin
Safflower

Sesame
Sunflower
Walnut

FEW
Butter (grass-fed)
Sesame

FORGET
None except for corn oil, lard, margarine,
   hydrogenated palm oil, safflower oil,
   shortening

Soups

FAVOR
Miso
Vegetable-based, legume-based, lean
   poultry with whole grains

FEW
Cream-based

FORGET
None

Spices

FAVOR
Black pepper
Cardamon
Cayenne (ground red) pepper
Cinnamon
Cumin
Garlic

Garlic-infused olive oil
Ginger, fresh or ground
Herbs
Mustard
Turmeric

FORGET
None

Sweet Additions

FAVOR
Chocolate (dark)*
Stevia

FEW
Agave syrup
Brown rice syrup
Chocolate (dark)
Cocoa products
Evaporated cane juice

Fruit sweeteners
Glucose
Honey
Maple syrup (pure)
Molasses, blackstrap
Sucrose (table sugar)

FORGET
None except limit (rare) artificial sweeteners,
   high-fructose corn syrup (in foods and
   beverages), mannitol, sorbitol, xylitol

Dark chocolate should be 70% or greater cocoa and be limited to 2 ounces per day.

Vegetables

FAVOR

Alfalfa
Artichokes (globe and Jerusalem)
Asparagus
Bamboo shoots
Beans (green)
Bean sprouts
Beets (nonpickled)
Bok choy
Brussels sprouts
Cabbage
Carrots
Cauliflower
Chard (Swiss)
Chicory root, raw
Chives
Choy sum
Cruciferous vegetables
Cucumber
Dandelion
Eggplant
Endive
Escarole
Fennel
Garlic
Green peas
Greens (collard, mustard, turnip)
Kabocha (Japanese pumpkin)
Kale
Leek
Lettuce
Mesclun greens
Mushrooms
Okra
Olives
Onion
Parsnips

Pickled foods:
  Fermented tofu
  Korean kimchi
  Miso
  Natto
  Pickled beets
  Pickled cabbage
  Pickled corn relish
  Pickled cucumbers
  Pickled garlic
  Pickled radish
  Sauerkraut
  Soy sauce
  Tempeh
Pumpkin
Radish
Shallots
Silverbeet
Snap peas
Snow peas
Spaghetti squash (baked)
Spinach
Spring onion (green part only)
Squash (yellow, zucchini, butternut)
Sweet corn
Sweet potato*
Tomato

FEW

All vegetables breaded, creamed, and
  fried
Overcooked tempura
Vegetable juices made with vegetables on
  Avoid list
White potato products

FORGET

None

Baked with skin—highly satiogenic, high fiber, anti-inflammatory.

PROTEIN/FAT SOURCES

Dairy

FAVOR

Butter

Cheese (Colby, Edam, feta, Gouda, mozzarella, Parmesan, Swiss)

Cheese, ripened (blue vein, Brie, Cheddar)

Cheese, soft (cottage, ricotta, cream cheese, mascarpone, crème fraîche)

Fromage fraise

Greek yogurt

Sour cream

Yogurt (cow's, sheep's, goat's), home-made preferred

Yogurt, nondairy

FEW

Cow's milk

Custard

Dairy desserts

Evaporated milk

Goat's milk

Ice cream

Lactose-free frozen yogurt

Milk powder

Sheep's milk

Sweetened condensed milk

FORGET

None except for processed cheeses

Fish

FAVOR

Wild-caught favored over sustainably farmed seafood. Salmon, tilapia, Atlantic or Pacific (US) cod, anchovy, butterfish, catfish, canned light tuna, flounder, haddock, herring, ocean perch, mussels, oysters, plaice, pollock, rainbow trout, rockfish, sardines, scallops, sea bass (black), shad (US), shrimp, sole, spiny lobster, striped bass, trout (freshwater), wild eastern oyster, whitefish, and whiting.

FEW

Striped bass, carp, Alaskan cod, halibut, lobster, mahi-mahi, monkfish, perch (freshwater), sablefish, skate, snapper, tuna (canned chunk white, skipjack), and weakfish (sea trout), albacore or Yellowfin tuna (1 time weekly)

FORGET

Shark, swordfish, king mackerel, or tilefish

Legumes

FAVOR

Chickpeas and other white beans (i.e., cannellini)

Kidney beans

Lentils

Mung beans

Soybeans

FORGET

None except for highly processed soy and legume foods (tofu hot dogs, soy chips, garbanzo bean chips, lentil chips, etc.), which are rarely consumed

(continued)

FOOD CHART   PHASE 3

Meat

FAVOR

Lean meats (beef, lamb, pork), grass-fed, organic favored

White-meat poultry

Wild game (deer, buffalo, bison)

FEW

Dark-meat poultry

Fatty cuts of meat (rib eye, lamb, duck)

Hamburger

Poultry with skin

FORGET

None except for processed meats (hot dogs, deli meats, canned meats like Spam), which are rarely consumed

Nuts

FAVOR

Almonds

Brazil nuts

Cashews

Hazelnuts

Macadamia nuts

Peanuts

Pecans

Pine nuts

Pistachios

Walnuts

FORGET

None except for processed nut and seed butters with hydrogenated oils and sweeteners

Other

FAVOR

Eggs (organic; whole, whites)

Soy

Seeds

FAVOR

Chia seeds

Flaxseeds (ground)

Hemp seeds

Poppy seeds

Pumpkin seeds (pepita)

Sesame seeds (tahini)

Sunflower seeds

THE GUT BALANCE REVOLUTION SUCCESS STORIES

Cindy Lindgren, 49
Scott Lindgren, 50

Looking for Cindy and Scott Lindgren on a Saturday? In the not-too-distant past, you'd find them sitting at their kitchen table with a cup of coffee and a box of Pop-Tarts. These days, though, you'll have a tough time tracking them down. They might be visiting the farmers' market or exploring a park or hanging out with friends. "Nowadays, if we switch on the TV," Cindy says, "we'll look at each other and say, 'Let's not watch this.' "

For Cindy and Scott, life has been transformed. Cindy, plagued by digestive issues in the wake of gallbladder surgery, struggled to find a solution to the constant nausea and diarrhea. "It really limited my life," she recalls. "I was exhausted all the time and constantly worried about what I could eat—and where the bathroom was." But that changed when she started on the Gut Balance Revolution.

Within 6 weeks, Cindy's symptoms were nearly gone. And there was an unexpected bonus. Her husband, Scott, who'd been trying to lose weight for years, dropped 19 pounds. "Both of us began feeling so much better," Cindy says, "just by eating healthy foods and getting rid of all that processed stuff. Instead of relying on takeout, it's amazing how quickly you can fix a meal that's delicious and healthy—without turning your kitchen into a science project."

Lots of other things changed, too. For Cindy, a quality assurance executive for a nonprofit organization, the business lunches are no longer a nightmare. And she and Scott can enjoy having dinner with friends, take in a movie, and even go to football parties. "Our world has opened up again," she says.

Best of all, Cindy and Scott have adopted a beagle puppy named Gunnar. "Taking care of a puppy can be overwhelming," Cindy says. "Gunnar is so full of energy and intellect, and before, we would've been way too sluggish to be able to deal with him. But we take him to puppy kindergarten, and we go on adventures with him—there's no way you can just sit on the couch with a puppy in the house. The Gut Balance Revolution has completely reinvigorated us!"

Here are the Gut Balance Revolution meal plans. For each phase, I've provided 2 weeks' worth of menus. You can repurpose these week after week or mix up the meals within them as you choose. The other options are simple "no cook" meals you can make by

	BREAKFAST	LUNCH
Monday	Blueberry Protein Smoothie (page 276)	Spiced Pumpkin Soup with chicken (page 283)
Tuesday	Eggs to Go (page 277)	Raspberry Mesclun Salad with Green Tea Dressing with chicken or shrimp (page 284)
Wednesday	2 scrambled eggs or 4 ounces scrambled tofu with 2 cups steamed broccoli	Green salad: mixed greens, tomatoes, celery, cucumbers, sliced or shredded almonds, grilled chicken, olive oil vinaigrette
Thursday	Power Breakfast Bar (page 279)	Crunchy Almond Tuna Salad (page 285)
Friday	Vanilla Spice Quinoa Breakfast Cereal (page 278)	Greek Village Salad (page 280)
Saturday	2 poached eggs on 2 cups raw spinach or arugula	Massaged Kale Salad with chicken or shrimp (page 286)
Sunday	Breakfast Roll-Up: ½ chicken sausage link or ¼ cup chicken cooked with 1 egg rolled in 1 corn tortilla	Leftover Slow-Cooker Chicken Piccata

combining the ingredients listed. If you prefer some recipes over others, or if you need to switch a "no cook" option for a recipe or vice versa, feel free to make those changes as needed.

SNACK	DINNER
¼ avocado mashed with 2 table-spoons onion-free salsa served with celery sticks or lettuce leaves	Orange Salmon with bok choy (page 281)
Fat-Burning Tea: ⅓ cup protein shake mixed with 1 cup hot water with a pinch of cinnamon and cayenne (ground red) pepper	Spiced Pork Roast with Cauliflower Mash (page 289)
2 hard-cooked eggs or 10 walnuts or almonds with Cilantro Green Drink or Basil Green Drink (page 336)	Pesto Baked Cod with spaghetti squash (page 282)
2 tablespoons chia seeds mixed with ½ cup plain, unsweetened coconut milk and a drizzle of vanilla extract	Chicken Lettuce Wraps: cubed cooked chicken served in lettuce leaves spritzed with fresh lime juice and topped with 2 tablespoons unsweetened shredded coconut
Ginger-Crusted Kale Chips (page 290)	Broiled cod or shrimp with black pepper and fresh lemon served over salad greens
4 teaspoons almond butter spread inside celery sticks	Slow-Cooker Chicken Piccata (page 287)
Coconut Joy Pudding (page 291)	Grilled cod kabobs with cubed veggies served over ½ cup cooked quinoa tossed with herbs

(continued)

	BREAKFAST	LUNCH
Monday	Power Breakfast Bar (page 279)	4 ounces smoked salmon over baby greens or grilled zucchini, peppers
Tuesday	Blueberry Protein Smoothie (page 276)	Fast Gazpacho: 1 tomato, ½ cucumber, ½ green or red bell pepper blended with lemon or lime juice and a pinch of salt, topped with 1 cup cubed cooked chicken or shrimp
Wednesday	¼ cup dried quinoa flakes cooked according to package directions with ⅓ cup whey protein powder stirred in and a pinch of cinnamon or cloves	1 can spring-water-packed tuna, drained, mixed with olive oil and paprika, served with cucumber and red bell pepper wedges or over greens
Thursday	Coffee- or Tea- Flavored Smoothie: 1 cup cold coffee or tea blended with ½ cup berries, ⅓ cup whey protein powder	Crunchy Almond Tuna Salad (page 285)
Friday	Vanilla Spice Quinoa Breakfast Cereal (page 278)	2 cups low-sodium canned chicken and vegetable soup (no noodles) or leftover Chicken Vegetable Soup
Saturday	Blueberry Protein Smoothie (page 276)	½ dozen oysters with lemon juice, green salad with olive oil vinaigrette
Sunday	2 poached eggs on 2 cups steamed broccoli or 1 cup sautéed spinach	Chicken Vegetable Soup (page 288)

SNACK	DINNER
1 cup frozen edamame pods steamed and sprinkled with spices of your choice, such as black pepper, cumin, paprika, or hot chili powder	Steamed veggies and stir-fried chicken (no sauce)
⅓ cup whey protein powder blended with cold green tea	Take-out or homemade steamed veggies (such as broccoli, peppers, zucchini, or spinach) with chicken or shrimp (no sauce)
2 hard-cooked eggs with Cilantro Green Drink or Basil Green Drink (page 336)	Take-out egg drop soup with a side of steamed broccoli
Unsweetened Iced Coffee: 1 cup cold coffee; 2 tablespoons plain, unsweetened coconut milk; pinch of cinnamon; 2 tablespoons whey protein powder	Roast chicken (skin discarded) with a side of green beans topped with nuts or olive oil
Ginger-Crusted Kale Chips (page 290)	Orange Salmon with Swiss Chard (page 281)
¼ cup blueberries with 10 plain almonds or walnuts and ginger tea	Chicken breast cooked in the slow cooker for 2 hours on low, topped with freshly grated ginger, 1 tablespoon tomato paste, spices of your choice; served over cooked greens, such as bok choy
Satay Veggie Dip: 2 tablespoons almond butter mixed with 2 tablespoons plain, unsweetened coconut milk and a pinch of cayenne (ground red) pepper; served with celery, sliced bell peppers, or cucumber wedges	Spiced Pork Roast with Cauliflower Mash (page 289)

(continued)

	BREAKFAST	LUNCH
Monday	Pumpkin Pie Yogurt Parfait (page 293)	Chicken Tikka Masala (page 297)
Tuesday	Pomegranate Margarita Smoothie (page 294)	1 cup three-bean salad dressed with olive oil vinaigrette over 2 cups greens; add 1 cup cooked cubed chicken or shrimp
Wednesday	⅓ cup dry buckwheat porridge cooked according to package directions with 1 tablespoon ground flaxseeds, ¼ sliced banana, 10 pecans or slivered almonds	Leftover Ginger Fried Rice
Thursday	Muffin-Size Frittatas (page 295)	Fish sushi (brown rice only) served over green salad tossed with sesame oil
Friday	2 scrambled eggs with 2 tablespoons chopped kimchi or pickle of your choice	Leftover Sautéed Apples and Chicken Sausage with Sauerkraut
Saturday	Berries and "Cream": ½ cup berries topped with ½ cup unsweetened kefir or yogurt whipped with 2 tablespoons plain, unsweetened coconut milk and optional stevia or vanilla	Arugula Salad with Creamy Avocado Dressing (page 302)
Sunday	Salsa and Eggs (page 292)	Creamy Asparagus Soup with chicken or shrimp (page 303)

SNACK	DINNER
Savory Yogurt Dip: ½ cup plain yogurt mixed with a pinch of cumin, hot chili powder, and black pepper; serve with sliced green bell pepper and celery	Tangy Buffalo Burger with Pickles and Slaw (page 299)
3 tablespoons store-bought hummus with celery and cucumber wedges	Ginger Fried Rice with chicken or shrimp or tofu (page 301)
½ cup plain yogurt with a few berries, ground flaxseeds, unsweetened cocoa powder, and/or coconut	Miso Soup with Seaweed Salad and salmon (page 300)
12 pistachios and 1 ounce chopped 85% dark chocolate	Sautéed Apples and Chicken Sausage with Sauerkraut (page 304)
Coconut Banana: ½ banana, cut into chunks, dipped in yogurt and rolled in 2 tablespoons unsweetened coconut	Pistachio-Chia Salmon with butternut squash (page 305)
Creamy Strawberry Sorbet (page 308)	Kimchi Pork Lo Mein (page 307)
Dark Chocolate Nut Clusters (page 309)	Cajun Cod (page 306) with beans

(continued)

	BREAKFAST	LUNCH
Monday	½ cup cooked old-fashioned rolled oats topped with 2 table-spoons canned pumpkin or berries or with 1 tablespoon nuts	Chicken Tikka Masala (page 297)
Tuesday	1 cup yogurt or kefir topped with ¼ cup fresh raspberries	1 cup three-bean salad dressed with olive oil vinaigrette over 2 cups greens; add 1 cup cooked cubed chicken or shrimp (opposite protein source from week 1)
Wednesday	Muffin-Size Frittatas (page 295)	Massaged Kale Salad (page 286) topped with 1 tablespoon chopped kimchi or pickles
Thursday	Pumpkin Pie Yogurt Parfait (page 293)	Leftover Zesty Lemon Chicken Salad
Friday	Salsa and Eggs (page 292)	Broiled shrimp or fish with grilled asparagus; Caesar salad (no croutons)
Saturday	½ cup cooked quinoa topped with ½ cup 2% plain kefir or yogurt, ½ teaspoon cinnamon	Creamy Asparagus Soup with chicken or shrimp (page 303)
Sunday	Pomegranate Margarita Smoothie (page 294)	1 cup shredded chicken with ½ cup cooked quinoa mixed with 2 tablespoons beans (any variety)

SNACK	DINNER
1 cup seaweed salad (homemade or store-bought)	Cool Cucumber-Avocado Soup with chicken or shrimp (page 296)
½ cup plain yogurt with a few berries, ground flaxseeds, unsweetened cocoa powder, and/or coconut	4 ounces extra-firm tofu sautéed in 1 tablespoon olive oil with ½ cup each broccoli florets and spinach; top with 1 teaspoon soy sauce or raw apple cider vinegar
2 tablespoons canned black beans mashed with 2 teaspoons olive oil and spices of your choice, served with celery and cucumber wedges	Zesty Lemon Chicken Salad (page 298)
1 cup leftover Cool Cucumber-Avocado Soup	Broiled cod with black pepper and fresh lemon served over salad greens
2 ounces store-bought spicy or mild seaweed chips	Grilled chicken with dill pickles over a plain salad
Frozen Berry Pops: ½ cup plain unsweetened kefir or yogurt blended with ¼ cup berries and optional stevia; freeze for 4 hours in ice pop molds or paper cups	Canned lentil soup topped with 1 cup cubed cooked chicken, shrimp, or tofu
10 macadamia nuts or hazelnuts and 1 ounce 85% dark chocolate	Pistachio-Chia Salmon with butternut squash (page 305)

(continued)

	BREAKFAST	LUNCH
Monday	Blueberry-Spice Waffles (page 313)	Quinoa Salad with Lemony Yogurt Dressing (page 315)
Tuesday	⅓ cup old-fashioned rolled oats cooked with 1 tablespoon flax-seeds and a pinch of cinnamon; stir in ⅓ cup whey protein powder	2 cups Minestrone Soup (page 316) sprinkled with Parmesan or Locatelli Pecorino Romano cheese
Wednesday	Fresh Cranberry-Spice Smoothie (page 311)	Dr. Gerry's Super Salmon Salad (page 317)
Thursday	Mediterranean Sunrise Surprise (page 310)	Leftover Turkey Chili
Friday	Lean Green Smoothie with Apple and Kale (page 312)	Smoked Salmon Salad (page 321)
Saturday	Leftover Blueberry Spice Waffles	Baked Zucchini Boats: zucchini, sliced in half lengthwise, each half topped with 2 tablespoons marinara and 2 tablespoons chopped cooked chicken, shrimp, or tofu
Sunday	Mocha Smoothie: 1 cup cold cof-fee blended with ½ cup 2% plain kefir or yogurt, ⅓ cup protein powder, 2 teaspoons unsweet-ened cocoa powder and optional stevia	Curried Red Lentil Soup with chicken or shrimp (page 320)

SNACK	DINNER
½ apple covered with 1 table-spoon almond butter and a pinch of cinnamon	Dr. Gerry's Super Salmon Salad (page 317), 1 cup Minestrone Soup (page 316)
Cucumber Salad: ½ thinly sliced cuke with 2 tablespoons yogurt or kefir and 1 tablespoon fresh lemon juice; add a pinch of spice	Zucchini Manicotti (page 325) with a side of tossed greens salad
½ apple with 1 square dark choc-olate	Turkey Chili (page 319)
½ cup 2% plain Greek yogurt with berries and/or shaved dark chocolate	Salmon Cakes with greens (page 323)
Dark Chocolate Flourless Cake (page 326)	Roasted Parmesan-Kale Lamb Chops (page 324)
½ apple with almond butter and a sprinkle of ground flaxseed	Roasted Rosemary Chicken with Brussels Sprouts (page 322)
Leftover Dark Chocolate Flourless Cake	Sunday Stew (page 318)

(continued)

	BREAKFAST	LUNCH
Monday	2 poached eggs over raw baby kale or kale roasted at 400°F for 10 minutes with 2 teaspoons olive oil	Quinoa Salad with Lemony Yogurt Dressing (page 315)
Tuesday	Fresh Cranberry-Spice Smoothie (page 311)	Leftover Wild Rice and Turkey Soup
Wednesday	Lean Green Smoothie with Apple and Kale (page 312) **or** Mediterranean Sunrise Surprise (page 310)	2 cups Minestrone Soup (page 316)
Thursday	Fresh Cranberry-Spice Smoothie (page 311)	Greek Village Salad (page 280)
Friday	Blueberry-Spice Waffles (page 313)	Chopped Salad: chicken, avocado, cucumber, tomato, and egg (no cheese) over greens
Saturday	Lean Green Smoothie with Apple and Kale (page 312)	Soup: 1 cup cooked cubed chicken warmed in a saucepan with 2 cups store-bought broth, 1 cup baby spinach, and 1 cup finely chopped broccoli florets
Sunday	Eggs Benedict: 2 poached eggs over greens topped with ½ cup yogurt whipped with herbs and 1 teaspoon lemon juice	Dr. Gerry's Super Salmon Salad (page 317)

SNACK	DINNER
10 nuts (such as walnuts, almonds, or macadamias) and ¼ cup berries, any variety	Wild Rice and Turkey Soup (page 314) with a side of tossed greens salad
2 tablespoons store-bought hummus mixed with 1 tablespoon ground flaxseeds and served with veggie sticks	Surf and Turf: broiled shrimp and small filet mignon (no sauce) served with sautéed greens or plain grilled salad
Fast Artichoke Dip: 3 thawed artichoke hearts blended with ½ cup 2% plain Greek yogurt and a pinch of cayenne or garlic powder and served with raw veggies	Simple Chicken Parm: 1 cup cooked cubed chicken with 2 tablespoons marinara and 1 tablespoon grated Parmesan cheese; warm in the oven and serve over 2 cups baby spinach
½ cup 2% plain Greek yogurt with berries and/or shaved dark chocolate	Zucchini Manicotti with tossed salad (page 325)
2 zucchini strips thinly sliced lengthwise, topped with 1 tablespoon yogurt or kefir and 2 slices smoked salmon	Salmon Cakes with greens (page 323)
½ apple with almond butter and a sprinkle of ground flaxseeds	Surf and Turf: broiled shrimp and small filet mignon (no sauce) served with sautéed greens or plain grilled salad
Almond Yogurt: ½ cup 2% plain kefir or yogurt mixed with 2 tablespoons chopped almonds and ¼ teaspoon almond extract	Roasted Parmesan-Kale Lamb Chops (page 324)

THE GUT BALANCE REVOLUTION SHOPPING LISTS

These shopping lists go along with the meal plans on pages 258–269. Assuming you stick to the meal plans, all you have to do is buy the ingredients on these lists. I have broken these out into weekly shopping lists. Try to shop a couple of days before you start a new week on the program.

SHOPPING LISTS	PHASE I WEEK I

PRODUCE

2 pounds baby spinach
2 pounds kale, any variety
2 bunches romaine or butterhead lettuce
2 pounds mesclun greens
1 bunch watercress or ½ pound arugula
1 pound bok choy or Swiss chard
½ pound sprouts, such as alfalfa
1 head cauliflower
3 heads broccoli
1 bunch celery
4 tomatoes
4 cucumbers
1 red bell pepper
2 avocados, preferably Hass
1 head garlic
1 spaghetti squash (about 1 pound)
4" piece fresh ginger
1 bunch cilantro
1 bunch basil
1 bunch parsley
1 bunch chives (optional)
1 pint blueberries
1 small horseradish root (optional)
1 large orange
2 limes
3 lemons

DAIRY

3 dozen eggs or 3 packages (14 ounces each) extra-firm tofu
½ gallon plain, unsweetened coconut milk
1 piece (6 ounces) Parmesan cheese
4 ounces Greek feta cheese

MEATS/PROTEINS

1 pound lean pork loin
4 pounds boneless, skinless chicken breasts
1 pound thinly sliced raw chicken cutlets
2 pounds medium peeled, deveined shrimp (about 22 per pound)
2 pounds salmon fillets, skin removed
2 pounds cod fillets
1 package (6 ounces) low-sodium chicken sausages (optional)

FROZEN

1 bag (12 ounces) frozen berries (any variety)
1 bag (12 ounces) frozen raspberries

OILS, CONDIMENTS, SPICES

1 can (5 ounces) olive oil cooking spray
1 bottle (25 ounces) extra-virgin olive oil
1 jar (14 ounces) coconut oil
1 jar (16 ounces) almond butter
1 jar (8 ounces) Dijon mustard
1 container (26 ounces) salt
1 container (2 ounces) black pepper
1 jar (2 ounces) mild chili powder or paprika
1 jar (2 ounces) ground cardamom
1 jar (2 ounces) ground cumin or cumin seeds
1 jar (2 ounces) dried oregano
1 jar (2 ounces) Italian herbs or rosemary
1 jar (2 ounces) ground turmeric
1 jar (2 ounces) ground coriander (optional)
1 jar (2 ounces) ground cinnamon
1 jar (2 ounces) ground cloves (optional)

1 jar (2 ounces) garlic powder
1 bottle (2 ounces) pure vanilla extract
1 bar (4 ounces) 70% cocoa chocolate bar
1 box (50 count or less) stevia packets
1 jar (12 ounces) onion-free salsa

GRAINS AND DRY GOODS
8 tortillas, 100% corn (6" diameter)
1 box (12 ounces) quinoa flakes
1 box (12 ounces) quinoa
1 bag (16 ounces) chia seeds
1 bag (16 ounces) ground flaxseeds
1 bag (16 ounces) hemp seeds
1 bag (8 ounces) shredded unsweetened
  flaked coconut
1 bag (8 ounces) walnuts

1 bag (8 ounces) almonds
1 bag (8 ounces) pecans or hazelnuts
1 container (12 ounces) vanilla whey
  protein powder
1 container (12 ounces) plain whey protein
  powder

CANNED/JARRED GOODS
1 can (15 ounces) pumpkin
2 cans (5 ounces each) light spring-water-
  packed tuna
1 jar (3 ounces) capers
2 containers (10 ounces each) pitted
  olives, such as kalamata
1 container (32 ounces) low-sodium
  chicken or vegetable broth
1 tube (2 ounces) wasabi paste (optional)

SHOPPING LISTS PHASE I WEEK 2

PRODUCE
1 pound mesclun greens
1 pound bok choy or Swiss chard
2 pounds kale, any variety
2 pounds baby spinach
2 heads broccoli
1 head cauliflower
1 bunch carrots
1 bunch celery
1 jalapeño chile pepper
1 zucchini
1 cucumber
2 red bell peppers
2 green bell peppers
1 bunch chives
1 bunch fresh rosemary (optional)
1 bunch cilantro
4" piece fresh ginger
2 lemons
1 lime

DAIRY
1 dozen eggs
½ gallon plain, unsweetened coconut milk

MEATS/PROTEINS
3 pounds boneless, skinless chicken
  breasts
4 bone-in chicken breasts
1 pound shrimp
1 pound lean pork loin
4 ounces smoked salmon

FROZEN
1 bag (10 ounces) frozen edamame pods
1 bag (12 ounces) frozen berries
1 bag (12 ounces) frozen blueberries

OILS, CONDIMENTS, SPICES
1 bottle (25 ounces) extra-virgin olive oil
1 jar (2 ounces) cayenne pepper or hot
  chili powder (optional)

GRAINS AND DRY GOODS
1 box (12 ounces) quinoa flakes
1 box (12 ounces) quinoa
1 container (12 ounces) vanilla whey
  protein powder
1 pound coffee, any roast

(continued)

CANNED/JARRED GOODS

3 cans (5 ounces each) light spring water–packed tuna

1 container (32 ounces) low-sodium chicken or vegetable broth

1 can (15 ounces) low-sodium chicken vegetable soup

1 can (5 ounces) tomato paste

SHOPPING LISTS — PHASE 2 WEEK 1

PRODUCE

1 pound kale, any variety

1 pound baby spinach

2 pounds arugula

1 head broccoli

1 pound Brussels sprouts

2 pounds asparagus

1 head romaine lettuce

2 heads bok choy

1 head cabbage, such as red, savoy, or napa

1 bunch celery

1 bag carrots

1 bunch beets

1 green bell pepper

2 red bell peppers

2 bulbs fennel

1 small butternut squash (about 1 pound)

2 avocados

1 bunch cilantro

1 bunch parsley

2 cucumbers

1 lemon

1 lime

1 kiwifruit

2 bananas

1 apple

DAIRY

1 dozen eggs or 1 package (14 ounces) extra-firm tofu

1 container (35 ounces) 2% plain Greek yogurt

1 bottle (32 ounces) 2% plain kefir

1 container (8 ounces) plain or spicy hummus

1 container (8 ounces) low-sodium miso paste

4 ounces Greek feta cheese

MEATS/PROTEINS

2 pounds boneless, skinless chicken breasts

2 pounds shrimp or tofu

1 pound salmon, skin intact

1 pound salmon or cod fillets, skin removed

1 pound cod fillets

1 pound ground buffalo meat

1 container (14 ounces) extra-firm tofu

8 low-sodium chicken sausages

4 lean pork chops

FROZEN

1 bag (12 ounces) frozen blueberries

1 bag (12 ounces) frozen strawberries

1 bag (12 ounces) shelled edamame

OILS, CONDIMENTS, SPICES

1 bottle (6 ounces) sesame oil

1 bottle (16 ounces) raw apple cider vinegar

1 jar (2 ounces) pumpkin pie spice (optional)

1 jar or can (2 ounces) curry powder, such as Madras

1 jar (2 ounces) celery seeds or caraway seeds

1 jar (2 ounces) low-sodium Cajun spices

1 jar (2 ounces) low-sodium steak seasoning or grilling spices

1 bottle (10 ounces) reduced-sodium, gluten-free soy sauce or tamari

GRAINS AND DRY GOODS

1-pound bag short-grain brown rice

1 canister (18 ounces) old-fashioned rolled oats

1 box (12 ounces) buckwheat porridge

1 container (12 ounces) vanilla whey protein powder

1 container (12 ounces) plain whey protein powder

1 bag (16 ounces) red lentils

1 container (5 ounces) macadamia nuts

1 bag (16 ounces) chia seeds

1 container (8 ounces) unsweetened cocoa powder

1 package (8 ounces) dried seaweed or nori

1 jar (2 ounces) sesame seeds

1 bag (6 ounces) pistachios

1 bar (4 ounces) 70% cocoa chocolate

1 bar (4 ounces) 85% cocoa chocolate

CANNED/JARRED GOODS

1 bottle (8 ounces) unsweetened pomegranate juice

1 can (15 ounces) 100% pure pumpkin

1 can (5 ounces) tomato paste

2 cans (5 ounces each) light spring water–packed tuna

3 cans (15 ounces each) assorted beans, such as black or kidney, or chickpeas

1 can (15 ounces) kidney beans

1 jar (16 ounces) low-sodium sauerkraut

1 jar (16 ounces) kimchi

1 container (10 ounces) pitted olives, such as kalamata

SHOPPING LISTS · PHASE 2 WEEK 2

PRODUCE

2 pounds spinach

1 pound mesclun greens

1 pound kale, any variety

1 pound arugula

1 pound asparagus

3 heads broccoli

1 cucumber

2 red bell peppers

1 bunch cilantro

1 bunch mint

1 bunch basil

1 head garlic

2 avocados

3 kiwis

2 lemons

2 limes

1 honeydew melon

1 pint raspberries

DAIRY

3 dozen eggs

2 containers (35 ounces each) 2% plain Greek yogurt

1 bottle (32 ounces) 2% plain kefir

4 ounces Greek feta cheese

MEATS/PROTEINS

4 pounds boneless, skinless chicken breasts

1 pound cod fillets

2 packages (14 ounces each) extra-firm tofu

FROZEN

2 pounds shrimp

1 bag (12 ounces) frozen blueberries

OILS, CONDIMENTS, SPICES

1 bottle (6 ounces) sesame oil

1 bottle (16 ounces) raw apple cider vinegar

1 jar (2 ounces) pumpkin pie spice (optional)

1 jar or can (2 ounces) curry powder, such as Madras

1 jar (2 ounces) celery seeds or caraway seeds

1 jar (2 ounces) low-sodium Cajun spices

1 jar (2 ounces) low-sodium steak seasoning or grilling spices

1 bottle (10 ounces) reduced-sodium, gluten-free soy sauce or tamari

(continued)

GRAINS AND DRY GOODS

1 bag (8 ounces) almonds
1 bag (8 ounces) hazelnuts

CANNED/JARRED GOODS

1 can (5 ounces) tomato paste
1 can (15 ounces) low-sodium black beans

1 can (15 ounces) low-sodium chickpeas
1 can (15 ounces) low-sodium lentil soup
1 container (32 ounces) low-sodium
   chicken or vegetable broth
2 packages (2 ounces each) seaweed
   chips, mild or spicy

SHOPPING LISTS   PHASE 3 WEEK 1

PRODUCE

2 pounds baby spinach
3 pounds mesclun greens
1 pound Swiss chard
1 pound kale
2 pounds Brussels sprouts
4 parsnips
1 head romaine lettuce
1 head cabbage, savoy or napa
1 head cauliflower
1 head broccoli
1 pound green beans
1 bunch celery
1 bulb fennel
1 medium tomato
1 bunch radishes
1 red bell pepper
1 bunch fresh rosemary (optional)
1 jalapeño chile pepper
4" piece fresh ginger
1 head garlic
1 bunch basil
1 bunch chives
1 bunch cilantro
1 bunch mint
6 medium zucchinis
1 cucumber
2 lemons
1 lime
3 apples
1 bag (8 ounces) fresh cranberries
½ pint raspberries

DAIRY

1 container (35 ounces) 2% plain Greek
   yogurt

1 bottle (32 ounces) 2% plain kefir
½ gallon plain, unsweetened coconut milk
2 dozen eggs
8 ounces Greek feta cheese
4 ounces soft goat cheese
1 piece (6 ounces) Parmesan or Pecorino
   Romano cheese
½ pint heavy cream
½ pound unsalted butter

MEATS/PROTEINS

3-pound roasting chicken
1 pound ground turkey
1 pound boneless, skinless chicken
   breasts
1 pound thinly sliced raw chicken cutlets
8 ounces smoked salmon
2 salmon fillets, skin removed (4 ounces
   each)
1 rack of lamb (about 1 pound)
1 pound beef stew cubes

FROZEN

1 package (8 ounces) frozen artichoke
   hearts
1 bag (8 ounces) frozen peas

OILS, CONDIMENTS, SPICES

1 bottle (25 ounces) extra-virgin olive oil
1 jar (14 ounces) raw honey
1 jar (2 ounces) red-pepper flakes
   (optional)
1 can (5 ounces) olive oil cooking spray

GRAINS AND DRY GOODS

1 bag (16 ounces) ground flaxseeds
1 bag (8 ounces) unsweetened coconut

1 container (7 ounces) baking powder

1 container (12 ounces) vanilla whey protein powder

1 bar (4 ounces) 70% cocoa chocolate

1 jar (4 ounces) instant espresso powder

CANNED/JARRED GOODS

2 containers (32 ounces each) low-sodium chicken or vegetable broth

1 jar (28 ounces) low-sodium marinara sauce

2 cans (15 ounces each) low-sodium beans, such as pinto or kidney, or chickpeas

1 can (15 ounces) low-sodium chicken or vegetable broth

2 cans (5 ounces each) tomato paste

1 jar (8 ounces) unsweetened pomegranate juice

1 container (10 ounces) pitted olives, such as kalamata

1 jar (14 ounces) coconut oil

SHOPPING LISTS   PHASE 3 WEEK 2

PRODUCE

2 pounds kale

1 pound spinach

1 pound arugula

3 pounds mesclun greens

1 bunch bok choy

1 bunch Swiss chard

1 pound green beans

2 heads broccoli

1 bulb fennel

2 bunches celery

1 bunch carrots

1 bunch radishes

4 tomatoes

3 cucumbers

1 zucchini

1 green or red bell pepper

1 avocado

4" piece fresh ginger

1 bunch mint

1 bag (8 ounces) fresh cranberries

1 apple

DAIRY

1 container (35 ounces) 2% plain Greek yogurt

1 bottle (32 ounces) 2% plain kefir

2 dozen eggs

1 piece (6 ounces) Parmesan or Pecorino Romano cheese

4 ounces Greek feta cheese

1 container (8 ounces) plain or spicy hummus

MEATS/PROTEINS

1 pound ground turkey

1 rack of lamb (about 1 pound)

2 pounds boneless, skinless chicken breasts

1 pound salmon fillets, skin removed

4 ounces smoked salmon

FROZEN

1 bag (12 ounces) frozen berries

1 bag (12 ounces) frozen blueberries

1 package (8 ounces) frozen artichoke hearts

OILS, CONDIMENTS, SPICES

1 jar (2 ounces) nutmeg

1 bottle (2 ounces) almond extract

GRAINS AND DRY GOODS

1 box (12 ounces) quinoa

1 package (8 ounces) walnuts

1 bag (4 ounces) wild rice

CANNED/JARRED GOODS

2 containers (32 ounces each) low-sodium chicken or vegetable broth

2 cans (15 ounces each) low-sodium beans, such as pinto or kidney, or chickpeas

1 container (5 ounces) tomato paste

1 bottle (8 ounces) unsweetened pomegranate juice

Blueberry Protein Smoothie

Tender and nutrient dense, spinach is a mild-tasting green to sneak into your breakfast foods. Blueberries and sweet-tasting stevia will mask any slight veggie taste, making it a good option to share with family members who don't always eat their veggies.

For Phase 2, replace the coconut milk with 2% plain kefir or yogurt. Or for a flavor swap, use ½ teaspoon almond extract in place of the cinnamon.

PREP TIME: 5 MINUTES ■ TOTAL TIME: 10 MINUTES

- 1 cup leftover brewed green tea (cold)
- 1 cup plain, unsweetened coconut milk
- ⅔ cup plain or vanilla whey protein powder
- ½ cup fresh or frozen blueberries
- ½ cup raw baby spinach
- 2 tablespoons ground flaxseeds or chia seeds (or chia-flax flour)
- 1 tablespoon coconut oil
- 2 teaspoons stevia powder
- ½ teaspoon ground cinnamon
- 8 ice cubes

In a blender, place the tea, coconut milk, protein powder, blueberries, spinach, ground seeds, oil, stevia, cinnamon, and ice. Process until smooth. Divide evenly into 2 glasses and serve immediately.

MAKES 2 SERVINGS

PER SERVING (2½ cups): 261 calories, 20 g protein, 18 g carbohydrates, 14 g total fat, 9 g saturated fat, 0 mg cholesterol, 6 g fiber, 115 mg sodium

HEALTHY KITCHEN TIPS

Shop for coconut milk in the dairy aisle—it's much lower in fat than canned coconut milk and a perfect sub for all your favorite breakfast recipes. My favorite brands: So Delicious, 365, Silk, and Almond Breeze.

Make your own "power powder" by grinding ½ cup flaxseeds with ½ cup chia seeds. Always purchase ground flaxseeds or grind the whole seeds yourself in a coffee grinder. Store flaxseeds in an airtight container in the fridge.

Eggs to Go

Eggs are not only a nutrient-dense source of vitamins such as B_{12} and B_2 but they also deliver choline that protects your nervous system and may boost your mood. Shop for omega-3-fortified or pasture-raised eggs.

For Phase 2, replace 1 cup of the greens with $\frac{1}{2}$ cup beans, thinly sliced asparagus, or $\frac{1}{2}$ cup pickled veggies.

PREP TIME: 10 MINUTES ■ TOTAL TIME: 15 MINUTES

4 eggs

4 egg whites

3 tablespoons plain whey protein powder

¼ teaspoon freshly ground black pepper

¼ teaspoon paprika or a pinch of ground cloves

2 tablespoons extra-virgin olive oil, divided

2 cups chopped greens, such as spinach or kale

4 soft corn tortillas (6" diameter)

1. In a small bowl, whisk together the eggs, egg whites, protein powder, pepper, and paprika or cloves. Set aside.

2. Warm a large ceramic-coated or cast-iron skillet over medium-high heat and add 1 tablespoon of the oil. Add the greens and cook for 1 to 2 minutes, turning often, or until the greens wilt. Transfer the greens to a plate.

3. Return the skillet to medium heat and add the remaining 1 tablespoon oil and then the egg mixture. Cook for 2 to 3 minutes, stirring often, or until the eggs start to scramble. Add the greens and stir, cooking for 1 minute, or until the eggs are cooked through.

4. Set each tortilla on an 8" x 8" sheet of foil. Divide the eggs between the tortillas. Fold the tortillas and wrap the foil around them. Serve within 1 hour or store, refrigerated, until ready to eat.

MAKES 4 SERVINGS

PER SERVING (1 tortilla, 1½ cups eggs and greens): 220 calories, 14 g protein, 13 g carbohydrates, 12 g total fat, 2 g saturated fat, 186 mg cholesterol, 2 g fiber, 168 mg sodium

HEALTHY KITCHEN TIP

Can't do eggs? Scramble protein-rich tofu instead. Cook the vegetables until tender, then crumble the tofu into the pan and warm through. Flavor the tofu with dried herbs or anti-inflammatory spices from page 243.

Vanilla Spice Quinoa Breakfast Cereal

Quinoa is a nutritious gluten-free seed. It's high in potassium, fiber, protein, and a long list of strength-building nutrients. Shop for prewashed quinoa, since saponin, a bitter-tasting compound, covers the outside of the seeds and needs to be thoroughly rinsed away.

For Phase 2, replace ½ cup of the quinoa with ½ cup prebiotic dry old-fashioned rolled oats. For a flavor swap for Phase 2 or 3, swap out the berries listed and add in the same amount of strawberries, plus a pinch of cardamom.

PREP TIME: 10 MINUTES ■ TOTAL TIME: 40 MINUTES

- ⅓ cup dry quinoa, rinsed under cold running water
- 2 cups water
- ⅔ cup plain or vanilla whey protein powder
- ½ cup shredded unsweetened coconut
- ¼ cup hemp seeds
- 1 teaspoon pure vanilla extract
- 1 teaspoon ground cinnamon
- ¼ teaspoon ground cardamom
- 2 tablespoons ground flaxseeds or chia seeds or chia-flax flour
- 1 cup fresh or frozen raspberries or blueberries
- ¼ cup chopped walnuts

1. In a large saucepan, place the quinoa and water and bring to a boil over high heat. Reduce to a simmer and cook for 15 to 20 minutes, or until the quinoa is tender and the centers of the grains are translucent.

2. Stir in the protein powder, coconut, hemp seeds, vanilla, cinnamon, and cardamom. Stir in the flaxseeds or chia seeds or seed flour. If the mixture is too thick, add another ¼ to ½ cup water to reach the desired consistency. Divide the quinoa mixture into 4 bowls and top each with ¼ cup berries and 1 tablespoon walnuts. Serve immediately.

MAKES 4 SERVINGS

PER SERVING (1 cup): 233 calories, 15 g protein, 19 g carbohydrates, 11 g total fat, 4 g saturated fat, 0 mg cholesterol, 7 g fiber, 47 mg sodium

Power Breakfast Bars

Store-bought protein bars can be a hidden haven for sugar—as much as in a candy bar. This version contains good-quality protein, like quinoa (high in iron) and chia (high in plant-based omega-3s).

For Phase 2, replace ½ cup of the quinoa with ½ cup prebiotic dry old-fashioned rolled oats. For a flavor swap for Phase 2 or 3, swap out the berries listed and add in the same amount of strawberries, plus a pinch of cardamom, or chopped cherries with chopped 85% dark chocolate.

PREP TIME: 15 MINUTES ■ TOTAL TIME: 25 MINUTES

½ cup fresh or frozen blueberries

⅓ cup almond butter

2 eggs

2 teaspoons stevia powder

1 cup quinoa flakes

1 cup unsweetened grated coconut

⅔ cup vanilla whey protein powder

¼ cup ground flaxseeds

1 teaspoon pure vanilla extract

½ teaspoon ground cinnamon

¼ teaspoon ground cloves or cardamom

1. Preheat the oven to 400°F. Line an 8" x 8" baking dish with foil. Coat the foil with cooking spray.

2. In a large bowl, combine the blueberries, almond butter, eggs, and stevia. Mash gently with the back of a spoon. Add the quinoa, coconut, protein powder, flaxseeds, vanilla, cinnamon, and cloves or cardamom. Mash well with a fork until a thick, crumbly mixture forms.

3. Transfer the mixture into the prepared baking dish, pressing it into an even layer with a rubber spatula. Bake for 8 to 10 minutes, or until the top begins to brown and the edges are firm to the touch. Cool completely before cutting into 8 bars.

MAKES 8 BARS

PER SERVING (1 bar): 218 calories, 10 g protein, 16 g carbohydrates, 13 g total fat, 4 g saturated fat, 46 mg cholesterol, 5 g fiber, 42 mg sodium

HEALTHY KITCHEN TIP

Looking to burn calories more efficiently? Look no further than your spice rack for tasty ways to perk up healthy ingredients and boost antioxidants in your diet. Think of your spice rack as a flavor savior that also helps you to burn more fat faster. Go to pages 270–275 for lists of the top spices. Pumpkin pie spice, for example, is a tasty, antioxidant-rich addition to breakfast cereals, bars, or smoothies.

Greek Village Salad

This fresh, summery salad is adapted from one by Alfred Himmelrich, owner of Stone Mill Bakery and Café in Lutherville, Maryland–Dr. Gerry's favorite eatery in the Baltimore area. This delicious and filling salad was a collaboration by Alfie and the Skinny Chef and features a tangy dressing you'll get hooked on. Use leftover chicken or even salmon from other recipes to make this a quick dinner.

PREP TIME: 10 MINUTES ■ TOTAL TIME: 20 MINUTES

¼ cup extra-virgin olive oil

¼ cup lemon juice

2 teaspoons dried oregano

1 teaspoon Dijon mustard

⅛ teaspoon freshly ground black pepper

½ pound cooked cubed chicken or medium shrimp

2 medium tomatoes, cut into 1" slices and quartered

1 large cucumber, cubed

1 red bell pepper, seeded and diced

2 ounces feta cheese, cut into ½" cubes (about ½ cup)

¼ cup pitted olives, such as kalamata

In a blender, combine the oil, lemon juice, oregano, mustard, and black pepper until smooth. In a large bowl, add the chicken or shrimp, tomatoes, cucumber, bell pepper, cheese, and olives. Pour in the dressing, toss well, and serve.

MAKES 4 SERVINGS

PER SERVING (1½ cups salad): 344 calories, 27 g protein, 9 g carbohydrates, 22 g total fat, 4 g saturated fat, 91 mg cholesterol, 2 g fiber, 365 mg sodium

Orange Salmon

If you're a fan of salty with sweet flavors, you'll adore this unique orange-olive combination that gives plain salmon something to sing about. Citrus not only adds plenty of flavor but also cuts the scent of fish for those who are salmon newbies.

PREP TIME: 10 MINUTES ▪ TOTAL TIME: 30 MINUTES

1 pound bok choy or Swiss chard, thinly sliced

4 salmon fillets (4 ounces each), skin removed

1 tablespoon extra-virgin olive oil

¼ cup black or green olives, chopped

½ teaspoon chili powder or ground coriander, mild or hot (optional)

½ teaspoon fennel seeds

1 large orange, peel grated, then thinly sliced

1. Preheat the oven to 400°F. In an 11" x 7" baking dish, spread the bok choy or chard and place the salmon on top.

2. In a small bowl, place the oil, olives, chili powder or coriander, fennel seeds, and orange peel and mash with the back of a spoon to combine. Spoon the mixture over the salmon and bake for 15 to 17 minutes, or until the fish is opaque and flakes easily. Top with the orange slices and serve immediately.

MAKES 4 SERVINGS

PER SERVING (1 salmon fillet, 1 cup greens): 307 calories, 25 g protein, 7 g carbohydrates, 20 g total fat, 4 g saturated fat, 62 mg cholesterol, 2 g fiber, 208 mg sodium

Pesto Baked Cod

Homemade pesto just takes minutes to whip together and tastes worlds above the jarred varieties. This basil pesto increases nutrition by 100 percent with the addition of spinach, a top superfood rich in vitamins A and C, folate, and fiber.

For Phase 2, replace 1 cup of the baby spinach with 1 cup fresh or frozen (and thawed) green peas.

PREP TIME: 15 MINUTES ■ TOTAL TIME: 45 MINUTES

2 cups baby spinach

2 cups basil leaves

½ cup grated Parmesan cheese

3 tablespoons extra-virgin olive oil

3 tablespoons walnuts

¼ teaspoon salt

4 cod fillets (4 ounces each)

1 spaghetti squash (about 1 pound), cut in half lengthwise

1. Preheat the oven to 400°F.

2. In a blender or food processor, combine the spinach, basil, cheese, oil, walnuts, and salt. Blend until a chunky mixture forms. Place the fish in an 11" x 17" baking dish. Spread the pesto in equal portions over each piece of fish. Bake for 15 to 18 minutes, or until the fish flakes easily.

3. While the fish is baking, prepare the spaghetti squash. Heat 4 inches of water in a large pot. Add a steamer basket and insert the squash. Steam for 10 to 15 minutes, adding ¼ cup water if the water level decreases, or until the squash is fork-tender. Transfer to a cutting board to cool. Remove the seeds and discard. Shred the flesh of the squash with 2 forks; you should have about 4 cups. Divide the squash between 4 plates, top each with a fillet, and serve immediately.

MAKES 4 SERVINGS

PER SERVING (1 cod with topping, 1 cup squash): 296 calories, 27 g protein, 10 g carbohydrates, 17 g total fat, 4 g saturated fat, 58 mg cholesterol, 3 g fiber, 402 mg sodium

HEALTHY KITCHEN TIP

Is your fishmonger out of cod this week? Then go for these two low-mercury choices: wild-caught pollack or freshwater trout. Both pollack and trout are sustainable fish and yummy!

Spiced Pumpkin Soup

It's easy to stick to your new eating plan when you feast on this velvety soup that's also appropriate for fall holidays. Rich-tasting, anti-inflammatory, fat-fighting spices like ginger, cinnamon, and coriander layer on serious flavor with hardly any calories and no sugar or salt.

For Phase 2, add ¼ cup old-fashioned rolled oats before blending, along with ¼ cup water to adjust the thickness.

PREP TIME: 10 MINUTES ▪ TOTAL TIME: 40 MINUTES

2 tablespoons extra-virgin olive oil or coconut oil, divided

4 chicken cutlets

1 clove garlic, minced

2 teaspoons minced ginger

¼ teaspoon freshly ground black pepper

1 quart low-sodium chicken broth

1 can (15 ounces) 100% pure pumpkin

½ teaspoon ground cinnamon or ground cloves

½ teaspoon ground coriander or garlic powder

¼ cup cilantro or parsley leaves (optional)

1. Heat a large pot over medium-high heat and add 1 tablespoon of the oil. Add the cutlets and sprinkle them with the garlic, ginger, and pepper. Cook for 4 to 5 minutes, turning occasionally, or until the chicken browns and the juices run clear. Transfer to a plate.

2. Reduce the heat to low and add the broth, pumpkin, cinnamon or cloves, coriander or garlic powder, and the remaining 1 tablespoon oil. Cover and simmer, stirring occasionally, until the soup thickens and becomes fragrant. Divide the soup among 4 bowls. Shred the chicken and divide it between the bowls. Garnish with the parsley or cilantro, if using, and serve immediately.

MAKES 4 SERVINGS

PER SERVING (1¾ cups made with olive oil): 235 calories, 24 g protein, 12 g carbohydrates, 10 g total fat, 2 g saturated fat, 54 mg cholesterol, 3 g fiber, 172 mg sodium

HEALTHY KITCHEN TIP

To give this soup a spring or summer makeover, use 15 ounces fresh spinach or zucchini in place of the pumpkin. For a vegetarian option, add 14 ounces extra-firm tofu instead of the chicken.

Raspberry Mesclun Salad
with Green Tea Dressing

Raspberries and green tea bring sweet-tart flavors along with fiber and antioxidants that can boost your calorie burn more efficiently. For serious gourmets, opt for the vanilla protein powder for a fragrant yet savory dressing.

For Phases 2 and 3, replace almonds with bright green pistachios, a fat-busting nut that also has visual appeal. Once you reach Phase 2, swap out the fresh radishes and cukes for the pickled equivalent.

PREP TIME: 10 MINUTES ■ TOTAL TIME: 40 MINUTES

6 cups baby mesclun greens

2 cups bean sprouts, such as alfalfa

1 cup thinly sliced radishes or cucumber

1 cup fresh or frozen raspberries, thawed

¼ cup chopped almonds

⅓ cup cold green tea

3 tablespoons plain or vanilla whey protein powder

3 tablespoons extra-virgin olive oil

1 teaspoon grated lime peel

2 tablespoons fresh lime juice

¼ teaspoon salt

12 ounces cooked chicken breast (2 breasts) or ½ pound cooked shrimp

1. In a large bowl, mix the greens, sprouts, radishes or cucumber, raspberries, and almonds.

2. In a blender, combine the tea, protein powder, oil, lime peel, lime juice, and salt. Blend until smooth. Drizzle over the greens. Top with the chicken or shrimp and serve immediately.

MAKES 4 SERVINGS

PER SERVING (2½ cups of salad with chicken): 288 calories, 25 g protein, 12 g carbohydrates, 16 g total fat, 2 g saturated fat, 54 mg cholesterol, 6 g fiber, 290 mg sodium

HEALTHY KITCHEN TIP

Save prep time but still get enough filling protein: Use 2 thinly sliced breasts of frozen cooked or grilled chicken without breading, added fat, or high amounts of salt. Or use 2 cups thawed cooked shrimp. For a vegetarian option, add 12 ounces drained tofu.

Crunchy Almond Tuna Salad

This crisp and refreshing tuna salad is made primarily from pantry staples that you'll have on hand. Look for light spring-water-packed tuna—it's lower in mercury levels.

For Phases 2 and 3, add ½ cup cooked quinoa or 1 cup pickled red cabbage.

PREP TIME: 10 MINUTES ■ TOTAL TIME: 15 MINUTES

2–3 teaspoons grated lemon peel

3 tablespoons fresh lemon juice

2 tablespoons plain, unsweetened coconut milk

2 tablespoons chia seeds

1 tablespoon coconut oil

¼ teaspoon salt

4 cups baby spinach or watercress, chopped

1 head broccoli, cut into florets (about 4 cups florets)

2 cans (5 ounces each) light spring-water-packed tuna, drained

¼ cup chopped pecans or hazelnuts

¼ cup chopped fresh chives (optional)

1. In a blender, combine the lemon peel, lemon juice, coconut milk, seeds, oil, and salt. Blend until smooth.

2. In a large bowl, place the spinach or watercress, broccoli, tuna, pecans or hazelnuts, and chives (if using). Drizzle with the dressing and toss well. Serve immediately.

MAKES 4 SERVINGS

PER SERVING (2½ cups): 244 calories, 24 g protein, 15 g carbohydrates, 11 g total fat, 1 g saturated fat, 21 mg cholesterol, 8 g fiber, 461 mg sodium

HEALTHY KITCHEN TIP

If you're on a low-sodium diet, omit the added salt in the dressing because tuna is naturally high in salt.

Massaged Kale Salad

Kale contains a world of nutrition, including incredibly high amounts of important anti-inflammatory nutrients like vitamins A and C. It also has lots of sulfur-based compounds that may combat several forms of cancers.

For a Phase 2 or 3 flavor swap, substitute the nuts with 3 tablespoons chia or sesame seeds. For a Phase 2 fiber boost, add 1 cup chickpeas, cooked lentils, or black beans.

PREP TIME: 10 MINUTES ▪ TOTAL TIME: 1 HOUR 10 MINUTES

- 1 bunch (10 ounces) kale, sliced into 1" chunks
- 2 tablespoons extra-virgin olive oil
- ¼ teaspoon ground cumin or freshly ground black pepper or ½ teaspoon cumin seeds
- ¼ cup green or black olives
- ¼ cup walnuts or almonds
- ¼ cup crumbled feta cheese or thinly shaved Parmesan cheese
- ¼ cup diced avocado
- 2 cooked chicken breasts, cubed or sliced, ½ pound cooked shrimp, or 10 ounces firm tofu

1. In a large bowl, place the kale, oil, and ground cumin or pepper or cumin seeds. Using clean hands, rub the oil into the kale leaves, gently squeezing the leaves to soften them.

2. Sprinkle on the olives, nuts, cheese, and avocado. Cover and refrigerate for at least 1 hour. Top with the chicken, shrimp, or tofu and serve immediately.

MAKES 4 SERVINGS

PER SERVING (2½ cups): 298 calories, 23 g protein, 10 g carbohydrates, 19 g total fat, 3 g saturated fat, 62 mg cholesterol, 3 g fiber, 366 mg sodium

HEALTHY KITCHEN TIP

This Mediterranean-inspired salad, with tangy feta and savory olives, is high in anti-inflammatory ingredients like spices and olive oil that are a perfect fit for Phase 3. This filling salad gets its rich taste from three good-quality, and antioxidant-rich fat sources—olives, nuts, and avocado—that also help you feel full.

Slow-Cooker Chicken Picatta

Tangy picatta relies on two great low-cal ingredients—fresh lemon and capers—to give it savory flavor. This simple slow-cooker recipe is the perfect way to make a lean protein juicy.

For Phase 2, replace 1 cup of the lettuce with 1 cup sliced asparagus or cooked artichokes.

PREP TIME: 10 MINUTES ▪ TOTAL TIME: 1 HOUR 30 MINUTES

2–3 teaspoons grated lemon peel

3 tablespoons fresh lemon juice

3 tablespoons extra-virgin olive oil

2 tablespoons capers, rinsed well under cold running water

¼ teaspoon freshly ground black pepper

1 teaspoon dried herbs, such as Italian seasoning, rosemary, or thyme

4 boneless, skinless chicken breasts

1 head romaine lettuce, thinly sliced

¼ cup thinly sliced Parmesan cheese

1. In a slow cooker, place the lemon peel, lemon juice, oil, capers, pepper, and dried herbs and stir well to combine. Add the chicken and turn to coat. Cover and cook on low for 1 to 1½ hours, or until a thermometer inserted in the thickest portion registers 165°F and the juices run clear. Transfer the chicken to a cutting board and cool for 5 minutes before slicing.

2. Divide the romaine between 4 plates and top each with 1 tablespoon of the cheese. Top with the chicken and juices from the slow cooker. Serve immediately.

MAKES 4 SERVINGS

PER SERVING (3 cups): 320 calories, 39 g protein, 5 g carbohydrates, 16 g total fat, 3 g saturated fat, 113 mg cholesterol, 2 g fiber, 406 mg sodium

HEALTHY KITCHEN TIP

Have limited space in your kitchen cabinets but still want to harness the flavor of herbs? Shop for premixed herbs such as Italian seasoning—a dried herb blend that's free of sugar and salt.

Chicken Vegetable Soup

Nothing is more soothing and nourishing than a hot bowl of soup, and this tasty version swaps out the customary onion for a gastrointestinal superfood, ginger. For a weekday shortcut, cook the veggies in the oil, then add shredded rotisserie chicken, the broth, and kale or spinach. Bring to a slow simmer, then serve.

For Phase 2, add $\frac{1}{2}$ cup prebiotic veggies such as asparagus. For Phase 3, stir in 1 cup cooked gluten-free brown rice noodles (al dente) or organic brown rice.

PREP TIME: 10 MINUTES ■ TOTAL TIME: 40 MINUTES

2 bone-in chicken breasts, skin on

$\frac{1}{4}$ teaspoon freshly ground black pepper

1 tablespoon extra-virgin olive oil

4 carrots, peeled and cut into 1" chunks

2 ribs celery, thinly sliced

1 jalapeño chile pepper, seeded and finely chopped (optional), wear plastic gloves when handling

2 cloves garlic, finely chopped

1 (1") piece fresh ginger, finely chopped

1 teaspoon fresh or dried rosemary leaves

1 quart low-sodium chicken broth

2 cups chopped kale or spinach

1. Sprinkle the chicken with the black pepper. Heat a large pot over medium heat. Add the oil and chicken, skin side down. Cook for 1 to 2 minutes, or until the skin starts to brown.

2. Scatter the carrots, celery, chile pepper (if using), garlic, ginger, and rosemary around the chicken and cook for 5 minutes. Turn the chicken and stir the vegetables. Increase the heat to high and add the chicken broth. Bring to a simmer, then reduce the heat to low and cover. Cook for 10 minutes, or until a thermometer inserted in the thickest portion registers 170°F and the juices run clear. Turn off the heat. Let stand for 20 minutes.

3. Transfer the chicken to a cutting board and cool slightly for 5 to 6 minutes. Discard the skin and shred the meat. Return the meat to the soup along with the kale or spinach and cover for 5 minutes to wilt the greens. Serve immediately.

MAKES 4 SERVINGS

PER SERVING (1½ cups): 194 calories, 20 g protein, 8 g carbohydrates, 8 g total fat, 1 g saturated fat, 113 mg cholesterol, 2 g fiber, 294 mg sodium

HEALTHY KITCHEN TIP

Kids love soups. To make this a complete kid's meal, add ½ cup cooked whole grain pasta or quinoa to each bowl. Out of kale or spinach? For Phase 2 or 3, add broccoli florets or Swiss chard.

Spiced Pork Roast with Cauliflower Mash

Pork loin is a lean, tender cut that makes a perfect weekend roast for a family gathering. Serve leftovers over salad greens or use as a fast no-cook lunch.

For Phase 2, replace 1 cup of the greens with 1 cup sauerkraut, your favorite pickled vegetable, or a few teaspoons of jarred prepared horseradish.

PREP TIME: 10 MINUTES ■ TOTAL TIME: 50 MINUTES

2 teaspoons grated fresh ginger

1 teaspoon chili powder, mild or hot

½ teaspoon ground turmeric

2 tablespoons extra-virgin olive oil, divided

1 pound lean pork loin, trimmed of excess fat

½ head cauliflower, cut into florets (about 3 cups florets)

¼ cup chopped cilantro

2 tablespoons wasabi powder or grated fresh horseradish

1. Preheat the oven to 400°F.

2. In a small bowl, place the ginger, chili powder, turmeric, and 1 tablespoon of the oil. Mix well with a spoon or small spatula.

3. Place the pork in an 11" x 7" baking dish. Spread the oil mixture over the loin and bake, uncovered, for 25 to 30 minutes. Let stand for 5 minutes on a cutting board before slicing.

4. While the pork is baking, prepare the cauliflower mash. Heat 4 inches of water in a large pot. Add a steamer basket and insert the florets. Steam for 5 to 6 minutes, or until fork-tender. Transfer to a large bowl and mash with the cilantro, wasabi or horseradish, and the remaining 1 tablespoon oil. Serve immediately with the pork.

MAKES 4 SERVINGS

PER SERVING (1½ cups): 213 calories, 26 g protein, 6 g carbohydrates, 10 g total fat, 2 g saturated fat, 74 mg cholesterol, 2 g fiber, 162 mg sodium

HEALTHY KITCHEN TIP

Don't have a steamer basket? Just add the cauliflower florets directly to the pot and steam. Add additional water as needed, ¼ cup at a time.

Ginger-Crusted Kale Chips

Kale chips are all the rage. They have a wonderful flaky texture and crunch that any chip lover will enjoy. These are crusted with a superroot—a heavy hitter when it comes to quenching inflammation.

For Phases 2 and 3, add 2 tablespoons ground flaxseed to boost the fiber.

PREP TIME: 5 MINUTES ■ TOTAL TIME: 15 MINUTES

1 bunch (10 ounces) curly kale, stems trimmed	2 tablespoons finely grated fresh ginger
¼ cup chopped pumpkin seeds or pecans	½ teaspoon chili powder or paprika
¼ cup chia seeds	¼ teaspoon salt
	2 egg whites

1. Preheat the oven to 400°F. Coat 2 baking sheets with olive oil cooking spray. Rinse the kale under cold water. Dry well with paper towels or a dry dishtowel.

2. On a sheet of waxed paper or a plate, place the pumpkin seeds or pecans, chia, ginger, chili powder or paprika, and salt. Mix well with your fingertips. It may clump slightly.

3. In a large bowl, whisk the egg whites with a wire whisk for about 10 seconds, or until foamy. Dip the edges of the kale leaves into the egg whites, then place on the prepared baking sheets. Sprinkle on the seed mixture. Spread the kale so the leaves don't touch. Coat the tops of the leaves with another spritz of cooking spray.

4. Bake for 10 to 12 minutes, or until the leaves are crisp and the seeds and nuts are golden. Cool for 2 minutes before serving.

MAKES 4 SERVINGS

PER SERVING (1 cup): 175 calories, 9 g protein, 13 g carbohydrates, 12 g total fat, 1 g saturated fat, 0 mg cholesterol, 4 g fiber, 212 mg sodium

Coconut Joy Pudding

No need to cook this sumptuous pudding, since protein-rich chia seeds swell when they come in contact with liquid. For a looser, creamier pudding, add an extra ¼ cup coconut milk to the oat and chia mixture before spooning into dessert dishes.

PREP TIME: 5 MINUTES ▪ TOTAL TIME: 1 HOUR 5 MINUTES

1 cup plain, unsweetened coconut milk

⅔ cup plain or vanilla whey protein powder

⅓ cup chia seeds

1 cup cold water

¼ cup + 4 tablespoons shredded unsweetened coconut

4 tablespoons chopped or shaved 70% (or higher) dark chocolate

1. In a large bowl, whisk together the coconut milk, protein powder, chia seeds, water, and ¼ cup shredded coconut. Combine well. Set out 4 parfait glasses or 4 small airtight containers and add ¾ cup of the coconut mixture to each.

2. Sprinkle each with 1 tablespoon shredded coconut and 1 tablespoon chocolate. Cover the glasses with plastic wrap or close the container lids. Place in the fridge and chill for 1 hour before serving.

MAKES 4 SERVINGS

PER SERVING (¾ cup): 201 calories, 12 g protein, 14 g carbohydrates, 14 g total fat, 6 g saturated fat, 0 mg cholesterol, 8 g fiber, 161 mg sodium

HEALTHY KITCHEN TIP

Normally, saturated fat is a red flag for your health, but the saturated fat in this filling pudding comes from anti-inflammatory, heart-healthy sources like coconut and dark chocolate—so indulge!

Salsa and Eggs

This tangy lime-laced salsa not only adds flavor to eggs but also gives you a good dose of two prebiotic superfoods: kiwifruit and beans. Use leftover salsa (or double the salsa recipe) to top salads, grilled chicken, or fish.

PREP TIME: 10 MINUTES ■ TOTAL TIME: 20 MINUTES

2 kiwifruit, peeled and finely chopped

2 cups low-sodium canned black beans, rinsed and drained

¼ cup packed cilantro

1–2 tablespoons fresh lime juice

4 eggs

4 egg whites

⅓ cup plain whey protein powder

¼ teaspoon freshly ground black pepper

¼ teaspoon ground cumin

1 tablespoon extra-virgin olive oil

½ cup 2% plain Greek yogurt

1. In a medium bowl, combine the kiwi, beans, cilantro, and lime juice. Set aside.

2. In a small bowl, whisk the eggs and egg whites. Gently whisk in the protein powder, pepper, and cumin. Set aside.

3. Warm a large ceramic-coated or cast-iron skillet over medium-high heat and add the oil. Add the egg mixture. Cook for 2 to 3 minutes, stirring, or until soft curds form and the eggs are cooked through. Divide the eggs among 4 plates and top each with ¾ cup of the salsa and 2 tablespoons yogurt.

MAKES 4 SERVINGS

PER SERVING (2¼ cups: 1½ cups eggs, ¾ cup salsa): 247 calories, 22 g protein, 23 g carbohydrates, 9 g total fat, 2 g saturated fat, 187 mg cholesterol, 7 g fiber, 395 mg sodium

Pumpkin Pie Yogurt Parfait

Store-bought parfaits can be bursting with carbs and fat, since they're typically made from white processed carbs and sugar. But this easy, homemade version, which can double as a snack, provides a huge hit of hunger-calming protein along with other key nutrients.

PREP TIME: 10 MINUTES ■ TOTAL TIME: 1 HOUR 5 MINUTES

2 cups 2% plain Greek yogurt

⅓ cup plain or vanilla whey protein powder

½ teaspoon pumpkin pie spice or ground cinnamon

¼ teaspoon ground cloves (optional)

2 tablespoons water

½ cup canned 100% pure pumpkin

¼ cup old-fashioned rolled oats

2 teaspoons stevia powder

1 teaspoon pure vanilla extract

1. In a medium bowl, place the yogurt, protein powder, pumpkin pie spice or cinnamon, and cloves, if using. Add the water and stir well. Distribute half of the yogurt mixture among 4 parfait glasses.

2. In a large bowl, place the pumpkin, oats, stevia, and vanilla. Stir well to combine. Divide half of the pumpkin mixture among the parfait glasses. Repeat with the yogurt and the pumpkin mixture. Cover each parfait glass with plastic wrap and refrigerate for at least 1 hour before serving.

MAKES 4 SERVINGS

PER SERVING (1¼ cups): 136 calories, 15 g protein, 13 g carbohydrates, 3 g total fat, 2 g saturated fat, 7 mg cholesterol, 2 g fiber, 54 mg sodium

HEALTHY KITCHEN TIP

For a flavor surprise, serve this healthy parfait topped with raspberries. For a spring version, substitute fresh or frozen berries in place of the pumpkin; in summer, try thinly sliced melon with fresh mint in place of the spices.

Pomegranate Margarita Smoothie

Blueberries and pomegranate make a strong anti-inflammatory pair, since antioxidants come from their vibrant color. You'll get hooked on the sweet-tart flavor of this delectable shake worthy of the name Margarita.

PREP TIME: 5 MINUTES ■ TOTAL TIME: 10 MINUTES

1 cup 2% plain Greek yogurt (or homemade yogurt, page 333) or kefir (or homemade kefir, page 334)

½ cup fresh or frozen blueberries

⅓ cup pomegranate juice

⅓ cup plain whey protein powder

2 tablespoons chopped macadamia nuts or walnuts

1 teaspoon grated lime peel

1–2 tablespoons fresh lime juice

2 tablespoons flaxseed, chia seed, or chia-flax flour

2 teaspoons stevia powder (optional)

½ cup water

8 ice cubes

In a blender, combine the yogurt or kefir, blueberries, pomegranate juice, protein powder, nuts, lime peel, lime juice, flaxseed or chia seed or chia-flax flour, stevia (if using), water, and ice cubes. Process until smooth. Divide into 2 glasses and serve immediately.

MAKES 2 SERVINGS

PER SERVING (1¼ cups): 272 calories, 21 g protein, 27 g carbohydrates, 12 g total fat, 3 g saturated fat, 8 mg cholesterol, 6 g fiber, 78 mg sodium

HEALTHY KITCHEN TIPS

Yearning for chocolate? Remove the lime juice and swap 2 tablespoons of 85% dark chocolate for the nuts.

Mix ½ cup pomegranate juice with ½ cup water and freeze in an ice cube tray. You'll love the convenience of using "pom cubes" for smoothies or in sparkling water, and you will have lowered calories and carbs by using the juice-water blend.

Muffin-Size Frittatas

Make these tasty frittatas in a muffin pan—they'll cook quickly and look elegant enough for a special brunch. Enjoy them at room temperature as finger food—they travel well, too.

For Phase 3, add a few teaspoons of salsa or add in $1/2$ cup diced cherry tomatoes with 2 tablespoons finely chopped chives.

PREP TIME: 10 MINUTES ▇ TOTAL TIME: 25 MINUTES

1 red bell pepper, seeded and thinly sliced

2 cups chopped spinach

¼ cup chopped fresh parsley and/or cilantro

¼ teaspoon dried herbs, such as thyme or rosemary (optional)

6 eggs

1 cup canned beans, such as black or kidney, rinsed and drained

¼ cup crumbled feta cheese

4 cups greens, such as arugula or dandelion greens

1. Preheat the oven to 400°F. Coat a 12-cup muffin pan with cooking spray and set it aside.

2. Coat a large skillet with cooking oil and place over medium heat. Add the bell pepper, spinach, parsley or cilantro, and dried herbs, if using. Cook for 3 to 4 minutes, stirring occasionally, or until the vegetables start to soften. Transfer to a plate.

3. In a large bowl, whisk together the eggs, beans, cheese, and cooked veggies. Pour the mixture into 8 muffin cups, filling them three-quarters full. Bake for 10 to 12 minutes, or until the eggs are firm and cooked through. Run a knife along the inside edge of each muffin cup and pull out the frittatas. Serve them over the greens.

MAKES 4 SERVINGS

PER SERVING (2 muffin frittatas, 1 cup greens): 218 calories, 16 g protein, 16 g carbohydrates, 10 g total fat, 4 g saturated fat, 287 mg cholesterol, 7 g fiber, 407 mg sodium

Cool Cucumber-Avocado Soup

Raw apple cider vinegar and kiwifruit give this creamy chilled soup a prebiotic boost. The perfect dish to take to your next cookout, serve it in paper cups for sipping or omit the water and use it as a dip for shrimp or thinly sliced raw celery and radishes.

PREP TIME: 5 MINUTES ▪ TOTAL TIME: 10 MINUTES

1 large cucumber, peeled and quartered

1 ripe Hass avocado, peeled

1 kiwifruit, peeled and quartered

½ cup almonds

¼ cup fresh mint leaves or fresh dill

2 tablespoons raw apple cider vinegar

¼ teaspoon garlic powder or chili powder

1 cup cold water or cold green tea

1 pound frozen precooked shrimp, thawed

In a food processor, place the cucumber, avocado, kiwi, almonds, mint or dill, vinegar, garlic or chili powder, and water or tea. Pulse the mixture until smooth. Top individual servings with the shrimp and serve immediately or chill, covered, in an airtight container for at least 1 hour or up to 2 days.

MAKES 4 SERVINGS

PER SERVING (1½ cups with shrimp): 266 calories, 20 g protein, 12 g carbohydrates, 16 g total fat, 1 g saturated fat, 186 mg cholesterol, 5 g fiber, 649 mg sodium

HEALTHY KITCHEN TIPS

Stop at your local fish market or counter and ask for precooked cocktail shrimp to make this soup a no-cook feast.

All the sodium in this dish comes from the shrimp. You can decrease the sodium by decreasing the amount of shrimp, but note that the protein count will go down, too. For a low-sodium version, swap in chicken instead.

Chicken Tikka Masala

Tikka Masala gets its flavorful sauce from ginger, cilantro, and sweet-tasting tomato paste. Restaurants douse this dish in heavy cream, but this lighter version, with less sauce, adds more protein by swapping cream for yogurt.

PREP TIME: 15 MINUTES ■ TOTAL TIME: 40 MINUTES

2 boneless, skinless chicken breasts, cubed

4 ounces tomato paste (¼ cup)

½ cup chopped cilantro

1 clove garlic, minced

2 teaspoons curry powder, such as Madras

1 cup 2% plain Greek yogurt or kefir, divided

1 tablespoon coconut oil

1 head broccoli, cut into florets (about 4 cups florets)

¼ cup red lentils

½ cup water

1. In a resealable plastic bag, place the chicken, tomato paste, cilantro, garlic, curry, and ½ cup of the yogurt or kefir. Seal the bag and shake well to coat. Refrigerate for at least 30 minutes or overnight.

2. Heat the oil in a large skillet over medium heat. Add the broccoli. Cook for 3 to 4 minutes, stirring occasionally, or until the broccoli starts to brown. Reduce the heat to low. Add the chicken and marinade. Cook for 2 to 3 minutes, turning the chicken, or until it starts to brown around the edges. Add the lentils along with the water. Cover and cook for 6 to 8 minutes, stirring occasionally, or until the chicken is no longer pink and the broccoli and lentils are tender. Stir in the remaining ½ cup yogurt or kefir. Serve immediately.

MAKES 4 SERVINGS

PER SERVING (1½ cups): 254 calories, 29 g protein, 19 g carbohydrates, 7 g total fat, 4 g saturated fat, 58 mg cholesterol, 4 g fiber, 276 mg sodium

HEALTHY KITCHEN TIP

To make a cooling cucumber raita side dish: In the bowl of a food processor, place 1 small cucumber, cut in thirds, with ¼ cup cilantro and ¼ cup mint. Add 1 cup plain kefir or yogurt and a pinch of cumin. Pulse until a chunky mixture forms, then serve immediately with the Tikka Masala.

Zesty Lemon Chicken Salad

Herbs, citrus, and spices are your one-way ticket to flavor without packing on the sugar, fat, or salt. Miso is the secret probiotic flavor booster that gives normally bland-tasting chicken extra-zesty appeal. Look for miso in the dairy aisle of your local health food store.

PREP TIME: 1 HOUR 10 MINUTES ■ TOTAL TIME: 1 HOUR 40 MINUTES

4 boneless, skinless chicken breasts

¼ cup chopped cilantro

1 tablespoon extra-virgin olive oil

2–3 teaspoons grated lemon peel

3 tablespoons fresh lemon juice

¼ teaspoon freshly ground black pepper

¼ teaspoon ground turmeric

½ cup 2% plain Greek yogurt

1 tablespoon low-sodium miso paste

1 red bell pepper, finely chopped

2 tablespoons chopped almonds or macadamia nuts

6 cups mixed greens, such as mesclun and baby kale

1. In a resealable plastic bag, place the chicken, cilantro, oil, lemon peel, lemon juice, black pepper, and turmeric. Shake well to coat the chicken. Marinate in the refrigerator for at least 1 hour or overnight.

2. Heat a grill or grill pan over medium-high heat. Grill the chicken for 8 to 10 minutes, turning occasionally, or until a thermometer inserted in the thickest portion registers 165°F and the juices run clear. Set aside.

3. In a large bowl, whisk the yogurt and miso to combine. Add the bell pepper and nuts. Chop the chicken and add it to the bowl. Toss well to coat and serve immediately over the mixed greens.

MAKES 4 SERVINGS

PER SERVING (2½ cups): 297 calories, 43 g protein, 17 g carbohydrates, 8 g total fat, 2 g saturated fat, 111 mg cholesterol, 4 g fiber, 265 mg sodium

Tangy Buffalo Burgers with Pickles and Slaw

Dry steak seasoning or grilling spices, often found tucked in the back of your spice rack, are another way to flavor your burger with antioxidant-rich spices. Look for low-sodium options and mixes without MSG. If you can't locate ground buffalo (also known as ground bison), try ground chicken or grass-fed beef instead.

PREP TIME: 20 MINUTES ■ TOTAL TIME: 40 MINUTES

Slaw

- 1 bulb fennel, trimmed and grated
- 4 carrots, peeled and grated
- ½ small red cabbage, grated (about 3 cups)
- 2–3 teaspoons lemon peel
- 3 tablespoons fresh lemon juice
- 1 cup 2% plain Greek yogurt
- 1 teaspoon celery seeds or caraway seeds

Burgers

- 1 pound ground buffalo meat
- ½ teaspoon dry steak seasoning or grilling spices
- ¼ teaspoon ground turmeric
- 1 avocado, sliced
- 8 thinly sliced low-sodium pickles or Pickled Cucumbers (page 331)

1. *To make the slaw:* In a large bowl, place the fennel, carrots, red cabbage, lemon peel, lemon juice, yogurt, and celery or caraway seeds. Toss well to combine and set aside.

2. *To make the burgers:* In a large bowl, place the buffalo meat, steak seasoning or grilling spices, and turmeric. Mix well and form into 4 burgers. Coat a large skillet or grill rack with cooking spray. Heat over medium-high heat and add the burgers. Cook or grill for 10 to 12 minutes, turning once or twice, or until the burgers are still slightly pink in the center.

3. Divide the slaw among 4 plates. Place a burger on top of each plate and top with avocado slices and 2 pickles each. Serve immediately.

MAKES 4 SERVINGS

PER SERVING (1 burger, 1 cup slaw): 284 calories, 31 g protein, 24 g carbohydrates, 9 g total fat, 2 g saturated fat, 56 mg cholesterol, 8 g fiber, 362 mg sodium

HEALTHY KITCHEN TIP

Buffalo meat is an excellent high-protein (and high-iron) substitution for corn-fed beef. Order it frozen online—try these sites: jhbuffalomeat.com, northstarbison.com, or wildideabuffalo.com.

Miso Soup with Seaweed Salad

You don't have to go to your favorite Japanese restaurant to enjoy a hot bowl of miso soup. Make this easy, protein-rich version at home that has the addition of fish.

PREP TIME: 15 MINUTES ■ TOTAL TIME: 40 MINUTES

Soup

- 8 cups water
- 1 tablespoon shredded nori or wakami seaweed
- 3 cups chopped greens, such as Swiss chard, kale, or bok choy
- ¼ cup low-sodium miso paste
- 1 block (4 ounces) firm tofu, cut into ½" cubes
- 4 salmon or cod fillets, cut into 1" cubes
- ¼ cup cilantro (optional)

Seaweed Salad

- 4 ounces dried seaweed
- 1 tablespoon raw apple cider vinegar
- 1 tablespoon sesame oil
- 1 teaspoon reduced-sodium soy sauce
- 1 tablespoon white or black sesame seeds

1. *To make the soup:* In a large saucepan, bring the water to a slow simmer and add the nori or wakami. Simmer for 5 to 6 minutes to flavor the water. Add the greens and cook for 1 minute. Reduce the heat to low and add the miso and tofu. Stir until the miso is well dissolved. Stir in the fish chunks and cilantro (if using), cover, and remove the saucepan from the heat. Let stand for 5 to 6 minutes, or until the fish is opaque and cooked through.

2. *To make the seaweed salad:* Put the dried seaweed in a large bowl and fill it with cold water. Soak for 10 to 12 minutes, or until tender.

3. Meanwhile, in a small bowl, whisk together the vinegar, oil, and soy sauce.

4. Drain the seaweed and use your hands to squeeze out excess water. Wipe out any water in the bowl, then return the seaweed. Add the dressing and sesame seeds. Toss well, then serve alongside the miso soup.

MAKES 4 SERVINGS

PER SERVING (2 cups soup, 1 cup seaweed salad): 340 calories, 29 g protein, 8 g carbohydrates, 21 g total fat, 4 g saturated fat, 62 mg cholesterol, 2 g fiber, 439 mg sodium

HEALTHY KITCHEN TIP

Carry the delicious seaweed salad into Phase 3 for a satisfying snack that gives you a fat-burning boost in the afternoon when the munchies strike.

Ginger Fried Rice

Take-out fried rice isn't only high in MSG, it's also made with white rice that can send your blood sugar skyrocketing. This version has plenty of vegetables and protein that can help anchor your appetite. You'll enjoy the base of brown rice, which is higher in fiber and has a pleasant, chewy texture.

PREP TIME: 10 MINUTES ■ TOTAL TIME: 15 MINUTES

½ cup dry short-grain brown rice

3 tablespoons coconut oil

2 boneless, skinless chicken breasts, cubed, or ½ pound shelled shrimp

1 head bok choy, chopped (about 4 cups)

2 cups frozen shelled edamame

2 tablespoons minced fresh ginger

2 cloves garlic, minced

½ teaspoon Chinese five-spice powder

¼ teaspoon ground turmeric

2 tablespoons reduced-sodium, gluten-free soy sauce or tamari sauce (optional)

1. Cook the rice according to package directions and set aside.

2. Heat a large skillet over medium heat. Add the coconut oil. Add the chicken or shrimp, bok choy, and edamame at once and increase the heat to medium-high. Cook for 3 to 4 minutes, stirring often, or until the chicken and vegetables begin to brown. Add the ginger, garlic, five-spice powder, and turmeric. Cook for 2 to 3 minutes, stirring well, or until the chicken is no longer pink and the juices run clear or the shrimp are opaque.

3. Reduce the heat to medium and stir in the rice and soy or tamari sauce, if using. Serve immediately.

MAKES 4 SERVINGS

PER SERVING (1½ cups): 376 calories, 28 g protein, 23 g carbohydrates, 16 g total fat, 10 g saturated fat, 54 mg cholesterol, 4 g fiber, 131 mg sodium

HEALTHY KITCHEN TIP

Top with probiotic Pickled Ginger (page 327) or serve ginger on the side.

Arugula Salad with Creamy Avocado Dressing

This salad has a one-two punch of superingredients–tangy kiwifruit and creamy avocado. Kiwi is low glycemic and a perfect prebiotic for the colon, while avocado, high in fiber, adds just the right kind of fat. For a vegetarian option, replace the tuna with 2 cups edamame.

PREP TIME: 20 MINUTES ■ TOTAL TIME: 25 MINUTES

Dressing

- 1 ripe avocado, cubed
- ¼ cup 2% plain Greek yogurt
- 1 kiwifruit, peeled
- 1 teaspoon garlic powder
- 1 teaspoon grated lime peel
- 2 tablespoons fresh lime juice
- 2 tablespoons water

Salad

- 1 teaspoon cumin seed
- 6 cups arugula
- 1 bulb fennel, shredded or thinly sliced
- 2 cans (5 ounces each) light spring-water-packed tuna, drained
- ¼ cup dry lentils, cooked according to package directions
- ¼ cup pitted olives, such as kalamata or Cerignola
- ¼ cup chopped almonds
- ½ cup Pickled Beets (page 328)

1. *To make the dressing:* In a blender, combine the avocado, yogurt, kiwi, garlic powder, lime peel, lime juice, and water until smooth.

2. *To make the salad:* Place the cumin in a small, dry skillet over medium-low heat. Toast the seeds in the skillet for 1 to 2 minutes, stirring often, or until the seeds are fragrant. Place the arugula and fennel in a large bowl or on a platter and scatter the seeds on top. Top with the tuna, lentils, olives, almonds, and beets. Drizzle with the dressing and serve immediately.

MAKES 4 SERVINGS

PER SERVING (3 cups with tuna): 264 calories, 24 g protein, 19 g carbohydrates, 12 g total fat, 1 g saturated fat, 22 mg cholesterol, 7 g fiber, 460 mg sodium

HEALTHY KITCHEN TIP

Trim your food budget by shopping for avocados in bulk. If your avocados aren't soft to the touch, store them on the countertop for 2 days to ripen, then transfer to the fridge to use throughout the week.

Creamy Asparagus Soup

Looking to make this soup more indulgent for Phase 3? Make your own Parmesan croutons. Preheat the oven to 400°F. Cover a baking sheet with parchment paper. Make 1-tablespoon mounds of grated Parmesan cheese on the baking sheet. Bake for 4 to 5 minutes, or until the Parmesan melts into crisp disks.

PREP TIME: 15 MINUTES ■ TOTAL TIME: 25 MINUTES

2 tablespoons extra-virgin olive oil

1 pound asparagus, trimmed and cut into 1" pieces

2 cloves garlic, minced

½ teaspoon ground cloves or ¼ teaspoon freshly grated nutmeg

¼ teaspoon freshly ground black pepper

32 ounces low-sodium chicken broth or vegetable broth

1 cup canned chickpeas, rinsed

¼ cup fresh basil leaves

2 cups diced cooked chicken or shrimp or 2 cups edamame

1. Heat a heavy stockpot over medium heat. Add the oil. Add the asparagus, garlic, cloves or nutmeg, and pepper. Cook for 3 to 4 minutes, stirring occasionally, or until the asparagus starts to brown lightly.

2. Add the broth and chickpeas. Bring to a simmer, then reduce the heat to medium-low. Cover and cook for 10 minutes, or until the asparagus is tender. Add the basil.

3. Using an immersion blender, puree the soup for about 1 minute, or until smooth. Alternatively, to puree in a standard blender, cool the soup for about 10 minutes, then work in batches. Puree half of the soup, transfer to bowls or an airtight container, then blend the remaining half. To serve, top with the chicken, shrimp, or edamame.

MAKES 4 SERVINGS

PER SERVING (2 cups): 242 calories, 22 g protein, 16 g carbohydrates, 11 g total fat, 2 g saturated fat, 36 mg cholesterol, 5 g fiber, 308 mg sodium

HEALTHY KITCHEN TIP

Buy whole nutmeg, with antioxidants still intact, for the freshest taste and the biggest nutritional punch. Grate it with a Microplane or on the fine grating side of a box grater.

Sautéed Apples and Chicken Sausage with Sauerkraut

Sweet, prebiotic apples pair perfectly with bok choy, another nutrient-dense fall food. Chicken sausages vary quite a bit in fat and sodium content, so double-check labels. If you can't find bok choy, substitute kale or spinach.

PREP TIME: 20 MINUTES ■ TOTAL TIME: 25 MINUTES

2 tablespoons extra-virgin olive oil

1 apple, thinly sliced

1 head bok choy, thinly sliced

½ teaspoon ground cinnamon

¼ teaspoon freshly ground black pepper

2 tablespoons white vinegar or raw apple cider vinegar

8 low-sodium chicken sausage links

8 ounces low-sodium sauerkraut, room temperature

1. Warm a large skillet over medium heat. Add the oil, apple, bok choy, cinnamon, and pepper. Cook for 4 to 5 minutes, or until the apple starts to soften and brown. Reduce the heat to low. Cover and cook for 2 minutes, or until the bok choy is very tender. Turn off the heat and stir in the vinegar.

2. In another skillet, add the sausage and cook over medium-high heat for 4 to 5 minutes, or until the sausage starts to brown. Reduce the heat to low and cover. Cook for 2 to 3 minutes, or until no longer pink. Serve immediately with the sauerkraut and apple mixture.

MAKES 4 SERVINGS

PER SERVING (2 sausage links, 1 cup apples with bok choy, ¼ cup sauerkraut): 254 calories, 24 g protein, 15 g carbohydrates, 12 g total fat, 2 g saturated fat, 40 mg cholesterol, 3 g fiber, 661 mg sodium

Pistachio-Chia Salmon

The pistachio is one skinny nut! Not only is it the lowest in calories, but new research shows that pistachios supercharge your body for weight loss while anchoring your hunger.

PREP TIME: 15 MINUTES ■ TOTAL TIME: 25 MINUTES

2 tablespoons shelled pistachios

¼ cup chia seeds

1 teaspoon fennel seeds or cumin seeds

4 salmon fillets (4 ounces each)

¼ cup dry quinoa, rinsed under cold running water

2 cups cubed butternut squash

½ teaspoon salt

3 cups water

1. Preheat the oven to 400°F.

2. In a food processor, place the pistachios, chia, and fennel or cumin seeds. Pulse 15 to 20 times, or until the pistachios are finely chopped.

3. Place the salmon in an 11" x 7" baking dish, skin side down. Coat each fillet with cooking spray. Sprinkle the pistachio mixture over the top. Bake on a bottom oven rack for 14 to 16 minutes, or until the fish is opaque.

4. While the salmon is baking, in a medium saucepan, place the quinoa, squash, salt, and water. Bring to a boil over high heat, then reduce to a simmer. Cover and cook for 20 to 25 minutes, or until the quinoa is tender and the squash is cooked through. Serve immediately with the salmon.

MAKES 4 SERVINGS

PER SERVING (1 crusted fillet, ¾ cup butternut-quinoa side dish): 364 calories, 27 g protein, 19 g carbohydrates, 20 g total fat, 4 g saturated fat, 62 mg cholesterol, 5 g fiber, 363 mg sodium

HEALTHY KITCHEN TIP

Many grocery chains are now peeling and cubing butternut squash and other squash for easy cooking. Ask your produce manager during your next grocery trip.

Cajun Cod

Cajun food often incorporates cayenne and black peppers as mainstay spices. Red bell pepper and celery are considered a must-have in Louisiana Creole cooking, and they make a flavorful addition to kidney or black beans.

PREP TIME: 10 MINUTES ■ TOTAL TIME: 30 MINUTES

4 cod fillets (4 ounces each)

1 teaspoon salt-free Cajun spice mix

1 pound asparagus, ends trimmed, cut into thirds

1 red bell pepper, seeded and chopped

2 ribs celery, chopped

2 cups canned kidney or black beans, rinsed and drained

2 tablespoons extra-virgin olive oil

2 tablespoons chopped cilantro or flat-leaf parsley

¼ teaspoon salt

1. Preheat the oven to 400°F.

2. Place the cod in an 11" x 7" baking dish. Sprinkle with the Cajun spice and coat the tops of the fillets with cooking spray. In a second baking disk, place the asparagus, bell pepper, celery, and beans. Drizzle with the oil and sprinkle on the cilantro or parsley and salt. Bake both dishes for 10 to 15 minutes, or until the fish flakes easily and the asparagus is tender.

MAKES 4 SERVINGS

PER SERVING (1 Cajun fillet, 1½ cups vegetables): 280 calories, 29 g protein, 24 g carbohydrates, 5 g total fat, 1 g saturated fat, 49 mg cholesterol, 9 g fiber, 538 mg sodium

HEALTHY KITCHEN TIP

Not a fan of spicy chiles? Start with just a pinch of pepper and work your way up to gradually build your tolerance for the hot stuff.

Kimchi Pork Lo Mein

Kimchi is a spicy pickled Korean cabbage that adds rich flavor to stir-fries and soups. Find it in your local health food store in the refrigerated aisle, where you'll also find miso.

PREP TIME: 10 MINUTES ■ TOTAL TIME: 30 MINUTES

3 tablespoons extra-virgin olive oil or coconut oil

4 lean pork chops, trimmed of excess fat, cut into thin 2"-long strips (about 12 ounces)

1 pound Brussels sprouts or cabbage, shredded

½ pound asparagus, thinly sliced

2 tablespoons reduced-sodium soy sauce

¼ cup kimchi, chopped

1 orange, peel grated, then thinly sliced

1. Heat the oil in a large skillet over medium heat. Add the pork strips. Cook for 2 to 3 minutes, stirring often, or until the pork begins to brown. Transfer to a plate. Reduce the heat to medium-low and add the Brussels sprouts or cabbage and asparagus. Cook for 2 to 3 minutes, stirring often, or until the sprouts or cabbage browns.

2. Return the pork to the skillet and add the soy sauce. Toss well to coat. Turn off the heat and stir in the kimchi and orange peel. Top with the orange slices and serve immediately.

MAKES 4 SERVINGS

PER SERVING (1½ cups): 265 calories, 24 g protein, 17 g carbohydrates, 12 g total fat, 2 g saturated fat, 40 mg cholesterol, 6 g fiber, 575 mg sodium

HEALTHY KITCHEN TIP

The traditional version of this recipe uses high-carb white noodles. Here, thinly sliced Brussels sprouts or cabbage takes their place, chopping calories by 75 percent and adding nutrients along the way. To make this a Phase 3 meal, add 2 ounces cooked soba noodles.

Creamy Strawberry Sorbet

Studies show that brightly colored vegetables and fruits reduce risk of chronic disease. But here's the really sweet news: Polyphenol-rich berries have even more antioxidant power when paired with dark chocolate, the perfect flavor mate.

PREP TIME: 10 MINUTES ■ TOTAL TIME: 4+ HOURS

2 pints fresh or frozen strawberries

½ cup pecans or walnuts

1 tablespoon coconut oil

2 egg whites or ¼ cup pasteurized egg whites from a carton

4 teaspoons stevia powder

1 teaspoon pure vanilla extract

¼ cup chopped 70% (or higher) dark chocolate (about 1½ ounces)

In a blender, combine the berries, nuts, oil, egg whites, stevia, and vanilla until smooth. Stir in the chocolate chunks. Transfer to an airtight container and freeze for at least 4 hours or overnight.

MAKES 8 SERVINGS

PER SERVING (½ cup): 101 calories, 2 g protein, 9 g carbohydrates, 7 g total fat, 3 g saturated fat, 0 mg cholesterol, 2 g fiber, 14 mg sodium

HEALTHY KITCHEN TIPS

If eating raw eggs concerns you, go for pasteurized egg whites from the carton for better food safety.

Berries and dark chocolate make an irresistible dessert pairing, but, since they're prebiotic, they're also a good match for your friendly gut bacteria.

Dark Chocolate Nut Clusters

Are you a fan of chocolate-covered pretzels or chocolate nut bark? Then these crunchy, high-protein nut clusters will hit the spot. Make an extra batch to take to parties or holiday events as the perfect hostess gift.

PREP TIME: 10 MINUTES ■ TOTAL TIME: 40 MINUTES

2 egg whites

½ teaspoon ground cinnamon

½ cup assorted nuts, such as pistachios, macadamias, and almonds

⅓ cup plain or vanilla whey protein powder

2 tablespoons ground flaxseeds

¼ cup chopped 70% dark chocolate

2 tablespoons plain, unsweetened coconut milk

1. Preheat the oven to 300°F. Coat a baking sheet with cooking spray.

2. In a large bowl, whisk the egg whites and cinnamon until frothy. Add the nuts, protein powder, and flaxseeds and toss well. Spread on the baking sheet. Bake for 18 to 20 minutes, stirring once, or until lightly browned.

3. In a small saucepan over low heat, place the dark chocolate and coconut milk. Cook for 3 to 4 minutes, stirring often, just until the chocolate is melted and smooth. Drizzle over the nuts to cover. Cool for 4 to 5 minutes on a rack, then transfer to a plate and cool for at least 10 minutes before serving. Transfer to an airtight container and store, refrigerated, for up to 1 week.

MAKES 4 SERVINGS

PER SERVING (2 clusters): 177 calories, 11 g protein, 11 g carbohydrates, 12 g total fat, 3 g saturated fat, 0 mg cholesterol, 4 g fiber, 50 mg sodium

Mediterranean Sunrise Surprise

These herby eggs, flavored with fresh basil, make the perfect brunch treat served with a pot of green tea or black coffee. Are you a newbie at cooking eggs? Then this easy recipe is for you–the eggs cook directly in the sauce, with no expertise required.

PREP TIME: 10 MINUTES ■ TOTAL TIME: 20 MINUTES

1 tablespoon extra-virgin olive oil

4 medium tomatoes (about 1½ pounds)

1 large zucchini, thinly sliced

½ cup water

¼ cup chopped black olives, such as kalamata

8 eggs

¼ cup basil leaves

1. Heat a large skillet over medium heat and add the oil. Add the tomatoes and zucchini. Cook for 2 to 3 minutes, stirring often, or until the tomatoes give off their juices and the zucchini softens. Add the water and olives and stir well.

2. Crack the eggs on top of the vegetables. Reduce the heat to low and cover. Cook for 3 to 4 minutes, or until the whites of the eggs are cooked through. Scatter the basil leaves over the top, then serve immediately.

MAKES 4 SERVINGS

PER SERVING (2 eggs, ½ cup sauce): 215 calories, 14 g protein, 7 g carbohydrates, 14 g total fat, 3 g saturated fat, 372 mg cholesterol, 2 g fiber, 217 mg sodium

Fresh Cranberry-Spice Smoothie

Dried cranberries are high in sugar and carbs, so go fresh with fresh cranberries, available in the produce aisle during the fall holiday season. If you find yourself falling in love with this smoothie, prepare for the summer months and freeze fresh cranberries in a large resealable bag for 3 months or more.

PREP TIME: 5 MINUTES ■ TOTAL TIME: 10 MINUTES

1 cup 2% plain Greek yogurt or kefir

1 cup fresh cranberries (about 3 ounces)

½ cup pomegranate juice

⅓ cup plain or vanilla whey protein powder

¼ cup ground flaxseeds

2 tablespoons chia seeds

1 teaspoon ground cinnamon

1 teaspoon pure vanilla extract (optional)

4 teaspoons stevia powder

8 ice cubes

In a blender, combine the yogurt or kefir, cranberries, pomegranate juice, protein powder, flaxseeds, chia seeds, cinnamon, vanilla (if using), stevia, and ice. Blend until smooth. Serve immediately.

MAKES 2 SERVINGS

PER SERVING (1½ cups): 174 calories, 11 g protein, 18 g carbohydrates, 6 g total fat, 1 g saturated fat, 3 mg cholesterol, 5 g fiber, 58 mg sodium

HEALTHY KITCHEN TIP

For a summer twist, try substituting raspberries or strawberries for the cranberries.

Lean Green Smoothie with Apple and Kale

Minty and refreshing, this lean and green breakfast smoothie is a great way to get a dose of veggies fast. If you're not a mint lover, substitute a pinch of cinnamon.

PREP TIME: 5 MINUTES ■ TOTAL TIME: 10 MINUTES

1 cup plain, unsweetened coconut milk

1 cup 2% plain Greek yogurt

1 cup baby spinach

½ apple, cubed

½ cup fresh mint leaves

2 teaspoons stevia powder

2 teaspoons grated fresh ginger

½ cup cold water

8 ice cubes

In a blender, combine the coconut milk, yogurt, spinach, apple, mint, stevia, ginger, water, and ice. Blend until smooth. Serve immediately.

MAKES 2 SERVINGS

PER SERVING (1½ cups): 170 calories, 12 g protein, 21 g carbohydrates, 5 g total fat, 4 g saturated fat, 21 mg cholesterol, 3 g fiber, 76 mg sodium

Blueberry-Spice Waffles

These tender waffles will defy the notion that whole grain waffles have a tough texture. Make a double batch and cool them before freezing half for future fast, toaster-friendly breakfasts.

PREP TIME: 10 MINUTES ■ TOTAL TIME: 35 MINUTES

⅓ cup old-fashioned rolled oats

⅓ cup ground flaxseeds

⅔ cup plain or vanilla whey protein powder

¼ cup shredded unsweetened coconut

2 teaspoons stevia powder

½ teaspoon baking powder

1 cup plain, unsweetened coconut milk

2 eggs

1 cup blueberries

1. In a food processor, grind the oats and flaxseeds for about 10 seconds, or until you have a chunky flour. Transfer to a large bowl. Add the protein powder, shredded coconut, stevia, and baking powder. Stir well. Whisk in the coconut milk and eggs. Gently stir in the blueberries.

2. Heat a waffle iron according to manufacturer's directions. Coat with cooking spray. Add ½ cup of the batter and spread it with the back of a spoon. Close the lid and cook for 2 to 3 minutes, or until the waffle is firm and lightly browned. Repeat with the remaining batter. Serve immediately.

MAKES 4 SERVINGS

PER SERVING (1 waffle): 221 calories, 11 g protein, 21 g carbohydrates, 10 g total fat, 4 g saturated fat, 93 mg cholesterol, 6 g fiber 101 mg sodium

Wild Rice and Turkey Soup

You won't have to wait until Thanksgiving to make this delicious, filling soup that uses fall superfoods like turkey and wild rice. You'll find lean turkey breast cutlets in the poultry section of your meat department. Alfred Himmelrich, owner of Stone Mill Bakery and Café, serves up this hearty soup for hungry lunchtime patrons. You can enjoy it in your own kitchen. Shop for wild rice, or more affordable wild rice mixes, in the grain aisle.

PREP TIME: 10 MINUTES ■ TOTAL TIME: 30 MINUTES

2 tablespoons extra-virgin olive oil, divided

2 ribs celery, chopped

2 carrots, chopped

½ cup wild rice

2 cloves garlic, chopped

1 pound turkey breast cutlets (about 2 pieces), cubed

1 tablespoon paprika

1 teaspoon dried oregano or thyme

½ teaspoon freshly grated nutmeg (optional)

1 head broccoli, cut into florets (about 4 cups florets)

1 quart low-sodium turkey or chicken broth

1 can (15 ounces) no-salt-added diced tomatoes

1. Warm 1 tablespoon of the oil in a large pot over medium heat. Add the celery, carrots, wild rice, and garlic. Cook for 4 to 5 minutes to allow the veggies to soften.

2. Sprinkle the turkey with the paprika, oregano or thyme, and nutmeg, if using. Push the veggies to the side of the pot. Add the remaining 1 tablespoon oil. Add the turkey and increase the heat to medium-high. Cook for 2 to 3 minutes, turning the cubes, until they brown. Add the broccoli, broth, and tomatoes. Bring to a simmer, then cover. Reduce the heat to low and cook for 8 to 10 minutes, or until the turkey is cooked through and the broccoli is tender. Serve immediately.

MAKES 4 SERVINGS

PER SERVING (2½ cups): 324 calories, 36 g protein, 24 g carbohydrates, 9 g total fat, 2 g saturated fat, 70 mg cholesterol, 6 g fiber, 305 mg sodium

HEALTHY KITCHEN TIP

Don't toss the last of the Thanksgiving Day turkey! Shred it and add it to this soup. Just sauté your vegetables and add the turkey at the end, before serving.

Quinoa Salad with Lemony Yogurt Dressing

If you enjoy Greek salad or Mediterranean flavors, you'll be right at home with this lemony salad that has two high-quality protein sources–egg and quinoa. Pack the dressing separately if you transport this filling salad for a work or school lunch.

PREP TIME: 10 MINUTES ■ TOTAL TIME: 40 MINUTES

4 eggs

2–3 teaspoons lemon peel

3 tablespoons fresh lemon juice

¼ cup crumbled feta cheese

2 tablespoons extra-virgin olive oil

6 cups mixed greens, such as watercress, mesclun, and baby kale

1 bulb fennel, shredded or grated

1 cup artichoke hearts

½ cup quinoa, cooked according to package directions

1 cup Pickled Radishes (page 329) or Pickled Cucumbers (page 331)

1. Place the eggs in a small saucepan and cover with cold water. Bring to a boil over high heat. As soon as the water comes to a boil, cover the pan, remove from the heat, and let stand for 15 minutes. Run the eggs under cold water and peel. Cut the eggs in quarters and set aside.

2. In a blender, combine the lemon peel, lemon juice, cheese, and oil until smooth. In a large bowl, place the greens, fennel, artichoke hearts, quinoa, and radish or cucumber pickle. Drizzle with the dressing. Toss well, top with the eggs, and serve immediately.

MAKES 4 SERVINGS

PER SERVING (2 cups): 232 calories, 11 g protein, 17 g carbohydrates, 14 g total fat, 4 g saturated fat, 194 mg cholesterol, 5 g fiber, 239 mg sodium

Minestrone Soup*

This hearty Italian soup will give you a prebiotic boost from the beans. Beans with red or black skins also boost your antioxidant levels–and provide a wonderful creamy texture.

PREP TIME: 10 MINUTES ■ TOTAL TIME: 40 MINUTES

2 tablespoons extra-virgin olive oil

2 cloves garlic, minced

2 teaspoons Italian seasoning or dried herbs

½ teaspoon red-pepper flakes (optional)

4 ribs celery, thinly sliced

2 cups thinly sliced cabbage or bok choy

2 tablespoons tomato paste

32 ounces low-sodium chicken broth

2 cups low-sodium canned beans, such as kidney or pinto, rinsed and drained

6 ounces Swiss chard, thinly sliced

¼ cup grated Parmesan cheese

1. In a large pot over medium heat, place the olive oil, garlic, seasoning or herbs, and red-pepper flakes, if using. Cook for 1 to 2 minutes, or until the garlic becomes golden. Add the celery and cabbage or bok choy. Cover and reduce the heat to low. Cook for 3 to 4 minutes, stirring often, or until the vegetables start to soften. Add the tomato paste and broth. Bring to a simmer, then reduce the heat to low.

2. Add the beans and the Swiss chard. Cook for 1 minute, or until the beans are warmed through. Sprinkle with the cheese and serve immediately.

MAKES 4 SERVINGS

PER SERVING (2 cups): 224 calories, 13 g protein, 24 g carbohydrates, 9 g total fat, 2 g saturated fat, 9 mg cholesterol, 6 g fiber, 587 mg sodium

HEALTHY KITCHEN TIP

For low-sodium diets, opt for no-salt-added beans. Kitchen Basics makes an all-natural, good-tasting, no-salt-added broth. Or make your own cooked beans by starting with sodium-free dried beans and cooking them in a slow cooker for 5 to 6 hours on low heat with water to cover.

Also good for Phase 2 and for meal plans.

Dr. Gerry's Super Salmon Salad

This Phase 3 favorite is one of Stone Mill Bakery's most popular menu items. They slightly modified it for me and then made it part of the menu. I'm sharing this omega-3 fatty acid–rich, health-promoting, and weight-maintenance special recipe designed by Alfie Himmelrich and prepared by chefs Sarah Pigott and Toby Willse. This also serves as a nice Phase 1 low-carb, high-protein option.

PREP TIME: 15 MINUTES ■ TOTAL TIME: 25 MINUTES

1 medium cucumber, peeled and thinly sliced

2 tablespoons raw apple cider vinegar

2 tablespoons chopped dill, parsley, or basil

10 ounces salad greens, such as mesclun, baby spinach, arugula, or red leaf lettuce

4 ounces organic alfalfa sprouts (about 3 cups)

1 head broccoli, cut into florets (about 4 cups florets)

¼ cup extra-virgin olive oil + 1 tablespoon for grilling the salmon

¼ cup fresh lemon juice (from about 1 large lemon)

½ teaspoon salt

¼ teaspoon freshly ground black pepper

4 salmon fillets (4 ounces each), skin removed

1. In a medium bowl, place the cucumber, vinegar, and herbs. Toss well and set aside.

2. Chop the greens, sprouts, and broccoli florets. Place them in a bowl. Add the ¼ cup oil, lemon juice, salt, and pepper. Toss well.

3. Warm a grill or grill pan over medium-high heat. Rub the salmon fillets with the remaining 1 tablespoon oil. Grill the salmon for 6 to 8 minutes, turning once or twice, or until the fish is opaque. Divide the salad onto 4 plates and top each with a piece of salmon. Serve immediately along with the cucumbers.

MAKES 4 SERVINGS

PER SERVING (1 salmon fillet, 4 cups salad): 371 calories, 27 g protein, 11 g carbohydrates, 24 g total fat, 3 g saturated fat, 62 mg cholesterol, 4 g fiber, 467 mg sodium

HEALTHY KITCHEN TIP

For larger appetites, shop for 6-ounce salmon fillets, which add only 45 calories per serving.

Sunday Stew

Paprika is a flavorful Hungarian chili powder that comes in both "sweet" (mild) or hot varieties that you can find in the spice aisle. To protect the health benefits and flavor of spices, store them in a dark, cool drawer or cabinet, since heat and light can damage them.

PREP TIME: 10 MINUTES ■ TOTAL TIME: 4 HOURS

1 pound cubed beef stew meat

1 red bell pepper, finely chopped

4 ribs celery, chopped

2 tablespoons tomato paste

2 cloves garlic, chopped

1 teaspoon mild chili powder or paprika, sweet or hot

¼ teaspoon salt

2 tablespoons dry quinoa, rinsed under cold running water

1 cup frozen peas or edamame

4 cups salad greens, such as mesclun or baby romaine

3 tablespoons fresh lemon or lime juice

1. In a slow cooker, stir together the beef, bell pepper, celery, tomato paste, garlic, chili powder or paprika, salt, and quinoa. Cook on high for 3 to 3½ hours, stirring once or twice, or until the meat is tender. Stir in the peas or edamame and cover. Let stand for 5 to 6 minutes, or until the peas or edamame thaw.

2. Place the salad greens in a large bowl and sprinkle with the lemon or lime juice. Divide the stew into 4 portions and serve immediately with the salad.

MAKES 4 SERVINGS

PER SERVING (1 cup beef stew with 1 cup salad): 263 calories, 30 g protein, 21 g carbohydrates, 7 g total fat, 2 g saturated fat, 75 mg cholesterol, 7 g fiber, 354 mg sodium

Turkey Chili

Zesty turkey chili benefits from the tangy taste of seeded jalapeños that aren't overly spicy. If you have leftover chicken breast on hand, don't run to the store for ground turkey–just grind your chicken in a food processor for about 15 pulses until smooth.

PREP TIME: 10 MINUTES ■ TOTAL TIME: 40 MINUTES

1 tablespoon extra-virgin olive oil

1 pound ground turkey

2 tablespoons chili powder, mild or hot

2 teaspoons ground cumin

2 cloves garlic, minced

1 jalapeño chile pepper, seeded and chopped (optional—wear plastic gloves when handling)

3 ounces canned tomato paste

2 cups low-sodium chicken broth

¼ cup dry quinoa, rinsed under cold running water

½ cup water

4 cups chopped greens, such as spinach or kale

1 cup canned beans, any variety, rinsed and drained

1. Heat a large pot over medium heat. Add the oil and turkey and sear for 1 to 2 minutes without stirring, then sprinkle the chili powder and cumin over the meat. Add the garlic, jalapeño (if using), and tomato paste. Cook for 1 minute, stirring once or twice, or until the paste and garlic become fragrant.

2. Add the broth, quinoa, and water. Cover and reduce the heat to low. Simmer for 20 to 25 minutes, or until the quinoa is cooked through. Add the greens and beans and cook for 2 to 3 minutes, or until the greens are tender. Serve immediately.

MAKES 4 SERVINGS

PER SERVING (2½ cups): 333 calories, 31 g protein, 24 g carbohydrates, 13 g total fat, 4 g saturated fat, 80 mg cholesterol, 8 g fiber, 526 mg sodium

HEALTHY KITCHEN TIP

Sensitive to salt? Select no-salt-added beans and broth.

Curried Red Lentil Soup

Curry powder is an antioxidant-rich spice mix that powers up the flavor of healthy foods like lentils and cauliflower. Search out brands without added salt or sugar and with the superspice turmeric in the ingredient list.

PREP TIME: 10 MINUTES ■ TOTAL TIME: 40 MINUTES

4 thinly sliced chicken cutlets (about 1 pound) or 1 pound shrimp

2 teaspoons curry powder, such as Madras

1 tablespoon extra-virgin olive oil

1 tablespoon butter

2 cloves garlic, thinly sliced

½ cup chopped cilantro

½ head cauliflower, cut into florets (about 3 cups)

½ cup dried brown or green lentils

32 ounces low-sodium chicken broth or vegetable broth

2 tablespoons chia seeds

1. Sprinkle the chicken or shrimp with the curry powder. Warm the oil in a large pot over medium heat. Add the chicken or shrimp and cook for 4 to 5 minutes, turning once or twice, or until the chicken or shrimp starts to brown, the spices become fragrant, and the chicken is no longer pink and the juices run clear or the shrimp is opaque. Transfer the chicken or shrimp to a plate.

2. To the same pot, add the butter, garlic, and cilantro. Reduce the heat to low and cook for 1 to 2 minutes, or until the garlic becomes fragrant. Add the cauliflower and lentils. Add the broth and cook, covered, for 10 to 15 minutes, or until the lentils and cauliflower are tender. Shred the chicken and return it to the pot or add the shrimp. Sprinkle with the chia seeds and serve immediately.

MAKES 4 SERVINGS

PER SERVING (2 cups): 336 calories, 31 g protein, 26 g carbohydrates, 12 g total fat, 3 g saturated fat, 62 mg cholesterol, 7 g fiber, 201 mg sodium

Smoked Salmon Salad

Smoked salmon isn't just for brunch-time bagels, it also makes a protein-rich topping for this salad. You'll enjoy the sweet, tangy dressing that features chives in place of the scallions you'd normally pair with smoked salmon.

PREP TIME: 10 MINUTES ■ TOTAL TIME: 20 MINUTES

2 tablespoons extra-virgin olive oil

1 tablespoon raw honey

2 tablespoons chopped chives

2 teaspoons dried herbs, such as Italian seasoning

1 teaspoon chili powder or ⅛ teaspoon cayenne (ground red) pepper

¼ teaspoon freshly ground black pepper

6 cups salad greens, such as mesclun, baby spinach or kale, or romaine

½ head broccoli, cut into florets (about 2 cups florets)

8 ounces smoked salmon, thinly sliced

½ cup fresh goat cheese (about 2 ounces) or crumbled feta cheese

1. In a small bowl, whisk the oil, honey, chives, dried herbs, chili powder or cayenne pepper, and black pepper until smooth. Set aside.

2. In a large bowl, place the greens, broccoli, salmon, and cheese. Drizzle with the dressing and serve immediately.

MAKES 4 SERVINGS

PER SERVING (2 cups): 322 calories, 18 g protein, 25 g carbohydrates, 15 g total fat, 4 g saturated fat, 19 mg cholesterol, 6 g fiber, 555 mg sodium

Roasted Rosemary Chicken
with Brussels Sprouts

Nothing warms up the house—and your dinner guests—like a homey roast chicken. Coating your bird with tomato paste may seem novel, but you'll enjoy the sweet, savory flavor it lends to tender white meat.

PREP TIME: 15 MINUTES ▪ TOTAL TIME: 1 HOUR 45 MINUTES

2 pounds Brussels sprouts, cut in half

4 parsnips, peeled and cut into 1" chunks

1 (3-pound) roasting chicken

1 tablespoon tomato paste

1 tablespoon extra-virgin olive oil

2 tablespoons chopped fresh rosemary

½ teaspoon garlic powder

¼ teaspoon ground turmeric

¼ teaspoon salt

1. Preheat the oven to 400°F. Place the oven rack at its lowest setting.

2. In an 11" x 9" baking dish, scatter the Brussels sprouts and parsnips. Rub the surface of the chicken with the tomato paste and oil, then sprinkle with the rosemary, garlic powder, turmeric, and salt.

3. Place the chicken on top of the vegetables. Cover loosely with a piece of foil. Roast for 1½ hours (stirring the veggies around the chicken once or twice), or until a thermometer inserted in a breast registers 180°F and the juices run clear. Let stand for 10 minutes before carving. Slice and serve immediately with the vegetables.

MAKES 6 SERVINGS

PER SERVING (½ pound chicken, 1 cup vegetables): 299 calories, 37 g protein, 25 g carbohydrates, 7 g total fat, 1 g saturated fat, 98 mg cholesterol, 8 g fiber, 276 mg sodium

Salmon Cakes

If you have a hankering for crab cakes, you'll dig this similar seafood cake made with omega-rich salmon. To prep ahead, simply bread the patties and chill them in the refrigerator for up to 3 hours before pan cooking.

PREP TIME: 20 MINUTES ■ TOTAL TIME: 35 MINUTES

2 salmon fillets (4 ounces each)

¼ cup old-fashioned rolled oats

2 teaspoons Dijon mustard

½ teaspoon Cajun spices or dried herbs such as thyme or rosemary

⅓ cup 2% plain Greek yogurt

½ cup ground flaxseeds or chia-flax flour

¼ teaspoon salt

4 cups greens, such as arugula, mesclun, or baby romaine

1. Coat the salmon with olive oil cooking spray. Heat a medium skillet over medium-high heat and add the fillets. Cook for 5 to 7 minutes, turning occasionally, or until the salmon flakes easily but is still slightly pink in the center. Transfer to a large bowl and let cool slightly.

2. To the same bowl with the salmon, add the oats, mustard, and spices or herbs. Toss to coat the salmon, breaking the fish into chunks. Add the yogurt and toss. Place the flaxseeds or chia-flax flour and salt on a plate and mix with your fingertips. Set aside.

3. Form the salmon mixture into 8 equal patties. Press each patty into the flax mixture and transfer to a baking sheet. Coat the tops of the patties with cooking spray and bake for 10 to 15 minutes, or until the patties are hot and the tops are crisp. Serve immediately over the greens.

MAKES 4 SERVINGS

PER SERVING (2 cakes, 1 cup greens): 338 calories, 25 g protein, 18 g carbohydrates, 18 g total fat, 4 g saturated fat, 127 mg cholesterol, 8 g fiber, 302 mg sodium

HEALTHY KITCHEN TIP

Mustard brings savory flavor to the fish in these cakes, and its spicy taste means it's thermogenic, helping you to burn more calories faster.

Roasted Parmesan-Kale Lamb Chops

This easy-to-prepare yet elegant meal will wow your family and friends even as you stick to your healthy-eating plan. Keep the recipe secret and feast on the compliments! For a splendid holiday or special-occasion meal, serve an additional vegetable side like roasted Brussels sprouts or the Massaged Kale Salad (page 286).

PREP TIME: 10 MINUTES ■ TOTAL TIME: 40 MINUTES

1 cup torn kale leaves

½ cup grated Parmesan cheese

1 tablespoon extra-virgin olive oil, divided

1 rack of lamb (about 1 pound), trimmed of excess fat

1 pound green beans, stemmed and cut into 1" pieces

1 teaspoon cumin seeds or fennel seeds

2 tablespoons chopped almonds

3 tablespoons ground flaxseeds

⅛ teaspoon salt

1. Preheat the oven to 400°F.

2. Place the kale in a food processor and pulse for about 20 seconds, or until finely chopped. Add the cheese and ½ tablespoon of the oil and process until smooth. Place the lamb in an 11" x 7" baking dish. Coat the top with the kale mixture. Bake, uncovered, for 40 to 45 minutes, or until a thermometer inserted in the center registers 145°F for medium-rare. Let stand for 10 minutes before slicing.

3. Meanwhile, warm the remaining ½ tablespoon oil in a large skillet over medium heat. Add the green beans and cumin or fennel seeds. Cook for 4 to 5 minutes, or until the beans start to brown and the seeds become fragrant. Add a few tablespoons of water and cover. Steam through for 1 minute. Remove the lid and toss in the almonds, flaxseeds, and salt. Serve immediately with the lamb.

MAKES 4 SERVINGS

PER SERVING (2 chops, 1 cup green beans): 355 calories, 31 g protein, 12 g carbohydrates, 20 g total fat, 5 g saturated fat, 81 mg cholesterol, 5 g fiber, 242 mg sodium

Zucchini Manicotti

Here's an Italian favorite redesigned to fit the new you. It still has the same flavors you long for, like marinara and Parmesan, but it ups the ante with fat-burning fuel like high-protein Greek yogurt and high-fiber spinach.

PREP TIME: 15 MINUTES ■ TOTAL TIME: 40 MINUTES

1 cup low-sodium jarred marinara sauce

1 pound zucchini, trimmed and thinly sliced lengthwise (about 2 medium)

1 cup 2% plain Greek yogurt

½ cup crumbled feta cheese or soft goat cheese

½ cup frozen peas, thawed

½ cup fresh basil (optional)

1 teaspoon garlic powder

½ cup grated Parmesan cheese

8 cups baby spinach

1. Preheat the oven or a toaster oven to 400°F. Spread ½ cup of the marinara sauce inside an 8" x 8" baking dish and set aside.

2. Heat a large skillet over medium heat. Pull the skillet off the heat and coat with cooking spray. Add the slices of zucchini, return the skillet to the heat, and cook for 2 to 3 minutes per side, or until the slices start to brown. Reduce the heat to low and cover. Cook for 2 to 3 minutes, or until the slices are tender. Remove the lid and let cool slightly while you prepare the filling.

3. In a large bowl, place the yogurt, feta or goat cheese, peas, basil, and garlic powder. Mix with a rubber spatula until smooth. Spoon 2 tablespoons of the yogurt mixture in the center of each zucchini slice, fold over, and place the pieces seam side down in the baking dish. Top with the remaining ½ cup marinara. Sprinkle the Parmesan over the top and bake for 15 to 20 minutes, or until the Parmesan is melted and brown. Serve immediately over the baby spinach.

MAKES 4 SERVINGS

PER SERVING (3 manicotti, 2 cups baby spinach): 224 calories, 17 g protein, 18 g carbohydrates, 9 g total fat, 5 g saturated fat, 30 mg cholesterol, 5 g fiber, 606 mg sodium

HEALTHY KITCHEN TIP

Shop for low-sodium or "sensitive formula" sauces that contain half the salt and no onions.

Dark Chocolate Flourless Cake

This cake is a protein burst in the guise of a tasty dessert. It is pretty enough for the grand finale of a dinner party or simply an end to a light meal of soup or salad.

PREP TIME: 5 MINUTES ■ TOTAL TIME: 30 MINUTES

¼ cup coconut oil

4 ounces 70% (or higher) dark chocolate, chopped

¼ cup stevia powder

1–2 teaspoons espresso powder (optional)

1 teaspoon pure vanilla extract

3 large eggs

⅓ cup plain or vanilla whey protein powder

¼ cup unsweetened cocoa powder

1 teaspoon baking powder

¼ cup heavy cream

¼ teaspoon ground cinnamon

½ teaspoon ground coriander

½ cup raspberries

1. Preheat the oven to 350°F. Lightly grease an 8" round cake pan. Cut a piece of parchment or waxed paper to fit, grease it, and lay it in the bottom of the pan.

2. In a microwaveable bowl, microwave the oil and chocolate for about 30 seconds, or until the chocolate is almost melted. Stir until the chocolate completely melts. Alternatively, place the coconut oil and chocolate in a small saucepan over very low heat and melt the chocolate, stirring often, for about 1 minute.

3. Transfer the melted mixture to a large mixing bowl and let cool slightly, for about 5 minutes. Add the stevia, espresso powder (if using), and vanilla and stir until smooth. Add the eggs, beating just until smooth. Add the protein powder, cocoa, and baking powder and mix just to combine. Spoon the batter into the prepared pan.

4. Bake for 7 to 10 minutes, or until the top forms a thin crust but is still soft to the touch in the center. Cool in the pan for 5 minutes. Loosen the edges of the pan with a butter knife and turn the cake out onto a serving plate.

5. Place the cream in a large mixing bowl. Add the cinnamon and coriander. Beat for about 2 minutes, or until fluffy. Stir in the raspberries. Spoon on the cake and serve.

MAKES 8 SERVINGS

PER SERVING (4" wedge with 1 heaping tablespoon whipped cream): 207 calories, 6 g protein, 10 g carbohydrates, 18 g total fat, 11 g saturated fat, 80 mg cholesterol, 3 g fiber, 39 mg sodium

Pickled Ginger

Use pickled ginger on cooked fish, chicken, or vegetables or blend it with olive oil to make a tasty dressing.

PREP TIME: 30 MINUTES ■ TOTAL TIME: 3 TO 7 DAYS

1 teaspoon whole cloves

¼ teaspoon salt

½ pound fresh ginger, peeled and thinly sliced

1. Place the cloves and salt in an airtight glass container. Fill the container halfway with warm water and stir well to dissolve the salt. Add the ginger and add more water if necessary to cover. Leave 1" of space between the top of the water and the top of the jar.

2. Cover loosely with a kitchen towel or cheesecloth. Leave on your counter for 3 to 7 days. Check daily. The brine will begin to get cloudy and slightly bubbly. When the pickles taste tangy, cover tightly and refrigerate. Store in the fridge for up to 3 weeks.

MAKES ABOUT 2 CUPS

PER SERVING (2 tablespoons): 11 calories, 0 g protein, 2 g carbohydrates, 0 g total fat, 0 g saturated fat, 2 mg cholesterol, 0 g fiber, 38 mg sodium

Pickled Beets

Serve pickled beets with their flavor mates–nuts, greens, and even raspberries–over fresh greens. Pickled beets are also delicious with lean white meats like roasted chicken or roast pork.

PREP TIME: 30 MINUTES ■ TOTAL TIME: 3 TO 7 DAYS

1 teaspoon black peppercorns

1 teaspoon lavender blossoms or Italian herbs

½ teaspoon ground cardamom

¼ teaspoon salt

½ pound beets, peeled and thinly sliced

1. In an airtight glass container, place the peppercorns, lavender or Italian herbs, cardamom, and salt. Fill the container halfway with warm water and stir well to dissolve the salt. Add the beets and add more water if necessary to cover. Leave 1" of space between the top of the water and the top of the jar.

2. Cover loosely with a kitchen towel or cheesecloth. Leave on your counter for 3 to 7 days. Check daily. The brine will begin to get cloudy and slightly bubbly. When the pickles taste tangy, cover tightly and refrigerate. Store in the fridge for up to 3 weeks.

MAKES ABOUT 2 CUPS

PER SERVING (2 tablespoons): 6 calories, 0 g protein, 1 g carbohydrates, 0 g total fat, 0 g saturated fat, 0 mg cholesterol, 0 g fiber, 47 mg sodium

Pickled Radishes

Tangy pickled radishes are perfect paired with black beans or lentils, as a side dish for soups or stews, or incorporated into salsas.

PREP TIME: 30 MINUTES ■ TOTAL TIME: 3 TO 7 DAYS

1 tablespoon chopped fresh or dried rosemary

1 clove garlic, thinly sliced

½ teaspoon cumin seeds or fennel seeds

½ teaspoon crushed red-pepper flakes

¼ teaspoon salt

½ pound radishes, stems removed and quartered

1. In an airtight glass container, place the rosemary, garlic, seeds, red-pepper flakes, and salt. Fill the container halfway with warm water and stir well to dissolve the salt. Add the radishes and add more water if necessary to cover. Leave 1" of space between the top of the water and the top of the jar.

2. Cover loosely with a kitchen towel or cheesecloth. Leave on your counter for 3 to 7 days. Check daily. The brine will begin to get cloudy and slightly bubbly. When the pickles taste tangy, cover tightly and refrigerate. Store in the fridge for up to 3 weeks.

MAKES ABOUT 2 CUPS

PER SERVING (2 tablespoons): 3 calories, 0 g protein, 1 g carbohydrates, 0 g total fat, 0 g saturated fat, 0 mg cholesterol, 0 g fiber, 42 mg sodium

Pickled Horseradish

Served with lean turkey sausage links or even rack of lamb, pickled horseradish adds flavor with hardly any calories. Blend with low-sodium tomato juice for a healthful virgin Bloody Mary.

PREP TIME: 30 MINUTES ■ TOTAL TIME: 3 TO 7 DAYS

2 cloves garlic, minced

1 teaspoon mustard seeds (optional)

¼ teaspoon salt

½ pound horseradish, peeled and grated

1. In an airtight glass container, place the garlic, mustard seeds (if using), and salt. Fill the container halfway with warm water and stir well to dissolve the salt. Add the horseradish and add more water if necessary to cover. Leave 1" of space between the top of the water and the top of the jar.

2. Cover loosely with a kitchen towel or cheesecloth. Leave on your counter for 3 to 7 days. Check daily. The brine will begin to get cloudy and slightly bubbly. When the pickles taste tangy, cover tightly and refrigerate. Store in the fridge for up to 3 weeks.

MAKES ½ POUND

PER SERVING (2 tablespoons): 13 calories, 0 g protein, 2 g carbohydrates, 0 g total fat, 0 g saturated fat, 0 mg cholesterol, 0 g fiber, 37 mg sodium

Pickled Cucumbers

This low-sodium pickle recipe is an ideal swap for high-sodium jarred kosher or dill pickles. Use on meats, burgers, or alongside coleslaw.

PREP TIME: 30 MINUTES ■ TOTAL TIME: 3 TO 7 DAYS

2 tablespoons chopped dill

2 cloves garlic, minced

1 teaspoon mustard seeds (optional)

¼ teaspoon salt

½ pound cucumbers, any variety, trimmed and cut into ½" slices

1. In an airtight glass container, place the dill, garlic, mustard seeds (if using), and salt. Fill the container halfway with warm water and stir well to dissolve the salt. Add the sliced cucumbers and add more water if necessary to cover. Leave 1" of space between the top of the water and the top of the jar.

2. Cover loosely with a kitchen towel or cheesecloth. Leave on your counter for 3 to 7 days. Check daily. The brine will begin to get cloudy and slightly bubbly. When the pickles taste tangy, cover tightly and refrigerate. Store in the fridge for up to 3 weeks.

MAKES ABOUT 2 CUPS

PER SERVING (2 tablespoons): 3 calories, 0 g protein, 0 g carbohydrates, 0 g total fat, 0 g saturated fat, 0 mg cholesterol, 0 g fiber, 36 mg sodium

Sauerkraut

Homemade kraut has a fresher flavor than the canned version, and the caraway seeds give it a savory burst you'll love. Use red cabbage to cash in on the antioxidants found in plant pigments.

PREP TIME: 30 MINUTES ■ TOTAL TIME: 3 TO 7 DAYS

2 cloves garlic, minced

½ pound cabbage (about ½ head), any variety, thinly sliced

½ teaspoon salt

1 teaspoon caraway seeds (optional)

1. In a large bowl, place the garlic, cabbage, salt, and caraway seeds (if using). Squeeze the cabbage with your fingers for 2 to 3 minutes to release some of its liquid. Transfer the mixture to a quart container. Press down on the cabbage occasionally with a spoon, pushing the cabbage under the liquid that it gives off. If it isn't covered with liquid after 24 hours, add ¼ cup water.

2. Cover loosely with a kitchen towel or cheesecloth. Leave on your counter for 3 to 7 days. Check daily. The brine will begin to get cloudy and slightly bubbly. Continue to press the cabbage beneath the liquid it generates. When the kraut tastes tangy, cover tightly and refrigerate. Store in the fridge for up to 3 weeks.

MAKES ABOUT 4 CUPS

PER SERVING (2 tablespoons): 3 calories, 0 g protein, 0 g carbohydrates, 0 g total fat, 0 g saturated fat, 0 mg cholesterol, 0 g fiber, 36 mg sodium

Homemade Dairy-Based Yogurt

Yogurt made at home has a superior flavor and a softer texture than store-bought. You'll savor its mild taste, which makes it an easier sell to kids.

PREP TIME: 30 MINUTES ■ TOTAL TIME: 6 HOURS 30 MINUTES

1 quart 2% milk, preferably from grass-fed cows

1 tablespoon raw honey

¼ cup store-bought low-fat plain yogurt or 2% plain yogurt (standard or Greek) with live cultures

1. In a heavy saucepan or 2-quart Dutch oven, heat the milk over medium-low heat for 6 to 7 minutes, or until it reaches 180°F and the milk is steamy and foamy. Do not let it boil. Stir the milk gently as it heats to make sure the bottom doesn't scorch. Add the honey and whisk well.

2. Let the milk cool for 12 to 14 minutes, or until it is just hot to the touch and measures 112° to 115°F. To speed the cooling process, fill a large bowl with ice and enough water to cover. Set the saucepan or Dutch oven into the ice water.

3. Pour about a cup of the warm milk into a small bowl and whisk it with the yogurt. Add the mixture to the warm milk.

4. Preheat the oven or toaster oven to 150°F for 4 minutes. Turn the heat off and allow the oven to cool for 5 minutes to drop the temperature to 112°F. Cover the top of the saucepan or the Dutch oven with foil, wrap in a clean dishtowel, and transfer to the warm oven, being sure the heat is off. Let stand, without turning the oven on, for 4 hours (for mild-tasting yogurt) to 6 hours (for tangier yogurt) to allow the bacteria to multiply. The texture should resemble a soft custard.

5. Remove the towel and secure the foil. Store the yogurt in the refrigerator for about 2 weeks.

MAKES 1 QUART

PER SERVING (½ cup): 78 calories, 5 g protein, 8 g carbohydrates, 2 g total fat, 1 g saturated fat, 9 mg cholesterol, 0 g fiber, 223 mg sodium

HEALTHY KITCHEN TIP

Homemade yogurt is definitely worth the 30-minute prep. It offers a mild taste and a silky texture, and once you've tried homemade you might not go back to store-bought. This low-sugar homemade recipe doesn't have the bitter tang of plain commercial yogurt. Flavor it with antioxidant-rich toppings like chopped 70% dark chocolate, dried cherries, or nuts.

Homemade Dairy-Based Kefir Made from Kefir Crystals

Shop for kefir crystals at your local health food store or online. While they're a little expensive, you'll save money in the long run by preparing your own kefir at home. And there isn't a simpler ferment you can make. Store unused crystals in a dark, cool cabinet until ready to use; they'll keep for a long time.

1 quart 2% milk, preferably from grass-fed cows	1 tablespoon kefir grains

Place the milk and the kefir grains in a glass jar and cover tightly. Set out at room temperature for 12 to 14 hours, or up to 24 hours, depending on the temperature of your home. Shake the jar gently a few times. When the kefir is ready, it will thicken. If the kefir grains coagulate on the top, strain the grains to use in the next batch. For a sourer, thicker kefir, let it ferment longer. For one less sour and thick, strain sooner. Experiment to see what works for you. Store the kefir, refrigerated, for 3 to 4 weeks.

Optional: There are many dairy-free kefir variations made by using other milks such as nuts (almond, walnut, and so on), coconut, rice, hemp, or organic, (non-GMO) soy, but the process of fermentation is less consistent than animal milks, which provide an ideal culture medium for the kefir grains to thrive and reproduce.

MAKES 1 QUART KEFIR

PER SERVING (½ cup): 68 calories, 5 g protein, 6 g carbohydrates, 2 g total fat, 1 g saturated fat, 9 mg cholesterol, 0 g fiber, 82 mg sodium

Dairy-Free Yogurt

Yogurt is one of the world's most popular fermented food. Store-bought yogurt is light on bacterial counts and just doesn't make a dent in restoring our gut flora. Homemade yogurt has billions of robust friendly flora to put us back into balance. Potent dairy-free yogurts are not commercially available.

2 cups cashew milk*

4 cups canned unsweetened coconut milk

1 tablespoon honey or coconut sugar

¼ teaspoon vanilla creme–flavored liquid stevia

1½ tablespoons gelatin or 1½ teaspoons agar powder dissolved in ½ cup boiling water

9 probiotic capsules containing 25 billion to 30 billion CFUs of any dairy-free probiotic

1. In a large saucepan over medium heat, place the milks, honey or coconut sugar, and stevia. Bring to a simmer. Watch carefully so it doesn't boil over. Once it begins to simmer, turn off the heat. Whisk in the dissolved gelatin or agar powder.

2. Pour the mixture into a large bowl. Put that bowl into a larger one of cold (but not iced) tap water and let the mixture stand until it cools to 92°F. If you used gelatin, you can whisk the mixture to cool it faster. Omit this step if you used agar powder, as whisking could make the agar powder lumpy.

3. When the mixture reaches about 92°F, add the contents of the probiotic capsules. Whisk them in well. Ladle into jars and keep warm for about 10 hours.†

4. If there is a clear pool at the bottom after 10 hours, secure the lids tightly and shake the yogurt to mix it in before refrigerating. (*Note:* For the agar option, shaking isn't necessary.) Refrigerate for 8 hours.

Optional: Put a drop or two of lemon extract on a spoon and stir into your jar of yogurt just before eating it.

MAKES 6 CUPS

PER SERVING (½ cup): 37 calories, 0 g protein, 4 g carbohydrates, 6 g total fat, 1 g saturated fat, 0 mg cholesterol, 0 g fiber, 29 mg sodium

* *Organic (non-GMO) soy and coconut are suitable substitutes while other milks such as hemp, rice, and nut milks have a consistency that is too thick.*

† *Keep warm with a yogurt maker or by putting it in a gas oven with a pilot light, in a cooler with warm water, or even into a hot tub.*

Cilantro Green Drink

Mojito lovers will adore this booze-free herb-y drink made with lime. It quenches your thirst with hardly any calories, a refreshing break from plain water. To make a whole pitcher, simply quadruple the ingredients and then store in your fridge for up to 3 days.

2 lime wedges	2 cups filtered water
1 handful cilantro	1 or 2 ice cubes (optional)

In a large glass, place the lime, cilantro, water, and ice (if using). Stir and serve immediately.

MAKES 1 SERVING

PER SERVING (2½ cups): 4 calories, 0 g protein, 1 g carbohydrates, 0 g total fat, 0 g saturated fat, 0 mg cholesterol, 0 g fiber, 0 mg sodium

Basil Green Drink

Ideal for those who don't love cilantro, basil is a fragrant flavor booster that pairs surprisingly well with lime. If fresh basil isn't available in your local grocery store, use mint instead.

2 lemon wedges	2 cups water
1 handful fresh basil	1 to 2 ice cubes (optional)

In a large glass, place the lemon, basil, water, and ice (if using). Stir and serve immediately.

MAKES 1 SERVING

PER SERVING (2½ cups): 5 calories, 0 g protein, 1 g carbohydrates, 0 g total fat, 0 g saturated fat, 0 mg cholesterol, 0 g fiber, 0 mg sodium

THE GUT BALANCE REVOLUTION SUCCESS STORIES

Jennifer Metevia, 37

What's normal, anyway? For Jennifer Metevia, it meant chronic sinus infections, constant courses of antibiotics, and tummy troubles that never seemed to go away. "I was continually getting sick," she recalls, "and after a while, I just figured that was how everybody felt—maybe it was just part of getting older." But swollen stomach that "freaked me out" and sent her on a late-night visit to the emergency room, and the eventual diagnosis of celiac disease, changed the way Jennifer looked at the world—and at her health. "I finally realized that living in pain wasn't normal, and I learned that there was something I could do to change it."

The solution? Though Jennifer had to take strong antibiotics to eliminate the overgrowth of the bacteria in the small intestine that were making her sick, an equally important part of her treatment was the eating plan of the Gut Balance Revolution. Within a few weeks, her symptoms began to disappear. And healing her gut came with a surprising side effect—the weight she'd been trying to lose for years began to literally melt away. Within just 2 weeks, she'd dropped 15 pounds.

Now, Jennifer insists, "I feel so much better, so much healthier. By eating differently, I'm noticing things about food that I'd never been aware of before. I used to crave sweets, but now I think my taste buds have changed—if I cheat a little bit and have a bite of cake, I can taste the chemicals and just spit it out. So I pretty much stay away from that stuff—I've learned that it's just not worth it."

Along with renewed health and a trim new figure, these days Jennifer has more energy than ever. Instead of coming home from work and crashing on the couch, she heads out to Zumba or takes a brisk walk. She had the fun of shopping for a new wardrobe, and her colleagues at work—she's an office manager—comment on her new appearance. "Everybody wants to know how I've done it," Jennifer says. "I've become a Gut Balance Revolution evangelist!"

CONCLUSION:
THE REAL SECRET TO WEIGHT LOSS

Before I close this book, I want to share the real secret to weight loss with you.

After reading hundreds of pages outlining the science behind good diet and gut microbiome health, you may be surprised that I would tell you there is yet another secret to weight loss. But there is, and it can be described in a single word.

Perseverance.

It's not sexy and it's not simple, but it's the truth. Despite the endless infomercials and advertisements that promise easy, dramatic results overnight, there are no magic solutions that will automatically and effortlessly cause you to lose weight. No single pill or supplement will allow you to burn away fat for the long term if you don't change what you eat and how you live. No one-size-fits-all diet will work for every person in every circumstance. Any claim to the contrary is simply a lie.

Of course, you probably already know this. If you've been on the path toward weight loss, if you've tried other diets and failed, if you've watched the pounds pile up around your waist yet can't figure out for the life of you why, then you know the real truth. Weight loss is not always easy. After all, life is challenging and it keeps on changing and moving forward. People fall off the diet wagon or get derailed due to life circumstances. They have difficulty changing their eating and exercise habits. Sometimes, medical issues, sleep disturbances, chronic stress, emotional problems, and other factors make it nearly impossible to lose weight.

Losing weight–and getting healthy–is not a bed of roses. It takes work. It takes persistence. It takes bravery to look yourself in the mirror, pull yourself up by your bootstraps, and get back to living a life that supports your weight and your health.

Lord knows I've been there. Losing 120 pounds was not easy for me, nor was recovering from a disabling illness. But through these experiences, I learned that when life knocks you down, you've got to pick yourself up and keep going.

If I can do it, you can do it.

Achieving your optimal weight and excellent health probably won't be a straightforward path. It may take twists and turns. You may have to dig in and do a little investigating, to see what works for you. Occasionally, sticking to your eating plan may be a challenge, and you may slip from time to time. But I'm living proof that you *can* lose weight and keep it off long term, *if* you persevere.

Winston Churchill, the famous British prime minister, was well known for statements like, "We shall never surrender," "Never give in," and "Withhold no sacrifice." After he finished his Upper Sixth Form (not the same thing as sixth grade here; more like high school) at Harrow, it took him three attempts to pass the entrance exam to the Royal Military Academy, Sandhurst, where he graduated 8th out of a class of 150, then ultimately rose to become one of the greatest wartime figures and speakers of the 20th century. Abraham Lincoln lost virtually every congressional election he ran in and was passed over as a vice presidential candidate. After he was finally elected president, his son Willie died less than a year after he took office. Despite his setbacks, he stands among the greatest American leaders in history.

I don't bring up historical figures like these for whimsy. On the contrary. These individuals have a lot to teach us about what it means to persevere–and succeed–in even the most trying circumstances. If Lincoln could lose nearly every election he ran in and then lose his son only 11 months after becoming president yet *still* rise to become one of our nation's finest statesmen, then you can lose the weight and find the health you deserve.

It may seem odd for a doctor to hang a poster of the movie character Rocky on his office wall, but it's there for a reason: Rocky represents the kind of mind and heart I believe it takes to succeed in the world *and* to be healthy. You have to be a fighter. Life will knock you down. But it's not about how many times you get knocked down, it's about how many times you get back up. Illness and weight gain are two of the most difficult setbacks we face as individuals and as a society. Yet we can fight against the tide of chronic disease in this country, just as we can battle against our personal bulge.

To do this, we must persevere.

So you get knocked off your diet. Get back on it. So life pushes you out of your exercise routine. Push back. Don't give up. Stay in the fight. As Rocky said, "That's how winning's done."

I know you can do it.

So go for it!

APPENDIX:

Common Dietary Supplements and Their Purported Mechanism of Action, Eefficacy, and Adverse Effects

The following easy-to-use table includes supplement names, proposed mechanism of action, adverse effects (if there are any), and other information where appropriate.

For the recommendations, I have applied an A through F grading system, just like in school. These grades were adapted from the levels of evidence and grades of recommendations used by the National Guideline Clearinghouse (guideline.gov), a public resource for evidence-based health-care practice guidelines. Here is what each grade means.

SUPPLEMENT (RECOMMENDED DOSE)	PROPOSED MECHANISM OF ACTION (IF KNOWN)	
Calcium*	• Causes fat cell death • Increases fecal fat losses	• Increases fat oxidation
Capsaicin	• Increases fat oxidation • Increases thermogenesis	
Carulluma fimbriata	• Suppresses appetite	
Chitin/chitosan	• Blocks dietary fat absorption • Improves satiety	• Lowers appetite • Lowers food intake
Chlorogenic acid	• Blocks fat cell formation • Is anti-inflammatory	• Enhances insulin sensitivity • Lipolytic—breaks down fat
Chromium picolinate	• Enhances insulin sensitivity • Enhances satiety	• Increases thermogenesis • Stabilizes blood sugar
Cissus quadrangularis	• Blocks dietary fat and carbohydrate uptake by inhibiting lipase and amylase enzymes • Reduces oxidative stress	
Citrus aurantium	• Adrenergic agonist—stimulates stress response • Decreases gastric motility and lowers food intake	
Coleus forskohlii	• Lipolytic—breaks down fat cells	
Conjugated linoleic acid	• Reduces fat synthesis • Increases fat oxidation	
Epigallocatechin gallate (EGCG: green tea extract)	• Increases energy expenditure • Increases fat oxidation • Suppresses the fat-making enzyme fatty acid synthetase	

Recommended dosage is 600–1,000 mg daily.

A–Evidence from meta-analysis of randomized controlled trials or evidence from at least one controlled study without randomization

B–Evidence from at least one controlled study without randomization or evidence from at least one other type of quasi-experimental study

C–Evidence from nonexperimental descriptive studies, such as comparative studies, correlation studies, and case-control studies

D–Evidence from expert committee reports or opinions, or clinical experience of respected authorities, or both

F–No evidence it works, and/or evidence it could harm your health

ADVERSE EFFECT(S)	RECOMMENDATION (A–F)
None reported	**Level A** when taken while maintaining sufficient 25-hydroxy vitamin D blood levels
Strongly pungent	**Level B** • Some evidence • Food-based source preferred
None reported	**Level F** • No known evidence • NOT recommended
Gastrointestinal discomfort and bloating	**Level F** • Some weak evidence • NOT recommended
None	**Level B** • Some evidence
Accumulation in the kidneys	**Level F** • Weak evidence • NOT recommended
None known	**Level F** • Weak evidence • NOT recommended
There are concerns that it may act like ephedra, but none reported to date	**Level F** • Weak evidence • NOT recommended
None reported	**Level F** • No evidence • NOT recommended
No known adverse effects	**Level D** • Uncertain • NOT recommended
No known adverse effects from tea. Herbal extracts can cause hepatotoxicity.	**Level A/B for tea** **Level F for extract as a supplement** • Some evidence • Recommended as a beverage (1–3 cups of tea per day) • NOT recommended for supplementation as an herbal extract

(continued)

Appendix: Common Dietary Supplements (CONT.)

SUPPLEMENT (RECOMMENDED DOSE)	PROPOSED MECHANISM OF ACTION (IF KNOWN)	
Fenugreek	• Lipolytic—breaks down fat cells or adipocytes • Is an antioxidant • Improves glucose tolerance	• Enhances insulin sensitivity • Improves blood lipids
Fish oil	• Blocks adipogenesis fat-making • Enhances insulin sensitivity • Increases fat oxidation	• Increases energy expenditure • Suppresses appetite
Garcinia cambogia	• Inhibits de novo lipogenesis—new fat cell production • Reduces appetite • Suppresses fatty acid synthesis	
Ginseng	• Delays fat absorption by inhibiting pancreatic lipase activity • Modulates carbohydrate metabolism	
Guar gum	• Blocks dietary fat absorption • Improves satiety	• Lowers appetite • Lowers food intake
Hoodia gordonii	• Is anti-inflammatory • Increases ATP production and decreases food intake • Inhibits de novo lipogenesis—new fat cell production • Suppresses appetite	
Konjac root fiber	• Blocks dietary fat absorption • Improves satiety	• Lowers appetite • Lowers food intake
L-carnitine	• Increases fat oxidation • Decreases fat synthesis	
Melatonin	• Is an antioxidant • Activates brown fat • Enhances insulin sensitivity	• Regulates leptin, ghrelin • Regulates sleep • Regulates stress
Phaseolus vulgaris	• Inhibits digestive enzyme alpha amylase and inhibits starch absorption	
Probiotics	• Are anti-inflammatory • Regulate appetite • Improve energy metabolism • Enhance gut barrier	• Improve dysbiosis • Improve SIBO • Enhance insulin sensitivity • Increase satiety
Psyllium	• Blocks dietary fat absorption • Improves satiety	• Lowers appetite • Lowers food intake
Resveratrol	• Is anti-inflammatory • Is an antioxidant • Enhances insulin sensitivity	• Increases fatty acid oxidation • Inhibits lipid formation in fat cells • Is a prebiotic
Vitamin D	• Unknown	

Table adapted from Poddar et al. with permission from Sage Publications.[6,7]

ADVERSE EFFECT(S)	RECOMMENDATION (A–F)
Unknown	**Level B** • Some evidence
Burping Fishy taste, odor	**Level B** • Some evidence
No known adverse effects	**Level B** • Some evidence
None known	**Level F** • No known evidence • NOT recommended
Gastrointestinal discomfort and bloating	**Level F** • No evidence • NOT recommended
None known	**Level F** • No known evidence • NOT recommended
Gastrointestinal discomfort and bloating	**Level B** • Some evidence
No adverse effects	**Level F** • No evidence • NOT recommended
Drowsiness	**Level B** • Some evidence
None known	**Level B/C** • Some evidence
Bloating, flatus	**Level A/B** • Good evidence—appears to be strain specific
Gastrointestinal discomfort and bloating	**Level B/C** • Some evidence
None	**Level F** • No evidence • NOT recommended
Kidney stones at very high serum levels	**Level B** **Level A** when taken with 600–1,000 mg of elemental calcium daily

ACKNOWLEDGMENTS

As with every book, this one has its own story and its own unique journey. It encompasses all of those dedicated to educating and positively impacting the health and quality of life of you, the reader. I would like to acknowledge as many as possible of those who assisted and supported me during the creation of this book.

Two years ago, I was on the phone with Anne Egan of Rodale discussing *The Inside Tract*. At the tail end of our conversation—and well before the topic of gut microbiome health began making waves in the press—I pitched the notion that the Track 2 diet in that book was helping my patients lose weight and merited its own book. Unlike most publishers, Anne followed through and took a leadership role in moving this concept to the project level. Anne, many thanks for all you have done. Acquisitions Editor Nancy Fitzgerald of Rodale facilitated the proposal. Nancy has been a godsend and has my gratitude for her dedication in making *The Gut Balance Revolution* a reality. Jennifer Levesque from Rodale came onto the scene at the later stages of development, my deepest gratitude for your support. Chris DeMarchis, Brent Gallenberger, Evan Klonsky, and Emily Weber are absolute gems—brava! A big thank-you to Mary Ann Naples and to all the staff at Rodale for being a class act! I would also like to acknowledge Charles Frank Morgan of Baltimore for his counsel and guidance.

I would like to express my gratitude to the many experts whose exceptional contributions made this book possible: First and foremost, Spencer Smith for his outstanding developmental and editorial assistance. I cannot give him enough accolades—he's simply the best. Also, Jennifer Iserloh, the Skinny Chef, for her creativity and energy in helping to transform concepts into recipes and meal plans for this book.

The creation of a book takes long hours, and I've been blessed to have so many supporters to lean on. First, I drew inspiration from the loving memory of my parents, and I received continuing encouragement from my family—Patrick and Tatianna, Tim and Barbara, Maureen and Gwenn and their children. I am thankful to my godchild, Angela Girratano, whose energy and spirit brighten my life, and to Brian Veith though he actively posts anti–New York Knicks propaganda on Facebook. I'm grateful to Monsignors Arthur Bastress and Arthur Valenzano for their spiritual support and guidance, and to the staff at St. Alphonsus Church and the Basilica of the Assumption in Baltimore, Maryland.

I've been fortunate to have close friends who have been my backbone during the more-than-2-year odyssey of producing this book: Conchita, Miriam, and the Keena family, and the late Patrick Keena; Dr. Loren Marks, a cutting-edge nutritionist and integrative medicine expert in New York City; Dr. Christopher Houlihan, his wife Debbie, and their family; Dr. Laura Matarese, an international expert in nutrition support and a coeditor with me on many book projects, including *Integrative Weight Management*; plus so many good friends at Johns Hopkins. A special thank-you to Drs. Nina Victoria Gallagher in Fixby Park, Huddersfield, West Yorkshire, UK; Oxana Ormonova in Mount Shasta, California; and Mr. Abdul Aziz Al Ghurair of Dubai, United Arab Emirates, for their support and friendship.

Of course, I'd like to acknowledge everyone at Stone Mill Bakery, where I've spent many a lunch- and dinnertime nourishing my body and spirit with the wonderful food and kindred spirits I found there–thank you to Alfie and Dana Himmelrich, Sarah Pigott, Cris Janoff, Devin Adams, Toby Willse, and all the staff who make my food experience first-rate!

There are many people who have guided my career and sparked my interest in nutrition, integrative digestive health, and weight management, and I'd like to offer my gratitude to them as well.

Thank you to my mentors who have guided my career over the years, in particular Drs. Anthony Kalloo, Andrew Weil, and Victoria Maizes; and to the nutritionists whose collaborations have fostered career development and friendships, especially Drs. Carol Ireton-Jones, Mark DeLegge, Steve McClave, Kelly Tappenden, Jeanette Hasse, and Amy Brown. A special word of thanks to Kathie Swift, who coauthored *The Inside Tract* and introduced me to the FODMAPs–that was indeed a game changer for me. To Dr. Sue Shepherd and Dr. Peter Gibson, coauthors of the book *The Complete Low-FODMAP Diet* as well as many pivotal research articles that have revolutionized our approach to the role of food-based therapies in digestive health. Thank you to my great friend, colleague, and mentor in the area of weight management, Dr. Larry Cheskin, director of the Johns Hopkins Weight Management Center.

I would like to also thank my colleagues and friends at the Institute for Functional Medicine–a wonderful organization designed to promote the application of whole-systems practice to prevent and treat chronic disease emphasizing nutrition and lifestyle-based interventions. In particular, I would like to thank Dr. Patrick Hanaway, whose many inspiring lectures on the gut microbiome opened my mind to the mad, mad world of mighty microbes. Laurie Hofmann, Drs. Liz Lipski, Mark Hyman, David Jones, Dan Lukaczer, and support staff Sherrie Torgerson, Sally Priest, Wendy Baker, and so many more. I would like to acknowledge The Johns Hopkins administrative leaders in nutrition who have assisted me through the years, Sylvia McAdoo, Tiffani Hays and Susan Oh, for their collaboration over the years as we together advanced nutrition awareness at our institution.

Space prohibits me from naming everyone who has supported my clinical practice at Johns Hopkins, but among them I am grateful to my medical office assistant Julie McKenna-Thorpe; Erin O'Keefe and nurse clinicians Kimberly Kidd-Watkins, Julie Dennis, and Rose Fusco; administrators Lisa Bach-Burdsall and Nathan Smith; Eric Tomakin, Roseann Wagner, Jennifer Metevia, Helen McGrain, Dr. Lis Ishii, Christian Hartman, Kim Gerred, administrative director Tiffany Boldin and Dr. Linda A. Lee. Dr. Lee is the clinical director of the Johns Hopkins Division of Gastroenterology and Hepatology and director of the Johns Hopkins Center for Integrative Medicine and Digestive Health. Dr. Lee is a courageous and spirited champion of integrative medicine. To Dr. Myron Weisfeldt, chair of medicine at Johns Hopkins who, with Tony Kalloo, brought me to Hopkins to "reboot" my career and has nurtured me ever since–my heartfelt thanks.

Finally, to Dr. Paul Rothman, dean of the medical faculty; Dr. Ed Miller, dean emeritus; Mr. Ronald R. Peterson, president of The Johns Hopkins Hospital and Health System and executive vice-president of Johns Hopkins Medicine; Dr. Redonda Miller, Meg Garrett, Jeffrey Natterman, and the Johns Hopkins Medicine administration–thank you! You are truly the best of the best and the reason why Hopkins continues to be the world's leading medical institution.

Finally, I'd like to thank the great Sylvester Stallone for making the Rocky movies. They continue to inspire me to this day. I watched many a clip on YouTube during late nights writing this book to stay motivated. Thanks, Sly. You gave me the eye of the tiger.

–*Gerard E. Mullin, MD*
Baltimore, Maryland

ENDNOTES

Introduction

1   chicagotribune.com/health/sns-rt-us-girls-fattagreuters-com2014newsml-kbn0de1xq-20140428,0,6368122
    .story.

2   Kirk S et al. Blame shame and lack of support–a multilevel study on obesity management. *Qualitative Health Research* 2014;11:790-800.

3   You can see the Hippocratic Oath at nlm.nih.gov/hmd/greek/greek_oath.html. When we swear the oath as physicians, usually the first two paragraphs are omitted and we begin with "I will use those dietary regimens which will benefit my patients according to my greatest ability and judgment, and I will do no harm or injustice to them."

4   Flegal KM, Carroll MD, Kit BK, Ogden CL. Prevalence of obesity and trends in the distribution of body mass index among US adults, 1999-2010. *JAMA*. 2012;307:491-97. doi:10.1001/jama.2012.39.

5   Cawley J, Meyerhoefer C. The medical care costs of obesity: an instrumental variables approach. *Journal of Health Economics* 2012; 31:219-30.

6   usda.gov/factbook/chapter2.pdf

Chapter 1

1   Mann T, Tomiyama AJ, Westling E, Lew AM, Samuels B, Chatman J. Medicare's search for effective obesity treatments: diets are not the answer. *American Psychologist* 2007;62:220-33.

2   Farias MM, Cuevas AM, Rodriguez F. Set-point theory and obesity. *Metabolic Syndrome and Related Disorders* 2011;9:85-89.

3   Colmers WF. If there is a weight set point, how is it set? *Canadian Journal of Diabetes* 2013;37(Suppl 2):S250.

4   Ibid.

5   Farias MM, Cuevas AM, Rodriguez F. Set-point theory and obesity. *Metabolic Syndrome and Related Disorders* 2011;9:85-89.

6   Colmers WF. If there is a weight set point, how is it set? *Canadian Journal of Diabetes* 2013;37(Suppl 2):S250.

7   Ford ES, Dietz WH. Trends in energy intake among adults in the United States: findings from NHANES. *American Journal of Clinical Nutrition* 2013;97:848-53.

8   Dietz, quoted in Reuters News. reuters.com/article/2013/03/06/us-despite-obesity-rise
    -idUSBRE92518620130306.

9   Conlan S, Kong HH, Segre JA. Species-level analysis of DNA sequence data from the NIH Human Microbiome Project. *PLoS One* 2012;7:e47075.

10 Peterson J, Garges S, Giovanni M, McInnes P, Wang L, Schloss JA, et al. The NIH Human Microbiome Project. *Genome Research* 2009;19:2317-23.

11 Leblanc JG, Milani C, de Giori GS, Sesma F, van Sinderen D, Ventura M. Bacteria as vitamin suppliers to their host: a gut microbiota perspective. *Current Opinion in Biotechnology* 2013;24:160-68.

12 Layden BT, Angueira AR, Brodsky M, Durai V, Lowe WL, Jr. Short chain fatty acids and their receptors: new metabolic targets. *Translational Research* 2013;161:131-40.

13 Ivanov II, Honda K. Intestinal commensal microbes as immune modulators. *Cell Host and Microbe* 2012;12:496-508.

14 Rhee SH, Pothoulakis C, Mayer EA. Principles and clinical implications of the brain-gut-enteric microbiota axis. *Nature Reviews Gastroenterology & Hepatology* 2009;6:306-14.

15 Larsen N, Vogensen FK, van den Berg FW, Nielsen DS, Andreasen AS, Pedersen BK, et al. Gut microbiota in human adults with type 2 diabetes differs from non-diabetic adults. *PLoS One* 2010;5:e9085.

16 Weinstock LB, Fern SE, Duntley SP. Restless legs syndrome in patients with irritable bowel syndrome: response to small intestinal bacterial overgrowth therapy. *Digestive Diseases and Sciences* 2008;535(5):1252-56.

17 Jeffery IB, Quigley EM, Ohman L, Simren M, O'Toole PW. The microbiota link to irritable bowel syndrome: an emerging story. *Gut Microbes* 2012;3:572-76.

18 Stratiki Z, Costalos C, Sevastiadou S, Kastanidou O, Skouroliakou M, Giakoumatou A, et al. The effect of a bifidobacter supplemented bovine milk on intestinal permeability of preterm infants. *Early Human Development* 2007;83(9):575-79.

19 Patel RT, Shukla AP, Ahn SM, Moreira M, Rubino F. Surgical control of obesity and diabetes: the role of intestinal vs. gastric mechanisms in the regulation of body weight and glucose homeostasis. *Obesity (Silver Spring)* 2014;22(1):159-69.

20 Suez J, Korem T, Zeevi D, Zilberman-Schapira G, Thaiss CA, Maza O, et al. Artificial sweeteners induce glucose intolerance by altering the gut microbiota. *Nature* 2014;514;181-86.

21 nrdc.org/health/effects/mercury/guide.asp.

22 Hart AL, Hendy P. The microbiome in inflammatory bowel disease and its modulation as a therapeutic manoeuvre. *Proceedings of the Nutrition Society* 2014;1-5.

23 Ali BH, Blunden G, Tanira MO, Nemmar A. Some phytochemical, pharmacological and toxicological properties of ginger (Zingiber officinale Roscoe): a review of recent research. *Food and Chemical Toxicology* 2008;46(2):409-20.

24 Howitt MR, Garrett WS. A complex microworld in the gut: gut microbiota and cardiovascular disease connectivity. *Nature Medicine* 2012;18:1188-89.

25 Niers L, Martin R, Rijkers G, Sengers F, Timmerman H, van Uden N, et al. The effects of selected probiotic strains on the development of eczema (the PandA study). *Allergy* 2009;64:1349-58.

26 del Giudice MM, Leonardi S, Ciprandi G, Galdo F, Gubitosi A, La Rosa M, et al. Probiotics in childhood: allergic illness and respiratory infections. *Journal of Clinical Gastroenterology* 2012;46(Suppl):S69-72.

27 Neufeld KA, Kang N, Bienenstock J, Foster JA. Effects of intestinal microbiota on anxiety-like behavior. *Communicative and Integrative Biology* 2011;4:492-94.

28 Koletzko B, von Kries R, Closa R, Escribano J, Scaglioni S, Giovannini M, et al. Can infant feeding choices modulate later obesity risk? *American Journal of Clinical Nutrition* 2009;89:1502S-8S.

29 Li H, Ye R, Pei L, Ren A, Zheng X, Liu J. Caesarean delivery, caesarean delivery on maternal request and childhood overweight: a Chinese birth cohort study of 181,380 children. *Pediatric Obesity* 2014;19:10-16.

30 Bengmark S. Nutrition of the critically ill—a 21st century perspective. *Nutrients* 2013;5:162-207. doi:10.3390/nu5010162.

31 cnn.com/2007/HEALTH/diet.fitness/09/22/kd.gupta.column/.

32 Angelkais E, Armougom F, Million M, Raoult D. The relationship between gut microbiota and weight gain in humans. *Future Microbiology* 2012 Jan;7:91-109. doi:10.2217/fmb.11.142.

33 Blaser MJ. *Missing Microbes*. New York: Henry Holt & Co, 2014.

34 Sharland M. The use of antibacterials in children: a report of the Specialist Advisory Committee on Antimicrobial Resistance (SACAR) Paediatric Subgroup. *Journal of Antimicrobial Chemotherapy* 2007;60(Suppl 1):i15-26.

35 Bailey LC, Forrest CB, Zhang P, Richards TM, Livshïts A, DeRusso PA. Association of antibiotics in infancy with early childhood obesity. *JAMA Pediatrics* 2014; 168(11):1063-69.

Chapter 2

1 Turnbaugh PJ, Backhed F, Fulton L, Gordon JI. Diet-induced obesity is linked to marked but reversible alterations in the mouse distal gut microbiome. *Cell Host and Microbe* 2008;3:213-23.

2 Koren O, Goodrich JK, Cullender TC, Spor A, Laitinen K, Bäckhed HK, Gonzalez A, Werner JJ, Angenent LT, Knight R, Bäckhed F, Isolauri E, Salminen S, Ley RE. Host remodeling of the gut microbiome and metabolic changes during pregnancy *Cell* 2012 Aug 3;150(3):470-80. doi: 10.1016/j.cell.2012.07.008

3 sciencemag.org/content/341/6150/1241214

4 jama.jamanetwork.com/article.aspx?articleid=1916296

5 medicalnewstoday.com/articles/254864.php

6 Vrieze A, Holleman F, Zoetendal EG, de Vos WM, Hoekstra JB, Nieuwdorp M. The environment within: how gut microbiota may influence metabolism and body composition. *Diabetologia* 2010;53:606-13.

7 El-Matary W, Simpson R, Ricketts-Burns N. Fecal microbiota transplantation: are we opening a can of worms? *Gastroenterology* 2012;143:e19; author reply e-20.

8 cbsnews.com/news/fda-struggles-to-regulate-fecal-transplants/.

9 medicalnewstoday.com/articles/249584.php.

10 Azad MB, Konya T, Maughan H, Guttman DS, Field CJ, Chari RS, et al. Gut microbiota of healthy Canadian infants: profiles by mode of delivery and infant diet at 4 months. *CMAJ* 2013;185:385-94.

11 Dominguez-Bello MG, Costello EK, Contreras M, Magris M, Hidalgo G, Fierer N, et al. Delivery mode shapes the acquisition and structure of the initial microbiota across multiple body habitats in newborns. *Proceedings of the National Academy of Sciences of the USA* 2010;107:11971-75.

12 Salminen S, Gibson GR, McCartney AL, Isolauri E. Influence of mode of delivery on gut microbiota composition in seven year old children. *Gut* 2004;53:1388-89.

13 Negele K, Heinrich J, Borte M, von Berg A, Schaaf B, Lehmann I, et al. Mode of delivery and development of atopic disease during the first 2 years of life. *Pediatric Allergy and Immunology* 2004;15:48-54.

14 Bager P, Simonsen J, Nielsen NM, Frisch M. Cesarean section and offspring's risk of inflammatory bowel disease: a national cohort study. *Inflammatory Bowel Diseases* 2012;18:857-62.

15 de Weerth C, Fuentes S, Puylaert P, de Vos WM. Intestinal microbiota of infants with colic: development and specific signatures. *Pediatrics* 2013;131:e550-58.

16 Koletzko B, von Kries R, Closa R, Escribano J, Scaglioni S, Giovannini M, et al. Can infant feeding choices modulate later obesity risk? *American Journal of Clinical Nutrition* 2009;89:1502S-8S.

17 Taffel SM, Placek PJ, Liss T. Trends in the United States cesarean section rate and reasons for the 1980-85 rise. *American Journal of Public Health*1987;77:955-59.

18 Li H, Ye R, Pei L, Ren A, Zheng X, Liu J. Caesarean delivery, caesarean delivery on maternal request and childhood overweight: a Chinese birth cohort study of 181,380 children. *Pediatric Obesity* 2014;9:10-16.

19 Hamilton BE, Martin JA, Ventura SJ. Births: preliminary data for 2010. *National Vital Statistics Reports* 2011;60:1-25. cdc.gov/nchs/data/nvsr/nvsr60/nvsr60_02.pdf.

20 Akinbami LJ, Moorman JE, Bailey C, Zahran HS, King M, Johnson CA, et al. Trends in asthma prevalence, health care use, and mortality in the United States, 2001-2010. *NCHS Data Brief* 2012:1-8.

21 Radon K, Windstetter D, Solfrank S, von Mutius E, Nowak D, Schwarz HP. Chronic autoimmune disease and contact to animals (CAT) study group. Exposure to farming environments in early life and type 1 diabetes: a case-control study. *Diabetes* 2005;54:3212-16.

22 Miller, D. *Farmacology: What Innovative Family Farming Can Teach Us about Health and Healing.* New York: Harper Collins Publishers, 2013.

23 Ball TM, Castro-Rodriguez JA, Griffith KA, Holberg CJ, Martinez FD, Wright AL. Siblings, day-care attendance, and the risk of asthma and wheezing during childhood. *New England Journal of Medicine* 2000;343:538-43.

24 Ege M. et al. Exposure to environmental microorganisms and childhood asthma. *New England Journal of Medicine* 2011;364:701-9.

25 Reganold J. et al. Fruit and soil quality of organic and conventional strawberry agroecosystems. *PLoS One* 2010;5:e12346.

26 Koberl M, Muller H, Ramadan EM, Berg G. Desert farming benefits from microbial potential in arid soils and promotes diversity and plant health. *PLoS One* 2011;6:e24452.

27 Sheikh A, Strachan DP. The hygiene theory: fact or fiction? *Current Opinion in Otolaryngology & Head and Neck Surgery* 2004;12:232-36.

28 Fung I, Garrett JP, Shahane A, Kwan M. Do bugs control our fate? The influence of the microbiome on autoimmunity. *Current Allergy and Asthma Reports* 2012;12:511-19.

29 Hviid A, Svanstrom H, Frisch M. Antibiotic use and inflammatory bowel diseases in childhood. *Gut* 2011;60:49-54.

30 Strachan DP. Family size, infection and atopy: the first decade of the "hygiene hypothesis." *Thorax* 2000;55(Suppl 1):S2-S10.

31 news-medical.net/news/20121003/e28098Hygiene-hypothesise28099-updated-to-e28098Old-Friendse28099-hypothesis.aspx.

32 Sharland M, SACAR Paediatric Subgroup. The use of antibacterials in children: a report of the Specialist Advisory Committee on Antimicrobial Resistance (SACAR) Paediatric Subgroup. *Journal of Antimicrobial Chemotherapy* 2007; Aug; 60(Suppl 1):i15-i26.

33 Jernberg C, Lofmark S, Edlund C, Jansson JK. Long-term ecological impacts of antibiotic administration on the human intestinal microbiota. *ISME Journal* 2007;1:56-66.

34 Dethlefsen L, Relman DA. Incomplete recovery and individualized responses of the human distal gut microbiota to repeated antibiotic perturbation. *Proceedings of the National Academy of Sciences of the USA* 2011;108(Suppl 1):4554-61.

35 Jukes TH, Williams WL. Nutritional effects of antibiotics. *Pharmacological Reviews* 1953;5:381-420.

36 Cho I, Yamanishi S, Cox L, Methe BA, Zavadil J, Li K, et al. Antibiotics in early life alter the murine colonic microbiome and adiposity. *Nature* 2012;488:621–26.

37 Henao-Mejia J, Elinav E, Jin C, Hao L, Mehal WZ, Strowig T, et al. Inflammasome-mediated dysbiosis regulates progression of NAFLD and obesity. *Nature* 2012;482:179–85.

38 Machado MV, Cortez-Pinto H. Gut microbiota and nonalcoholic fatty liver disease. *Annals of Hepatology* 2012;11:440–49.

39 Wigg AJ, Roberts-Thomson IC, Dymock RB, McCarthy PJ, Grose RH, Cummins AG. The role of small intestinal bacterial overgrowth, intestinal permeability, endotoxaemia, and tumour necrosis factor alpha in the pathogenesis of non-alcoholic steatohepatitis. *Gut* 2001;48:206–11.

40 Lichtman SN, Keku J, Schwab JH, Sartor RB. Hepatic injury associated with small bowel bacterial overgrowth in rats is prevented by metronidazole and tetracycline. *Gastroenterology* 1991;100:513–19.

41 Miyake Y, Yamamoto K. Role of gut microbiota in liver diseases. *Hepatology Research* 2013;43:139–46.

42 Cani PD, Possemiers S, Van de Wiele T, Guiot Y, Everard A, Rottier O, et al. Changes in gut microbiota control inflammation in obese mice through a mechanism involving GLP-2-driven improvement of gut permeability. *Gut* 2009;58:1091–103.

43 Ding S, Lund PK. Role of intestinal inflammation as an early event in obesity and insulin resistance. *Current Opinion in Clinical Nutrition and Metabolic Care* 2011;14:328–33.

44 Creely SJ, McTernan PG, Kusminski CM, Fisher f M, Da Silva NF, Khanolkar M, et al. Lipopolysaccharide activates an innate immune system response in human adipose tissue in obesity and type 2 diabetes. *American Journal of Physiology: Endocrinology and Metabolism* 2007;292:E740–E747.

45 Yang RZ, Lee MJ, Hu H, Pollin TI, Ryan AS, Nicklas BJ, et al. Acute-phase serum amyloid A: an inflammatory adipokine and potential link between obesity and its metabolic complications. *PLoS Medicine* 2006;3:e287.

46 Al-Attas OS, Al-Daghri NM, Al-Rubeaan K, da Silva NF, Sabico SL, Kumar S, et al. Changes in endotoxin levels in T2DM subjects on anti-diabetic therapies. *Cardiovascular Diabetology* 2009;8:20.

47 Cani PD, Neyrinck AM, Fava F, Knauf C, Burcelin RG, Tuohy KM, et al. Selective increases of bifidobacteria in gut microflora improve high-fat-diet-induced diabetes in mice through a mechanism associated with endotoxaemia. *Diabetologia* 2007;50:2374–83.

48 Cani PD, Amar J, Iglesias MA, Poggi M, Knauf C, Bastelica D, et al. Metabolic endotoxemia initiates obesity and insulin resistance. *Diabetes* 2007;56:1761–72.

49 Ma X, Hua J, Li Z. Probiotics improve high fat diet-induced hepatic steatosis and insulin resistance by increasing hepatic NKT cells. *Journal of Hepatology* 2008;49:821–30.

50 Stratiki Z, Costalos C, Sevastiadou S, Kastanidou O, Skouroliakou M, Giankoumatou A, et al. The effect of a bifidobacter supplemented bovine milk on intestinal permeability of preterm infants. *Early Human Development* 2007;83(9):575–79.

51 Okeke F, Roland BC, Mullin GE. The role of gut microbiome in pathogenesis and treatment of obesity. *Global Advances in Health and Medicine* 2014;3:44–57. doi:10.7453/gahmj.2014.018.

52 Ley RE, Turnbaugh PJ, Klein S, Gordon JI. Microbial ecology: human gut microbes associated with obesity. *Nature* 2006;444:1022–23.

53 Ibid.

54 Turnbaugh PJ, Hamady M, Yatsunenko T, Cantarel BL, Duncan A, Ley RE, et al. A core gut microbiome in obese and lean twins. *Nature* 2009;457:480–84.

55 Patel RT, Shukla AP, Ahn SM, Moreira M, Rubino F. Surgical control of obesity and diabetes: the role of intestinal vs. gastric mechanisms in the regulation of body weight and glucose homeostasis. *Obesity (Silver Spring)* 2014;22(1):159–69.

56 Zhang H, DiBaise JK, Zuccolo A, Kudrna D, Braidotti M, Yu Y, et al. Human gut microbiota in obesity and after gastric bypass. *Proceedings of the National Academy of Sciences of the USA* 2009;106:2365–70.

57 Duncan SH, Lobley GE, Holtrop G, Ince J, Johnstone AM, Louis P, et al. Human colonic microbiota associated with diet, obesity and weight loss. *International Journal of Obesity* 2008;32:1720–24.

58 ncbi.nlm.nih.gov/pubmed/23712978

59 livescience.com/41954-gut-microbes-make-you-fat.html

60 cell.com/abstract/S0092-8674(14)01241-0

61 Turnbaugh PJ, Backhed F, Fulton L, Gordon JI. Diet-induced obesity is linked to marked but reversible alterations in the mouse distal gut microbiome. *Cell Host and Microbe* 2008;3:213–23.

62 Wu GD, Chen J, Hoffmann C, Bittinger K, Chen YY, et al. Linking long-term dietary patterns with gut microbial enterotypes. *Science* 2011;334:105–8. doi:10.1126/science.1208344.

63 britannica.com/EBchecked/topic/1368888/quorum-sensing.

64 Hehemann JH et al. Bacteria of the human gut microbiome catabolize red seaweed glycans with carbohydrate-active enzyme updates from extrinsic microbes. *Proceedings of the National Academy of Sciences of the USA* 2012;109:19786–91. doi: 10.1073/pnas.1211002109.

65 Hehemann JH, Correc G, Barbeyron T, Helbert W, Czjzek M, Michel G. Transfer of carbohydrate-active enzymes from marine bacteria to Japanese gut microbiota. *Nature* 2010;464:908–12.

66 sciencedaily.com/releases/2009/02/090205214418.htm.

67 Xu J, Gordon JI. Honor thy symbionts. *Proceedings of the National Academy of Sciences of the USA* 2003;100(18):10452-9.

68 Semova I, Carten JD, Stombaugh J, et al. Microbiota regulate intestinal absorption and metabolism of fatty acids in the zebrafish. *Cell Host and Microbe* 2012;12: 277–88.

69 Backhed F, Manchester JK, Semenkovich CF, Gordon JI. Mechanisms underlying the resistance to diet-induced obesity in germ-free mice. *Proceedings of the National Academy of Sciences of the USA* 2007;104:979–84.

70 Ibid.

71 Mandard S, Zandbergen F, van Straten E, Wahli W, Kuipers F, Muller M, et al. The fasting-induced adipose factor/angiopoietin-like protein 4 is physically associated with lipoproteins and governs plasma lipid levels and adiposity. *Journal of Biological Chemistry* 2006;281:934–44.

72 Quigley EM. Small intestinal bacterial overgrowth: what it is and what it is not. *Current Opinion in Gastroenterology* 2014;30:141–46.

73 Jeffery IB, Quigley EM, Ohman L, Simren M, O'Toole PW. The microbiota link to irritable bowel syndrome: an emerging story. *Gut Microbes* 2012;3:572–76.

74 Ford AC. Breath testing and antibiotics for possible bacterial overgrowth in irritable bowel syndrome. *Expert Review of Anti-Infective Therapy* 2010;8:855–57.

75 Pimentel M, Lembo A, Chey WD, Zakko S, Ringel Y, Yu J, et al. Rifaximin therapy for patients with irritable bowel syndrome without constipation. *New England Journal of Medicine* 2011;364:22–32.

76 Phatak UP, Pashankar DS. Prevalence of functional gastrointestinal disorders in obese and overweight children. *International Journal of Obesity* 2014 May 2. doi:1038/ijo.2014.67. [Epub ahead of print]

77 Sabate JM, Jouet P, Harnois F, Mechler C, Msika S, Grossin M, et al. High prevalence of small intestinal bacterial overgrowth in patients with morbid obesity: a contributor to severe hepatic steatosis. *Obesity Surgery* 2008;18:371–77.

78 Ilan Y. Leaky gut and the liver: a role for bacterial translocation in nonalcoholic steatohepatitis. *World Journal of Gastroenterology* 2012;18:2609–18.

79 Mathur R, Amichai M, Chua KS, Mirocha J, Barlow GM, Pimental M. Methane and hydrogen positivity on breath test is associated with great body mass index and body fat. *Journal of Clinical Endocrinology and Metabolism* 2013;98: E698–E702.

80 webmd.com/diet/news/20130326/breath-test-might-predict-obesity-risk.

81 Chedid V, Dhalla S, Clarke JO, Roland BC, Dunbar KB, Koh J, et al. Herbal therapy is equivalent to rifaximin for the treatment of small intestinal bacterial overgrowth. *Global Advances in Health and Medicine* 2014;3:16–24.

82 Gershon M. *The Second Brain*. New York: Harper Collins Publishers, 1999.

83 Sudo N, Chida Y, Aiba Y, Sonoda J, Oyama N, Yu XN, et al. Postnatal microbial colonization programs the hypothalamic-pituitary-adrenal system for stress response in mice. *Journal of Physiology* 2004;558(Pt 1):263–75.

84 Messaoudi M, Violle N, Bisson JF, Desor D, Javelot H, Rougeot C. Beneficial psychological effects of a probiotic formulation (Lactobacillus helveticus R0052 and Bifidobacterium longum R0175) in healthy human volunteers. *Gut Microbes* 2011;2:256–61.

85 Messaoudi M, Lalonde R, Violle N, Javelot H, Desor D, Nejdi A, et al. Assessment of psychotropic-like properties of a probiotic formulation (Lactobacillus helveticus R0052 and Bifidobacterium longum R0175) in rats and human subjects. *British Journal of Nutrition* 2011;105:755–64.

86 Cani PD, Possemiers S, Van de Wiele T, Guiot Y, Everard A, Rottier O, et al. Changes in gut microbiota control inflammation in obese mice through a mechanism involving GLP-2-driven improvement of gut permeability. *Gut* 2009;58:1091–103.

87 Cani PD, Hoste S, Guiot Y, Delzenne NM. Dietary non-digestible carbohydrates promote L-cell differentiation in the proximal colon of rats. *British Journal of Nutrition* 2007;98:32–37.

88 Reinhardt C, Reigstad CS, Backhed F. Intestinal microbiota during infancy and its implications for obesity. *Journal of Pediatric Gastroenterology and Nutrition* 2009;48:249–56.

89 Holst JJ. Glucagon and glucagon-like peptides 1 and 2. *Results and Problems in Cell Differentiation* 2010;50:121–35.

90 Parnell JA, Reimer RA. Weight loss during oligofructose supplementation is associated with decreased ghrelin and increased peptide YY in overweight and obese adults. *American Journal of Clinical Nutrition* 2009;89:1751–59.

Chapter 3

1   Di Gioia D, Aloisio I, Mazzola G, Biavati B. Bifidobacteria: their impact on gut microbiota composition and their applications as probiotics in infants. *Applied Microbiology and Biotechnology* 2014;98:563–77.

2   Tsai YT, Cheng PC, Pan TM. Anti-obesity effects of gut microbiota are associated with lactic acid bacteria. *Applied Microbiology and Biotechnology* 2014;98:1–10.

3   Francois F, Roper J, Joseph N, Pei Z, Chhada A, Shak JR, et al. The effect of H. pylori eradication on meal-associated changes in plasma ghrelin and leptin. *BMC Gastroenterology* 2011;11:37.

4   Chacko Y, Holtmann GJ. Helicobacter pylori eradication and weight gain: has it opened a Pandora's box? *Alimentary Pharmacology & Therapies* 2011;34:256.

5   Madrid AM, Poniachik J, Quera R, Defilippi C. Small intestinal clustered contractions and bacterial overgrowth: a frequent finding in obese patients. *Digestive Diseases and Sciences* 2011;56:155–60.

6   Clements RH, Gonzalez QH, Foster A, et al. Gastrointestinal symptoms are more intense in morbidly obese patients and are improved with laparoscopic Roux-en-Y gastric bypass. *Obesity Surgery* 2003;13:610–14.

7   Shai I, Schwarzfuchs D, Henkin Y, et al. Weight loss with a low-carbohydrate, Mediterranean, or low-fat diet. *New England Journal of Medicine* 2008;359:229–41.

8   Foster GD, Wyatt HR, Hill JO, et al. A randomized trial of a low-carbohydrate diet for obesity. *New England Journal of Medicine* 2003;348:2082–90.

9   Brehm BJ, Seeley RJ, Daniels SR, D'Alessio DA. A randomized trial comparing a very low carbohydrate diet and a calorie-restricted low fat diet on body weight and cardiovascular risk factors in healthy women. *Journal of Clinical Endocrinology and Metabolism* 2003;88:1617–23.

10 Gardner CD, Kiazand A, Alhassan S, et al. Comparison of the Atkins, Zone, Ornish, and LEARN diets for change in weight and related risk factors among overweight premenopausal women: the A TO Z Weight Loss Study: a randomized trial. *JAMA* 2007;297:969–77.

11 Yancy WS, Jr., Olsen MK, Guyton JR, Bakst RP, Westman EC. A low-carbohydrate, ketogenic diet versus a low-fat diet to treat obesity and hyperlipidemia: a randomized, controlled trial. *Annals of Internal Medicine* 2004;140:769–77.

12 Seshadri P, Iqbal N, Stern L, et al. A randomized study comparing the effects of a low-carbohydrate diet and a conventional diet on lipoprotein subfractions and C-reactive protein levels in patients with severe obesity. *American Journal of Medicine* 2004;117:398–405.

13 Nistal E, Caminero A, Vivas S, et al. Differences in faecal bacteria populations and faecal bacteria metabolism in healthy adults and celiac disease patients. *Biochimie* 2012;94:1724–29.

14 De Palma G, Nadal I, Collado MC, Sanz Y. Effects of a gluten-free diet on gut microbiota and immune function in healthy adult human subjects. *British Journal of Nutrition* 2009;102:1154–60.

15 Stern L, Iqbal N, Seshadri P, et al. The effects of low-carbohydrate versus conventional weight loss diets in severely obese adults: one-year follow-up of a randomized trial. *Annals of Internal Medicine* 2004;140:778–85.

16 De Palma G, Nadal I, Collado MC, Sanz Y. Effects of a gluten-free diet on gut microbiota and immune function in healthy adult human subjects. *British Journal of Nutrition* 2009;102:1154–60.

17 Nistal E, Caminero A, Herran AR, et al. Differences of small intestinal bacteria populations in adults and children with/without celiac disease: effect of age, gluten diet, and disease. *Inflammatory Bowel Diseases* 2012;18:649–56.

18 Nistal E, Caminero A, Vivas S, et al. Differences in faecal bacteria populations and faecal bacteria metabolism in healthy adults and celiac disease patients. *Biochimie* 2012;94:1724–29.

19 De Palma G, Nadal I, Collado MC, Sanz Y. Effects of a gluten-free diet on gut microbiota and immune function in healthy adult human subjects. *British Journal of Nutrition* 2009;102:1154–60.

20 Santacruz A, Marcos A, Warnberg J, et al. Interplay between weight loss and gut microbiota composition in overweight adolescents. *Obesity* 2009;17:1906–15.

21 Million M, Maraninchi M, Henry M, et al. Obesity-associated gut microbiota is enriched in Lactobacillus reuteri and depleted in Bifidobacterium animalis and Methanobrevibacter smithii. *International Journal of Obesity* 2012;36:817–25.

22 Kalliomaki M, Collado MC, Salminen S, Isolauri E. Early differences in fecal microbiota composition in children may predict overweight. *American Journal of Clinical Nutrition* 2008;87:534–38.

23 Schwiertz A, Taras D, Schafer K, et al. Microbiota and SCFA in lean and overweight healthy subjects. *Obesity* 2010;18:190–95.

24 Collado MC, Isolauri E, Laitinen K, Salminen S. Distinct composition of gut microbiota during pregnancy in overweight and normal-weight women. *American Journal of Clinical Nutrition* 2008;88:894–99.

25 Heine RG. Preventing atopy and allergic disease. *Nestlé Nutrition Institute Workshop Series* 2014;78: 141–53.

26 Owen CG, Martin RM, Whincup PH, Smith GD, Cook DG. Effect of infant feeding on the risk of obesity across the life course: a quantitative review of published evidence. *Pediatrics* 2005;115:1367–77.

27 Harder T, Bergmann R, Kallischnigg G, Plagemann A. Duration of breastfeeding and risk of overweight: a meta-analysis. *American Journal of Epidemiology* 2005;162:397–403.

Chapter 4

1 Haahtela T, Holgate S, Pawankar R, et al. The biodiversity hypothesis and allergic disease: World Allergy Organization position statement. *World Allergy Organization Journal* 2013;6:3.

2 Schnabl B, Brenner DA. Interactions between the intestinal microbiome and liver diseases. *Gastroenterology* 2014;146:1513–24.

3 Bengmark S. Nutrition of the critically ill–a 21st-century perspective. *Nutrients*. 2013;5:162–207.

4 Hold GL. Western lifestyle: a 'master' manipulator of the intestinal microbiota? *Gut* 2014;63:5–6.

5 Bengmark S. Nutrition of the critically ill–a 21st-century perspective. *Nutrients*. 2013;5:162–207.

6 Wu GD, Chen J, Hoffmann C, et al. Linking long-term dietary patterns with gut microbial enterotypes. *Science* 2011;334:105–8.

7 Pendyala S, Walker JM, Holt PR. A high-fat diet is associated with endotoxemia that originates from the gut. *Gastroenterology* 2012;142:1100–1 e2.

8 Hansen R, Russell RK, Reiff C, et al. Microbiota of de-novo pediatric IBD: increased Faecalibacterium prausnitzii and reduced bacterial diversity in Crohn's but not in ulcerative colitis. *American Journal of Gastroenterology* 2012;107:1913–22.

9 Martinez-Medina M, Denizot J, Dreux N, et al. Western diet induces dysbiosis with increased E. coli in CEABAC10 mice, alters host barrier function favouring AIEC colonisation. *Gut* 2014;63:116–24.

10 Devkota S, Wang Y, Musch MW, et al. Dietary-fat-induced taurocholic acid promotes pathobiont expansion and colitis in Il10-/- mice. *Nature* 2012;487:104–8.

11 Ghosh S, Molcan E, DeCoffe D, Dai C, Gibson DL. Diets rich in n-6 PUFA induce intestinal microbial dysbiosis in aged mice. *British Journal of Nutrition* 2013;110:515–23.

12 de La Serre CB, Ellis CL, Lee J, Hartman AL, Rutledge JC, Raybould HE. Propensity to high-fat diet-induced obesity in rats is associated with changes in the gut microbiota and gut inflammation. *American Journal of Physiology: Gastrointestinal and Liver Physiology* 2010;299:G440–48.

13 Ghosh S, Molcan E, DeCoffe D, Dai C, Gibson DL. Diets rich in n-6 PUFA induce intestinal microbial dysbiosis in aged mice. *British Journal of Nutrition* 2013;110:515–23.

14 usda.gov/factbook/2001–2002factbook.pdf.table 2–6, page 20.

15 usda.gov/factbook/chapter2.pdf.tables 2–6, page 20.

16 Cordain L, Eaton SB, Sebastian A, et al. Origins and evolution of the Western diet: health implications for the 21st century. *American Journal of Clinical Nutrition* 2005;81:341–54.

17 Cordain L. Implications for the role of diet in acne. *Seminars in Cutaneous Medicine and Surgery* 2005;24:84–91.

18 Yang Q, Zhang Z, Gregg EW, Flanders WD, Merritt R, Hu FB. Added sugar intake and cardiovascular diseases mortality among US adults. *JAMA Internal Medicine* 2014;17:516–24.

19 Schmidt LA. New unsweetened truths about sugar. *JAMA Internal Medicine* 2014;17:525–26.

20 usda.gov/factbook/chapter2.pdf.tables 2–6, page 20.

21 Yang Q, Zhang Z, Gregg EW, Flanders WD, Merritt R, Hu FB. Added sugar intake and cardiovascular diseases mortality among US adults. *JAMA Internal Medicine* 2014;17:516–24.

22 Johnson RK, Appel LJ, Brands M, et al. Dietary sugars intake and cardiovascular health: a scientific statement from the American Heart Association. *Circulation* 2009;120:1011-20.

23 Yang Q, Zhang Z, Gregg EW, Flanders WD, Merritt R, Hu FB. Added sugar intake and cardiovascular diseases mortality among US adults. *JAMA Internal Medicine* 2014;17:516–24.

24 Ibid.

25 Green AK, Jacques PF, Rogers G, Fox CS, Meigs JB, McKeown NM. Sugar-sweetened beverages and prevalence of the metabolically abnormal phenotype in the Framingham Heart Study. *Obesity* 2014;22:E157–63.

26 Turnbaugh PJ, Ridaura VK, Faith JJ, Rey FE, Knight R, Gordon JI. The effect of diet on the human gut microbiome: a metagenomic analysis in humanized gnotobiotic mice. *Science Translational Medicine* 2009;1:6ra14.

27 Ibid.

28 Kavanagh K, Wylie AT, Tucker KL, et al. Dietary fructose induces endotoxemia and hepatic injury in calorically controlled primates. *American Journal of Clinical Nutrition* 2013;98:349–57.

29 Nomura K, Yamanouchi T. The role of fructose-enriched diets in mechanisms of nonalcoholic fatty liver disease. *Journal of Nutritional Biochemistry* 2012;23:203–8.

30 Riveros MJ, Parada A, Pettinelli P. [Fructose consumption and its health implications; fructose malabsorption and nonalcoholic fatty liver disease]. *Nutrición hospitalaria* 2014;29:491–99.

31 usda.gov/factbook/2001–2002factbook.pdf.table 2–6, page 20.

32 usda.gov/factbook/chapter2.pdf.tables 2–6, page 20.

33 Nomura K, Yamanouchi T. The role of fructose-enriched diets in mechanisms of nonalcoholic fatty liver disease. *Journal of Nutritional Biochemistry* 2012;23:203–8.

34 Riveros MJ, Parada A, Pettinelli P. [Fructose consumption and its health implications; fructose malabsorption and nonalcoholic fatty liver disease]. *Nutrición hospitalaria* 2014;29:491–99.

35 Mager DR, Iniguez IR, Gilmour S, Yap J. The effect of a low fructose and low glycemic index/load (FRAGILE) dietary intervention on indices of liver function, cardiometabolic risk factors, and body composition in children and adolescents with nonalcoholic fatty liver disease (NAFLD). *JPEN: Journal of Parenteral and Enteral Nutrition* 2013 Aug 23. [Epub ahead of print]

36 Kelishadi R, Mansourian M, Heidari-Beni M. Association of fructose consumption and components of metabolic syndrome in human studies: a systematic review and meta-analysis. *Nutrition* 2014;30:503-10.

37 Ha V, Jayalath VH, Cozma AI, Mirrahimi A, de Souza RJ, Sievenpiper JL. Fructose-containing sugars, blood pressure, and cardiometabolic risk: a critical review. *Current Hypertension Reports* 2013;15:281–97.

38 Martin-Calvo N, Martinez-Gonzalez MA, Bes-Rastrollo M, et al. Sugar-sweetened carbonated beverage consumption and childhood/adolescent obesity: a case-control study. *Public Health Nutrition* 2014 Jan 31:1–9. [Epub ahead of print]

39 Nickelson J, Lawrence JC, Parton JM, Knowlden AP, McDermott RJ. What proportion of preschool-aged children consume sweetened beverages? *Journal of School Health* 2014;84:185–94.

40 Kavanagh K, Wylie AT, Tucker KL, et al. Dietary fructose induces endotoxemia and hepatic injury in calorically controlled primates. *American Journal of Clinical Nutrition* 2013;98:349–57.

41 Bleich SN, Wolfson JA, Vine S, Wang YC. Diet-beverage consumption and caloric intake among US adults, overall and by body weight. *American Journal of Public Health* 2014;104:e72-78.

42 Fowler SP, Williams K, Resendez RG, Hunt KJ, Hazuda HP, Stern MP. Fueling the obesity epidemic? Artificially sweetened beverage use and long-term weight gain. *Obesity* 2008;16:1894–900.

43 Sternini C. In search of a role for carbonation: is this a good or bad taste? *Gastroenterology* 2013;145:500–503.

44 Di Salle F, Cantone E, Savarese MF, et al. Effect of carbonation on brain processing of sweet stimuli in humans. *Gastroenterology* 2013;145:537–39 e3.

45 Soffritti M, Padovani M, Tibaldi E, Falcioni L, Manservisi F, Belpoggi F. The carcinogenic effects of aspartame: The urgent need for regulatory re-evaluation. *American Journal of Industrial Medicine* 2014;57:383–97.

46 Suez J, Korem T, Zeevi D, Zilberman-Schapira G, Thaiss CA, Mazo O, et al. Artificial sweeteners induce glucose intolerance by altering the gut microbiota. *Nature* 2014.

47 Wu GD, Chen J, Hoffmann C, et al. Linking long-term dietary patterns with gut microbial enterotypes. *Science* 2011;334:105–8.

48 Steinert RE, Frey F, Topfer A, Drewe J, Beglinger C. Effects of carbohydrate sugars and artificial sweeteners on appetite and the secretion of gastrointestinal satiety peptides. *British Journal of Nutrition* 2011;105:1320–28.

49 Piya MK, Harte AL, McTernan PG. Metabolic endotoxaemia: is it more than just a gut feeling? *Current Opinion in Lipidology* 2013;24:78–85.

50 Van Engelen M, Khodabandeh S, Akhavan T, Agarwal J, Gladanac B, Bellissimo N. Effect of sugars in solutions on subjective appetite and short-term food intake in 9- to 14-year-old normal weight boys. *European Journal of Clinical Nutrition* 2014;66(7):773–77.

51 Garcia-Caceres C, Tschop MH. The emerging neurobiology of calorie addiction. *eLife* 2014;3:e01928.

52 Malkusz DC, Banakos T, Mohamed A, et al. Dopamine signaling in the medial prefrontal cortex and amygdala is required for the acquisition of fructose-conditioned flavor preferences in rats. *Behavioural Brain Research* 2012;233:500–507.

53 Halmos EP, Christophersen CT, Bird AR, Shepherd SJ, Gibson PR, Muir JG. Diets that differ in their FODMAP content alter the colonic luminal microenvironment. *Gut* 2014 Jul 14. [Epub ahead of print]

54 Paoli A. Ketogenic diet for obesity: friend or foe? *International Journal of Environmental Research and Public Health* 2014;11:2092–107.

55 Ibid.

56 Paoli A, Rubini A, Volek JS, Grimaldi KA. Beyond weight loss: a review of the therapeutic uses of very-low-carbohydrate (ketogenic) diets. *European Journal of Clinical Nutrition* 2013;67:789–96.

57 Veldhorst M, Smeets A, Soenen S, et al. Protein-induced satiety: effects and mechanisms of different proteins. *Physiology & Behavior* 2008;94:300–307.

58 Westerterp-Plantenga MS, Nieuwenhuizen A, Tome D, Soenen S, Westerterp KR. Dietary protein, weight loss, and weight maintenance. *Annual Review of Nutrition* 2009;29:21–41.

59 Sumithran P, Prendergast LA, Delbridge E, et al. Ketosis and appetite-mediating nutrients and hormones after weight loss. *European Journal of Clinical Nutrition* 2013;67:759–64.

60 Veldhorst MA, Westerterp-Plantenga MS, Westerterp KR. Gluconeogenesis and energy expenditure after a high-protein, carbohydrate-free diet. *American Journal of Clinical Nutrition* 2009;90:519–26.

61 Fine EJ, Feinman RD. Thermodynamics of weight loss diets. *Nutrition & Metabolism* 2004;1:15.

62 Volek JS, Phinney SD, Forsythe CE, et al. Carbohydrate restriction has a more favorable impact on the metabolic syndrome than a low fat diet. *Lipids* 2009;44:297–309.

63 Volek JS, Sharman MJ, Forsythe CE. Modification of lipoproteins by very low-carbohydrate diets. *Journal of Nutrition* 2005;135:1339–42.

64 Lefevre F, Aronson N. Ketogenic diet for the treatment of refractory epilepsy in children: a systematic review of efficacy. *Pediatrics* 2000;105:E46.

65 Vining EP, Freeman JM, Ballaban-Gil K, et al. A multicenter study of the efficacy of the ketogenic diet. *Archives of Neurology* 1998;55:1433–37.

66 Thakur KT, Probasco JC, Hocker SE, et al. Ketogenic diet for adults in super-refractory status epilepticus. *Neurology* 2014;82:665–70.

67 Woolf EC, Scheck AC. The ketogenic diet for the treatment of malignant glioma. *Journal of Lipid Research* 2014 Feb 6. [Epub ahead of print]

68 Perez-Guisado J. [Ketogenic diets: additional benefits to the weight loss and unfounded secondary effects]. *Archivos latinoamericanos de nutrición* 2008;58:323–29.

69 Ibid.

70 Sacks FM, Bray GA, Carey VJ, et al. Comparison of weight-loss diets with different compositions of fat, protein, and carbohydrates. *New England Journal of Medicine* 2009;360:859–73.

71 Siri-Tarino PW, Sun Q, Hu FB, Krauss RM. Meta-analysis of prospective cohort studies evaluating the association of saturated fat with cardiovascular disease. *American Journal of Clinical Nutrition* 2010;91:535–46.

72 Lands B. Consequences of essential fatty acids. *Nutrients* 2012;4:1338–57

73 Cameron M, Gagnier JJ, Chrubasik S. Herbal therapy for treating rheumatoid arthritis. *Cochrane Database of Systematic Reviews* 2011:CD002948.

74 Galland L. Diet and inflammation. *Nutrition in Clinical Practice* 2010;25:634–40.

75 Palmer S. Fill in the fiber gaps—dietitians offer practical strategies to get clients to meet the daily requirements. *Today's Dietitian* 2012;14:40.

76 Roland BC, Ciarleglio MM, Clarke JO, et al. Low ileocecal valve pressure is significantly associated with small intestinal bacterial overgrowth (SIBO). *Digestive Diseases and Sciences* 2014;59:1269–77.

77 Bonilla S, Wang D, Saps M. Obesity predicts persistence of pain in children with functional gastrointestinal disorders. *International Journal of Obesity* 2011;35:517–21.

78   Halmos EP, Power VA, Shepherd SJ, Gibson PR, Muir JG. A diet low in FODMAPs reduces symptoms of irritable bowel syndrome. *Gastroenterology* 2014;146:67–75 e5.

79   Jouet P, Coffin B, Sabate JM. Small intestinal bacterial overgrowth in patients with morbid obesity. *Digestive Diseases and Sciences* 2011;56:615; author reply 616.

80   Sabate JM, Jouet P, Harnois F, et al. High prevalence of small intestinal bacterial overgrowth in patients with morbid obesity: a contributor to severe hepatic steatosis. *Obesity Surgery* 2008;18:371-77.

81   Madrid AM. Small intestinal bacterial overgrowth in patients with morbid obesity: reply. *Digestive Diseases and Sciences* 2011;56:615–16.

82   Madrid AM, Poniachik J, Quera R, Defilippi C. Small intestinal clustered contractions and bacterial overgrowth: a frequent finding in obese patients. *Digestive Diseases and Sciences* 2011;56:155–60.

83   Jouet P, Coffin B, Sabate JM. Small intestinal bacterial overgrowth in patients with morbid obesity. *Digestive Diseases and Sciences* 2011;56:615; author reply 616.

84   Ibid.

85   Madrid AM. Small intestinal bacterial overgrowth in patients with morbid obesity: reply. *Digestive Diseases and Sciences* 2011;56:615–16.

86   Madrid AM, Poniachik J, Quera R, Defilippi C. Small intestinal clustered contractions and bacterial overgrowth: a frequent finding in obese patients. *Digestive Diseases and Sciences* 2011;56:155–60.

87   Clements RH, Gonzalez QH, Foster A, et al. Gastrointestinal symptoms are more intense in morbidly obese patients and are improved with laparoscopic Roux-en-Y gastric bypass. *Obesity Surgery* 2003;13:610–14.

88   Foster A, Laws HL, Gonzalez QH, Clements RH. Gastrointestinal symptomatic outcome after laparoscopic Roux-en-Y gastric bypass. *Journal of Gastrointestinal Surgery* 2003;7:750–53.

89   Foster A, Richards WO, McDowell J, Laws HL, Clements RH. Gastrointestinal symptoms are more intense in morbidly obese patients. *Surgical Endoscopy* 2003;17:1766–68.

90   Levy RL, Linde JA, Feld KA, Crowell MD, Jeffery RW. The association of gastrointestinal symptoms with weight, diet, and exercise in weight-loss program participants. *Clinical Gastroenterology and Hepatology* 2005;3:992–96.

91   Ibid.

92   doctoroz.com/videos/botox-future-weight-loss.

93   Faria M, Pavin EJ, Parisi MC, et al. Delayed small intestinal transit in patients with long-standing type 1 diabetes mellitus: investigation of the relationships with clinical features, gastric emptying, psychological distress, and nutritional parameters. *Diabetes Technology & Therapeutics* 2013;15:32–38.

94   Staudacher HM, Irving PM, Lomer MC, Whelan K. Mechanisms and efficacy of dietary FODMAP restriction in IBS. *Nature Reviews Gastroenterology & Hepatology* 2014;11:256–66.

95   Halmos EP, Christophersen CT, Bird AR, Shepherd SJ, Gibson PR, Muir JG. Diets that differ in their FODMAP content alter the colonic luminal microenvironment. *Gut* 2014 Jul 14. [Epub ahead of print]

96   Kirby M, Danner E. Nutritional deficiencies in children on restricted diets. *Pediatric Clinics of North America* 2009;56:1085-103.

97   Nistal E, Caminero A, Vivas S, et al. Differences in faecal bacteria populations and faecal bacteria metabolism in healthy adults and celiac disease patients. *Biochimie* 2012;94:1724–29.

98   De Palma G, Nadal I, Collado MC, Sanz Y. Effects of a gluten-free diet on gut microbiota and immune function in healthy adult human subjects. *British Journal of Nutrition* 2009;102:1154–60.

99   Zhu W, Cai D, Wang Y, et al. Calcium plus vitamin D_3 supplementation facilitated fat loss in overweight and obese college students with very-low calcium consumption: a randomized controlled trial. *Nutrition Journal* 2013;12:8.

100 Tremblay A, Gilbert JA. Human obesity: is insufficient calcium/dairy intake part of the problem? *Journal of the American College of Nutrition* 2011;30:449S–53S.

101 Sun X, Zemel MB. Calcium and dairy products inhibit weight and fat regain during ad libitum consumption following energy restriction in Ap2-agouti transgenic mice. *Journal of Nutrition* 2004;134:3054–60.

102 Mozaffarian D, Hao T, Rimm EB, Willett WC, Hu FB. Changes in diet and lifestyle and long-term weight gain in women and men. *New England Journal of Medicine* 2011;364:2392–404.

103 Ross AC, Manson JE, Abrams SA, et al. The 2011 Dietary Reference Intakes for calcium and vitamin D: what dietetics practitioners need to know. *Journal of the American Dietetic Association* 2011;111:524–27.

104 Ibid.

105 Veldhorst M, Smeets A, Soenen S, et al. Protein-induced satiety: effects and mechanisms of different proteins. *Physiology & Behavior* 2008;94:300–307.

106 Lejeune MP, Kovacs EM, Westerterp-Plantenga MS. Additional protein intake limits weight regain after weight loss in humans. *British Journal of Nutrition* 2005;93:281–89.

107 Westerterp-Plantenga MS, Lejeune MP. Protein intake and body-weight regulation. *Appetite* 2005;45:187–90.

108 Westerterp-Plantenga MS, Lejeune MP, Nijs I, van Ooijen M, Kovacs EM. High protein intake sustains weight maintenance after body weight loss in humans. *International Journal of Obesity and Related Metabolic Disorders* 2004;28:57–64.

109 Westerterp-Plantenga MS, Nieuwenhuizen A, Tome D, Soenen S, Westerterp KR. Dietary protein, weight loss, and weight maintenance. *Annual Review of Nutrition* 2009;29:21–41.

110 Lejeune MP, Kovacs EM, Westerterp-Plantenga MS. Additional protein intake limits weight regain after weight loss in humans. *British Journal of Nutrition* 2005;93:281–89.

111 Westerterp-Plantenga MS, Lejeune MP. Protein intake and body-weight regulation. *Appetite* 2005;45:187–90.

112 Westerterp-Plantenga MS, Lejeune MP, Nijs I, van Ooijen M, Kovacs EM. High protein intake sustains weight maintenance after body weight loss in humans. *International Journal of Obesity and Related Metabolic Disorders* 2004;28:57–64.

113 Bowen J, Noakes M, Clifton PM. Appetite regulatory hormone responses to various dietary proteins differ by body mass index status despite similar reductions in ad libitum energy intake. *Journal of Clinical Endocrinology and Metabolism* 2006;91:2913–19.

114 Lejeune MP, Westerterp KR, Adam TC, Luscombe-Marsh ND, Westerterp-Plantenga MS. Ghrelin and glucagon-like peptide 1 concentrations, 24-h satiety, and energy and substrate metabolism during a high-protein diet and measured in a respiration chamber. *American Journal of Clinical Nutrition* 2006;83:89–94.

115 Batterham RL, Heffron H, Kapoor S, et al. Critical role for peptide YY in protein-mediated satiation and body-weight regulation. *Cell Metabolism* 2006;4:223–33.

116 Bowen J, Noakes M, Trenerry C, Clifton PM. Energy intake, ghrelin, and cholecystokinin after different carbohydrate and protein preloads in overweight men. *Journal of Clinical Endocrinology and Metabolism* 2006;91:1477–83.

117 Smeets AJ, Soenen S, Luscombe-Marsh ND, Ueland O, Westerterp-Plantenga MS. Energy expenditure, satiety, and plasma ghrelin, glucagon-like peptide 1, and peptide tyrosine-tyrosine concentrations following a single high-protein lunch. *Journal of Nutrition* 2008;138:698–702.

118 Holt SH, Miller JC, Petocz P, Farmakalidis E. A satiety index of common foods. *European Journal of Clinical Nutrition* 1995;49:675–90.

119 Uhe AM, Collier GR, O'Dea K. A comparison of the effects of beef, chicken and fish protein on satiety and amino acid profiles in lean male subjects. *Journal of Nutrition* 1992;122:467–72.

120 Pal S, Ellis V. The acute effects of four protein meals on insulin, glucose, appetite and energy intake in lean men. *British Journal of Nutrition* 2010;104:1241–48.

121 Rebello CJ, Liu AG, Greenway FL, Dhurandhar NV. Dietary strategies to increase satiety. *Advances in Food and Nutrition Research* 2013;69:105–82.

122 Douglas SM, Ortinau LC, Hoertel HA, Leidy HJ. Low, moderate, or high protein yogurt snacks on appetite control and subsequent eating in healthy women. *Appetite* 2013;60:117–22.

123 Hession M, Rolland C, Kulkarni U, Wise A, Broom J. Systematic review of randomized controlled trials of low-carbohydrate vs. low-fat/low-calorie diets in the management of obesity and its comorbidities. *Obesity Reviews* 2009;10:36–50.

124 Mozaffarian D, Hao T, Rimm EB, Willett WC, Hu FB. Changes in diet and lifestyle and long-term weight gain in women and men. *New England Journal of Medicine* 2011;364:2392–404.

125 Rosell M, Appleby P, Spencer E, Key T. Weight gain over 5 years in 21,966 meat-eating, fish-eating, vegetarian, and vegan men and women in EPIC-Oxford. *International Journal of Obesity* 2006;30:1389–96.

126 Cocate PG, Natali AJ, Oliveira AD, et al. Red but not white meat consumption is associated with metabolic syndrome, insulin resistance and lipid peroxidation in Brazilian middle-aged men. *European Journal of Preventive Cardiology* 2013 Oct 8. [Epub ahead of print]

127 Babio N, Sorli M, Bullo M, et al. Association between red meat consumption and metabolic syndrome in a Mediterranean population at high cardiovascular risk: cross-sectional and 1-year follow-up assessment. *Nutrition, Metabolism, and Cardiovascular Diseases* 2012;22:200–207.

128 Pan A, Sun Q, Bernstein AM, Manson JE, Willett WC, Hu FB. Changes in red meat consumption and subsequent risk of type 2 diabetes mellitus: three cohorts of US men and women. *JAMA Internal Medicine* 2013;173:1328–35.

129 Vergnaud AC, Norat T, Romaguera D, et al. Meat consumption and prospective weight change in participants of the EPIC-PANACEA study. *American Journal of Clinical Nutrition* 2010;92:398–407.

130 Cho I, Yamanishi S, Cox L, et al. Antibiotics in early life alter the murine colonic microbiome and adiposity. *Nature* 2012;488:621–26.

131 Jobin C. [Microbial dysbiosis, a new risk factor in colorectal cancer?]. *Médecine sciences* 2013;29:582–85.

132 cancerpreventionresearch.aacrjournals.org/content/7/11/1112

133 Wang Z, Klipfell E, Bennett BJ, et al. Gut flora metabolism of phosphatidylcholine promotes cardiovascular disease. *Nature* 2011;472:57–63.

134 Davidson S. Flagging flora: heart disease link. *Nature* 2011;477:162.

135 Ussher JR, Lopaschuk GD, Arduini A. Gut microbiota metabolism of L-carnitine and cardiovascular risk. *Atherosclerosis* 2013;231:456–61.

136 Levine ME, Suarez JA, Brandhorst S, et al. Low protein intake is associated with a major reduction in IGF-1, cancer, and overall mortality in the 65 and younger but not older population. *Cell Metabolism* 2014;19:407–17.

137 Thorpe DL, Knutsen SF, Beeson WL, Rajaram S, Fraser GE. Effects of meat consumption and vegetarian diet on risk of wrist fracture over 25 years in a cohort of peri- and postmenopausal women. *Public Health Nutrition* 2008;11:564–72.

138 Nicoll R, McLaren Howard J. The acid-ash hypothesis revisited: a reassessment of the impact of dietary acidity on bone. *Journal of Bone and Mineral Metabolism* 2014 Feb 21. [Epub ahead of print]

139 Calvez J, Poupin N, Chesneau C, Lassale C, Tome D. Protein intake, calcium balance and health consequences. *European Journal of Clinical Nutrition* 2012;66:281–95.

140 Wu GD, Chen J, Hoffmann C, et al. Linking long-term dietary patterns with gut microbial enterotypes. *Science* 2011;334:105–8.

141 David LA, Maurice CF, Carmody RN, et al. Diet rapidly and reproducibly alters the human gut microbiome. *Nature* 2014;505:559–63.

142 Tuohy KM, Fava F, Viola R. 'The way to a man's heart is through his gut microbiota'–dietary pro- and prebiotics for the management of cardiovascular risk. *Proceedings of the Nutrition Society* 2014:1–14.

143 Razquin C, Martinez JA, Martinez-Gonzalez MA, Fernandez-Crehuet J, Santos JM, Marti A. A Mediterranean diet rich in virgin olive oil may reverse the effects of the -174G/C IL6 gene variant on 3-year body weight change. *Molecular Nutrition & Food Research* 2010;54(Suppl 1):S75–S82.

144 Razquin C, Martinez JA, Martinez-Gonzalez MA, Salas-Salvado J, Estruch R, Marti A. A 3-year Mediterranean-style dietary intervention may modulate the association between adiponectin gene variants and body weight change. *European Journal of Nutrition* 2010;49:311–19.

145 Lucas L, Russell A, Keast R. Molecular mechanisms of inflammation. Anti-inflammatory benefits of virgin olive oil and the phenolic compound oleocanthal. *Current Pharmaceutical Design* 2011;17:754–68.

146 Wendland E, Farmer A, Glasziou P, Neil A. Effect of alpha linolenic acid on cardiovascular risk markers: a systematic review. *Heart* 2006;92:166–69.

147 Lin L, Allemekinders H, Dansby A, et al. Evidence of health benefits of canola oil. *Nutrition Reviews* 2013;71:370–85.

148 Hung HC, Joshipura KJ, Jiang R, et al. Fruit and vegetable intake and risk of major chronic disease. *Journal of the National Cancer Institute* 2004;96:1577–84.

149 Mattes R. Soup and satiety. *Physiology & Behavior* 2005;83:739–47.

150 Muckelbauer R, Sarganas G, Gruneis A, Muller-Nordhorn J. Association between water consumption and body weight outcomes: a systematic review. *American Journal of Clinical Nutrition* 2013;98:282–99.

151 usda.gov/factbook/chapter2.pdf.tables 2–6, page 20.

152 Nielsen SJ, Popkin BM. Changes in beverage intake between 1977 and 2001. *American Journal of Preventive Medicine* 2004;27:205–10.

153 Mullin GE. Red wine, grapes, and better health–resveratrol. *Nutrition in Clinical Practice* 2011;26:722–23.

154 Bertelli AA, Das DK. Grapes, wines, resveratrol, and heart health. *Journal of Cardiovascular Pharmacology* 2009;54:468–76.

155 Lekli I, Ray D, Das DK. Longevity nutrients resveratrol, wines and grapes. *Genes & Nutrition* 2010;5:55–60.

156 Wu GD, Bushmanc FD, Lewis JD. Diet, the human gut microbiota, and IBD. *Anaerobe* 2013;24:117–20.

157 coffeeconfidential.org/health/decaffeination/.

Chapter 5

1 Vander Wal JS, Marth JM, Khosla P, Jen KL, Dhurandhar NV. Short-term effect of eggs on satiety in overweight and obese subjects. *Journal of the American College of Nutrition* 2005;24:510–15.

2   Ibid.

3   Vander Wal JS, Gupta A, Khosla P, Dhurandhar NV. Egg breakfast enhances weight loss. *International Journal of Obesity* 2008;32:1545–51.

4   Ratliff J, Leite JO, de Ogburn R, Puglisi MJ, VanHeest J, Fernandez ML. Consuming eggs for breakfast influences plasma glucose and ghrelin, while reducing energy intake during the next 24 hours in adult men. *Nutrition Research* 2010;30:96–103.

5   Karra E, Chandarana K, Batterham RL. The role of peptide YY in appetite regulation and obesity. *Journal of Physiology* 2009;587:19–25.

6   Fallaize R, Wilson L, Gray J, Morgan LM, Griffin BA. Variation in the effects of three different breakfast meals on subjective satiety and subsequent intake of energy at lunch and evening meal. *European Journal of Nutrition* 2013;52:1353–59.

7   Vuksan V, Jenkins AL, Dias AG, et al. Reduction in postprandial glucose excursion and prolongation of satiety: possible explanation of the long-term effects of whole grain Salba (Salvia Hispanica L.). *European Journal of Clinical Nutrition* 2010;64:436–38.

8   Chicco AG, D'Alessandro ME, Hein GJ, Oliva ME, Lombardo YB. Dietary chia seed (Salvia hispanica L.) rich in alpha-linolenic acid improves adiposity and normalises hypertriacylglycerolaemia and insulin resistance in dyslipaemic rats. *British Journal of Nutrition* 2009;101:41–50.

9   Vuksan V, Jenkins AL, Dias AG, et al. Reduction in postprandial glucose excursion and prolongation of satiety: possible explanation of the long-term effects of whole grain Salba (Salvia Hispanica L.). *European Journal of Clinical Nutrition* 2010;64:436–38.

10 Chicco AG, D'Alessandro ME, Hein GJ, Oliva ME, Lombardo YB. Dietary chia seed (Salvia hispanica L.) rich in alpha-linolenic acid improves adiposity and normalises hypertriacylglycerolaemia and insulin resistance in dyslipaemic rats. *British Journal of Nutrition* 2009;101:41–50.

11 Vuksan V, Whitham D, Sievenpiper JL, et al. Supplementation of conventional therapy with the novel grain Salba (Salvia hispanica L.) improves major and emerging cardiovascular risk factors in type 2 diabetes: results of a randomized controlled trial. *Diabetes Care* 2007;30:2804–10.

12 Ayerza R, Jr., Coates W. Effect of dietary alpha-linolenic fatty acid derived from chia when fed as ground seed, whole seed and oil on lipid content and fatty acid composition of rat plasma. *Annals of Nutrition & Metabolism* 2007;51:27–34.

13 Ranasinghe P, Pigera S, Premakumara GA, Galappaththy P, Constantine GR, Katulanda P. Medicinal properties of 'true' cinnamon (Cinnamomum zeylanicum): a systematic review. *BMC Complementary and Alternative Medicine* 2013;13:275.

14 Bandara T, Uluwaduge I, Jansz ER. Bioactivity of cinnamon with special emphasis on diabetes mellitus: a review. *International Journal of Food Sciences and Nutrition* 2012;63:380–86.

15 Mullin GE. Nutraceuticals for diabetes: what is the evidence? *Nutrition in Clinical Practice* 2011;26:199–201.

16 Mullin GE, Clarke JO. Role of complementary and alternative medicine in managing gastrointestinal motility disorders. *Nutrition in Clinical Practice* 2010;25:85–87.

17 Hlebowicz J. Postprandial blood glucose response in relation to gastric emptying and satiety in healthy subjects. *Appetite* 2009;53:249–52.

18 Hlebowicz J, Darwiche G, Bjorgell O, Almer LO. Effect of cinnamon on postprandial blood glucose, gastric emptying, and satiety in healthy subjects. *American Journal of Clinical Nutrition* 2007;85:1552–56.

19 Mettler S, Schwarz I, Colombani PC. Additive postprandial blood glucose-attenuating and satiety-enhancing effect of cinnamon and acetic acid. *Nutrition Research* 2009;29:723–27.

20 Ranasinghe P, Pigera S, Premakumara GA, Galappaththy P, Constantine GR, Katulanda P. Medicinal properties of 'true' cinnamon (Cinnamomum zeylanicum): a systematic review. *BMC Complementary and Alternative Medicine* 2013;13:275.

21 Joseph SV, Edirisinghe I, Burton-Freeman BM. Berries: anti-inflammatory effects in humans. *Journal of Agricultural and Food Chemistry* 2014 Mar 17. [Epub ahead of print]

22 Rodriguez-Mateos A, Heiss C, Borges G, Crozier A. Berry (poly)phenols and cardiovascular health. *Journal of Agricultural and Food Chemistry* 2013 Oct 7. [Epub ahead of print]

23 Prior RL, S EW, T RR, Khanal RC, Wu X, Howard LR. Purified blueberry anthocyanins and blueberry juice alter development of obesity in mice fed an obesogenic high-fat diet. *Journal of Agricultural and Food Chemistry* 2010;58:3970–76.

24 Vuong T, Benhaddou-Andaloussi A, Brault A, et al. Antiobesity and antidiabetic effects of biotransformed blueberry juice in KKA(y) mice. *International Journal of Obesity* 2009;33:1166–73.

25 Vendrame S, Daugherty A, Kristo AS, Riso P, Klimis-Zacas D. Wild blueberry (Vaccinium angustifolium) consumption improves inflammatory status in the obese Zucker rat model of the metabolic syndrome. *Journal of Nutritional Biochemistry* 2013;24:1508–12.

26 Stoner GD, Wang LS, Seguin C, et al. Multiple berry types prevent N-nitrosomethylbenzylamine-induced esophageal cancer in rats. *Pharmaceutical Research* 2010;27:1138–45.

27 Song Y, Park HJ, Kang SN, et al. Blueberry peel extracts inhibit adipogenesis in 3T3-L1 cells and reduce high-fat diet-induced obesity. *PloS One* 2013;8:e69925.

28 Ibid.

29 Moghe SS, Juma S, Imrhan V, Vijayagopal P. Effect of blueberry polyphenols on 3T3-F442A preadipocyte differentiation. *Journal of Medicinal Food* 2012;15:448–52.

30 Khanal RC, Howard LR, Wilkes SE, Rogers TJ, Prior RL. Effect of dietary blueberry pomace on selected metabolic factors associated with high fructose feeding in growing Sprague-Dawley rats. *Journal of Medicinal Food* 2012;15:802–10.

31 Roopchand DE, Kuhn P, Rojo LE, Lila MA, Raskin I. Blueberry polyphenol-enriched soybean flour reduces hyperglycemia, body weight gain and serum cholesterol in mice. *Pharmacological Research* 2013;68:59–67.

32 Stull AJ, Cash KC, Johnson WD, Champagne CM, Cefalu WT. Bioactives in blueberries improve insulin sensitivity in obese, insulin-resistant men and women. *Journal of Nutrition* 2010;140:1764–68.

33 Takikawa M, Inoue S, Horio F, Tsuda T. Dietary anthocyanin-rich bilberry extract ameliorates hyperglycemia and insulin sensitivity via activation of AMP-activated protein kinase in diabetic mice. *Journal of Nutrition* 2010;140:527–33.

34 Puupponen-Pimia R, Nohynek L, Hartmann-Schmidlin S, et al. Berry phenolics selectively inhibit the growth of intestinal pathogens. *Journal of Applied Microbiology* 2005;98:991–1000.

35 Rosillo MA, Sanchez-Hidalgo M, Cardeno A, de la Lastra CA. Protective effect of ellagic acid, a natural polyphenolic compound, in a murine model of Crohn's disease. *Biochemical Pharmacology* 2011;82:737–45.

36 Torronen R, Kolehmainen M, Sarkkinen E, Poutanen K, Mykkanen H, Niskanen L. Berries reduce postprandial insulin responses to wheat and rye breads in healthy women. *Journal of Nutrition* 2013;143:430–36.

37 Hodgson JM, Croft KD. Tea flavonoids and cardiovascular health. *Molecular Aspects of Medicine* 2010;31:495–502.

38 Mullin GE. Comment on: black and green tea consumption and the risk of coronary artery disease: a meta-analysis. *Nutrition in Clinical Practice* 2011;26(3):356.

39 Larsson SC. Coffee, tea, and cocoa and risk of stroke. *Stroke* 2014;45:309–14.

40 Larsson SC, Virtamo J, Wolk A. Black tea consumption and risk of stroke in women and men. *Annals of Epidemiology* 2013;23:157–60.

41 Bogdanski P, Suliburska J, Szulinska M, Stepien M, Pupek-Musialik D, Jablecka A. Green tea extract reduces blood pressure, inflammatory biomarkers, and oxidative stress and improves parameters associated with insulin resistance in obese, hypertensive patients. *Nutrition Research* 2012;32:421-27.

42 Suliburska J, Bogdanski P, Szulinska M, Stepien M, Pupek-Musialik D, Jablecka A. Effects of green tea supplementation on elements, total antioxidants, lipids, and glucose values in the serum of obese patients. *Biological Trace Element Research* 2012;149:315–22.

43 Hursel R, Westerterp-Plantenga MS. Catechin- and caffeine-rich teas for control of body weight in humans. *American Journal of Clinical Nutrition* 2013;98:1682S–93S.

44 Hursel R, van der Zee L, Westerterp-Plantenga MS. Effects of a breakfast yoghurt, with additional total whey protein or caseinomacropeptide-depleted alpha-lactalbumin-enriched whey protein, on diet-induced thermogenesis and appetite suppression. *British Journal of Nutrition* 2010;103:775–80.

45 Hursel R, Viechtbauer W, Westerterp-Plantenga MS. The effects of green tea on weight loss and weight maintenance: a meta-analysis. *International Journal of Obesity* 2009;33:956–61.

46 Phung OJ, Baker WL, Matthews LJ, Lanosa M, Thorne A, Coleman CI. Effect of green tea catechins with or without caffeine on anthropometric measures: a systematic review and meta-analysis. *American Journal of Clinical Nutrition* 2010;91:73–81.

47 Axling U, Olsson C, Xu J, et al. Green tea powder and Lactobacillus plantarum affect gut microbiota, lipid metabolism and inflammation in high-fat fed C57BL/6J mice. *Nutrition & Metabolism* 2012;9:105.

48 Hodgson AB, Randell RK, Jeukendrup AE. The effect of green tea extract on fat oxidation at rest and during exercise: evidence of efficacy and proposed mechanisms. *Advances in Nutrition* 2013;4:129–40.

49 Hsu TF, Kusumoto A, Abe K, et al. Polyphenol-enriched oolong tea increases fecal lipid excretion. *European Journal of Clinical Nutrition* 2006;60:1330–36.

50 Conterno L, Fava F, Viola R, Tuohy KM. Obesity and the gut microbiota: does up-regulating colonic fermentation protect against obesity and metabolic disease? *Genes & Nutrition* 2011;6:241–60.

51 Josic J, Olsson AT, Wickeberg J, Lindstedt S, Hlebowicz J. Does green tea affect postprandial glucose, insulin and satiety in healthy subjects: a randomized controlled trial. *Nutrition Journal* 2010;9:63.

52 Ali BH, Blunden G, Tanira MO, Nemmar A. Some phytochemical, pharmacological and toxicological properties of ginger (Zingiber officinale Roscoe): a review of recent research. *Food and Chemical Toxicology* 2008;46(2):409–20.

53 Haniadka R, Saldanha E, Sunita V, Palatty PL, Fayad R, Baliga MS. A review of the gastroprotective effects of ginger (Zingiber officinale Roscoe). *Food & Function* 2013;4:845–55.

54 Shobana S, Naidu KA. Antioxidant activity of selected Indian spices. *Prostaglandins, Leukotrienes, and Essential Fatty Acids* 2000;62:107–10.

55 Grzanna R, Lindmark L, Frondoza CG. Ginger–an herbal medicinal product with broad anti-inflammatory actions. *Journal of Medicinal Food* 2005;8:125–32.

56 Shobana S, Naidu KA. Antioxidant activity of selected Indian spices. *Prostaglandins, Leukotrienes, and Essential Fatty Acids* 2000;62:107–10.

57 Ramadan G, El-Menshawy O. Protective effects of ginger-turmeric rhizomes mixture on joint inflammation, atherogenesis, kidney dysfunction and other complications in a rat model of human rheumatoid arthritis. *International Journal of Rheumatic Diseases* 2013;16:219–29.

58 Eldershaw TP, Colquhoun EQ, Dora KA, Peng ZC, Clark MG. Pungent principles of ginger (Zingiber officinale) are thermogenic in the perfused rat hindlimb. *International Journal of Obesity and Related Metabolic Disorders* 1992;16:755–63.

59 Ibid.

60 Sugita J, Yoneshiro T, Hatano T, et al. Grains of paradise (Aframomum melegueta) extract activates brown adipose tissue and increases whole-body energy expenditure in men. *British Journal of Nutrition* 2013;110:733–38.

61 Mansour MS, Ni YM, Roberts AL, Kelleman M, Roychoudhury A, St-Onge MP. Ginger consumption enhances the thermic effect of food and promotes feelings of satiety without affecting metabolic and hormonal parameters in overweight men: a pilot study. *Metabolism: Clinical and Experimental* 2012;61:1347–52.

62 Henry CJ, Piggott SM. Effect of ginger on metabolic rate. *Human Nutrition Clinical Nutrition* 1987;41:89–92.

63 Balliett M, Burke JR. Changes in anthropometric measurements, body composition, blood pressure, lipid profile, and testosterone in patients participating in a low-energy dietary intervention. *Journal of Chiropractic Medicine* 2013;12:3–14.

64 Mahmoud RH, Elnour WA. Comparative evaluation of the efficacy of ginger and orlistat on obesity management, pancreatic lipase and liver peroxisomal catalase enzyme in male albino rats. *European Review for Medical and Pharmacological Sciences* 2013;17:75–83.

65 Paniagua JA, de la Sacristana AG, Sanchez E, et al. A MUFA-rich diet improves posprandial glucose, lipid and GLP-1 responses in insulin-resistant subjects. *Journal of the American College of Nutrition* 2007;26:434–44.

66 Wien M, Haddad E, Oda K, Sabate J. A randomized 3x3 crossover study to evaluate the effect of Hass avocado intake on post-ingestive satiety, glucose and insulin levels, and subsequent energy intake in overweight adults. *Nutrition Journal* 2013;12:155.

67 Nagata C, Nakamura K, Wada K, et al. Association of dietary fat, vegetables and antioxidant micronutrients with skin ageing in Japanese women. *British Journal of Nutrition* 2010;103:1493–98.

68 Cho E, Hankinson SE, Rosner B, Willett WC, Colditz GA. Prospective study of lutein/zeaxanthin intake and risk of age-related macular degeneration. *American Journal of Clinical Nutrition* 2008;87:1837–43.

69 Berti C, Riso P, Monti LD, Porrini M. In vitro starch digestibility and in vivo glucose response of gluten-free foods and their gluten counterparts. *European Journal of Nutrition* 2004;43:198–204.

70 Gomez-Caravaca AM, Iafelice G, Lavini A, Pulvento C, Caboni MF, Marconi E. Phenolic compounds and saponins in quinoa samples (Chenopodium quinoa Willd.) grown under different saline and nonsaline irrigation regimens. *Journal of Agricultural and Food Chemistry* 2012;60:4620–27.

71 Ruales J, Nair BM. Nutritional quality of the protein in quinoa (Chenopodium quinoa, Willd) seeds. *Plant Foods for Human Nutrition* 1992;42:1–11.

72 Raghavendra RH, Naidu KA. Spice active principles as the inhibitors of human platelet aggregation and thromboxane biosynthesis. *Prostaglandins, Leukotrienes, and Essential Fatty Acids* 2009;81:73–78.

73 Sayin MR, Karabag T, Dogan SM, Akpinar I, Aydin M. A case of acute myocardial infarction due to the use of cayenne pepper pills. *Wiener klinische Wochenschrift* 2012;124:285–87.

74 Ibid.

75 Sogut O, Kaya H, Gokdemir MT, Sezen Y. Acute myocardial infarction and coronary vasospasm associated with the ingestion of cayenne pepper pills in a 25-year-old male. *International Journal of Emergency Medicine* 2012;5:5.

76 Peppin JF, Pappagallo M. Capsaicinoids in the treatment of neuropathic pain: a review. *Therapeutic Advances in Neurological Disorders* 2014;7:22–32.

77 Sawynok J. Topical analgesics for neuropathic pain: Preclinical exploration, clinical validation, future development. *European Journal of Pain* 2014;18:465–81.

78 Peppin JF, Pappagallo M. Capsaicinoids in the treatment of neuropathic pain: a review. *Therapeutic Advances in Neurological Disorders* 2014;7:22–32.

79 Cameron M, Chrubasik S. Topical herbal therapies for treating osteoarthritis. *Cochrane Database of Systematic Reviews* 2013;5:CD010538.

80 Lin CH, Lu WC, Wang CW, Chan YC, Chen MK. Capsaicin induces cell cycle arrest and apoptosis in human KB cancer cells. *BMC Complementary and Alternative Medicine* 2013;13:46.

81 Whiting S, Derbyshire E, Tiwari BK. Capsaicinoids and capsinoids. A potential role for weight management? A systematic review of the evidence. *Appetite* 2012;59:341–48.

82 Kovacs EM, Mela DJ. Metabolically active functional food ingredients for weight control. *Obesity Reviews* 2006;7:59–78

83 Mercader J, Wanecq E, Chen J, Carpene C. Isopropylnorsynephrine is a stronger lipolytic agent in human adipocytes than synephrine and other amines present in Citrus aurantium. *Journal of Physiology and Biochemistry* 2011;67:443–52.

84 Davies IR, Brown JC, Livesey G. Energy values and energy balance in rats fed on supplements of guar gum or cellulose. *British Journal of Nutrition* 1991;65:41533.

85 Yoshioka M, St-Pierre S, Drapeau V, et al. Effects of red pepper on appetite and energy intake. *British Journal of Nutrition* 1999;82:115–23.

86 Whiting S, Derbyshire EJ, Tiwari B. Could capsaicinoids help to support weight management? A systematic review and meta-analysis of energy intake data. *Appetite* 2014;73:183–38.

87 Reidy PT, Walker DK, Dickinson JM, et al. Protein blend ingestion following resistance exercise promotes human muscle protein synthesis. *Journal of Nutrition* 2013;143:410–16.

88 Bowen J, Noakes M, Trenerry C, Clifton PM. Energy intake, ghrelin, and cholecystokinin after different carbohydrate and protein preloads in overweight men. *Journal of Clinical Endocrinology and Metabolism* 2006;91:1477–83.

89 Morrison CD, Xi X, White CL, Ye J, Martin RJ. Amino acids inhibit Agrp gene expression via an mTOR-dependent mechanism. *American Journal of Physiology Endocrinology and Metabolism* 2007;293:E165–E171.

90 Franceschelli A, Cappello A, Cappello G. [Retrospective study on the effects of a whey protein concentrate on body composition in 262 sarcopenic tube fed patients]. *Minerva medica* 2013;104:103–12.

91 Coker RH, Miller S, Schutzler S, Deutz N, Wolfe RR. Whey protein and essential amino acids promote the reduction of adipose tissue and increased muscle protein synthesis during caloric restriction-induced weight loss in elderly, obese individuals. *Nutrition Journal* 2012;11:105.

92 Hall WL, Millward DJ, Long SJ, Morgan LM. Casein and whey exert different effects on plasma amino acid profiles, gastrointestinal hormone secretion and appetite. *British Journal of Nutrition* 2003;89:239–48.

93 Veldhorst MA, Nieuwenhuizen AG, Hochstenbach-Waelen A, et al. Effects of complete whey-protein breakfasts versus whey without GMP-breakfasts on energy intake and satiety. *Appetite* 2009;52:388–95.

94 ——. A breakfast with alpha-lactalbumin, gelatin, or gelatin + TRP lowers energy intake at lunch compared with a breakfast with casein, soy, whey, or whey-GMP. *Clinical Nutrition* 2009;28:147–55.

95 Bowen J, Noakes M, Clifton PM. Appetite regulatory hormone responses to various dietary proteins differ by body mass index status despite similar reductions in ad libitum energy intake. *Journal of Clinical Endocrinology and Metabolism* 2006;91:2913–19.

96 Meister D, Bode J, Shand A, Ghosh S. Anti-inflammatory effects of enteral diet components on Crohn's disease-affected tissues in vitro. *Digestive and Liver Disease* 2002;34:430–38.

97 Polk DB, Hattner JA, Kerner JA, Jr. Improved growth and disease activity after intermittent administration of a defined formula diet in children with Crohn's disease. *Journal of Parenteral and Enteral Nutrition* 1992;16:499–504.

98 Benjamin J, Makharia G, Ahuja V, et al. Glutamine and whey protein improve intestinal permeability and morphology in patients with Crohn's disease: a randomized controlled trial. *Digestive Diseases and Sciences* 2012;57:1000–12.

99 Munukka E, Pekkala S, Wiklund P, et al. Gut-adipose tissue axis in hepatic fat accumulation in humans. *Journal of Hepatology* 2014;61:132–38.

100 Trujillo-de Santiago G, Saenz-Collins CP, Rojas-de Gante C. Elaboration of a probiotic oblea from whey fermented using Lactobacillus acidophilus or Bifidobacterium infantis. *Journal of Dairy Science* 2012;95:6897–904.

Chapter 6

1 Million M, Angelakis E, Paul M, Armougom F, Leibovici L, Raoult D. Comparative meta-analysis of the effect of Lactobacillus species on weight gain in humans and animals. *Microbial Pathogenesis* 2012;53:100–108.

2 Kadooka Y, Sato M, Imaizumi K, et al. Regulation of abdominal adiposity by probiotics (Lactobacillus gasseri SBT2055) in adults with obese tendencies in a randomized controlled trial. *European Journal of Clinical Nutrition* 2010;64:636–43.

3 Aronsson L, Huang Y, Parini P, et al. Decreased fat storage by Lactobacillus paracasei is associated with increased levels of angiopoietin-like 4 protein (ANGPTL4). *PLoS One* 2010;5.

4 Takemura N, Okubo T, Sonoyama K. Lactobacillus plantarum strain No. 14 reduces adipocyte size in mice fed high-fat diet. *Experimental Biology and Medicine* 2010;235:849–56.

5 Kadooka Y, Sato M, Imaizumi K, et al. Regulation of abdominal adiposity by probiotics (Lactobacillus gasseri SBT2055) in adults with obese tendencies in a randomized controlled trial. *European Journal of Clinical Nutrition* 2010;64:636–43.

6 Andreasen AS, Larsen N, Pedersen-Skovsgaard T, et al. Effects of Lactobacillus acidophilus NCFM on insulin sensitivity and the systemic inflammatory response in human subjects. *British Journal of Nutrition* 2010;104:1831–38.

7 Mullin GE. Integrative weight management. In: Bendich A, ed. *Nutrition in Health*. New York: Springer, 2014:71–106.

8 Lee HY, Park JH, Seok SH, et al. Human originated bacteria, Lactobacillus rhamnosus PL60, produce conjugated linoleic acid and show anti-obesity effects in diet-induced obese mice. *Biochimica et biophysica acta* 2006;1761:736–44.

9 Naito E, Yoshida Y, Makino K, et al. Beneficial effect of oral administration of Lactobacillus casei strain Shirota on insulin resistance in diet-induced obesity mice. *Journal of Applied Microbiology* 2011;110:650–57.

10 O'Brien PE, McPhail T, Chaston TB, Dixon JB. Systematic review of medium-term weight loss after bariatric operations. *Obesity Surgery* 2006;16:1032–40.

11 Woodard GA, Encarnacion B, Downey JR, et al. Probiotics improve outcomes after Roux-en-Y gastric bypass surgery: a prospective randomized trial. *Journal of Gastrointestinal Surgery* 2009;13:1198–204.

12 Sharifi SD, Dibamehr A, Lotfollahian H, Baurhoo B. Effects of flavomycin and probiotic supplementation to diets containing different sources of fat on growth performance, intestinal morphology, apparent metabolizable energy, and fat digestibility in broiler chickens. *Poultry Science* 2012;91:918–27.

13 Cani PD, Lecourt E, Dewulf EM, et al. Gut microbiota fermentation of prebiotics increases satietogenic and incretin gut peptide production with consequences for appetite sensation and glucose response after a meal. *American Journal of Clinical Nutrition* 2009;90:1236–43.

14 Parnell JA, Reimer RA. Weight loss during oligofructose supplementation is associated with decreased ghrelin and increased peptide YY in overweight and obese adults. *American Journal of Clinical Nutrition* 2009;89:1751–59.

15 Jakobsdottir G, Nyman M, Fak F. Designing future prebiotic fiber to target the metabolic syndrome. *Nutrition* 2013;30:497–502.

16 Arora T, Singh S, Sharma RK. Probiotics: Interaction with gut microbiome and antiobesity potential. *Nutrition* 2013;29:591–96.

17 Lawton CL, Walton J, Hoyland A, et al. Short term (14 days) consumption of insoluble wheat bran fibre-containing breakfast cereals improves subjective digestive feelings, general wellbeing and bowel function in a dose dependent manner. *Nutrients* 2013;5:1436–55.

18 Delzenne NM, Neyrinck AM, Cani PD. Modulation of the gut microbiota by nutrients with prebiotic properties: consequences for host health in the context of obesity and metabolic syndrome. *Microbial Cell Factories* 2011;10(Suppl 1):S10.

19 Delzenne NM, Neyrinck AM, Backhed F, Cani PD. Targeting gut microbiota in obesity: effects of prebiotics and probiotics. *Nature Reviews Endocrinology* 2011;7:639–46.

20 Cani PD, Osto M, Geurts L, Everard A. Involvement of gut microbiota in the development of low-grade inflammation and type 2 diabetes associated with obesity. *Gut Microbes* 2012;3:279–88.

21 Fallucca F, Porrata C, Fallucca S, Pianesi M. Influence of diet on gut microbiota, inflammation and type 2 diabetes mellitus. First experience with macrobiotic Ma-Pi 2 diet. *Diabetes/Metabolism Research and Reviews* 2014;30(Suppl 1):48–54.

22 Xiao S, Fei N, Pang X, et al. A gut microbiota-targeted dietary intervention for amelioration of chronic inflammation underlying metabolic syndrome. *FEMS Microbiology Ecology* 2014;87:357–67.

23 Ray K. Gut microbiota: microbial metabolites feed into the gut-brain-gut circuit during host metabolism. *Nature Reviews Gastroenterology & Hepatology* 2014;11:76.

24 Umu OC, Oostindjer M, Pope PB, et al. Potential applications of gut microbiota to control human physiology. *Antonie van Leeuwenhoek* 2013;104:609–18.

25 Cani PD, Joly E, Horsmans Y, Delzenne NM. Oligofructose promotes satiety in healthy humans: a pilot study. *European Journal of Clinical Nutrition* 2006;60:567-72.

26 Davis W. *Wheat Belly.* New York: Rodale, 2011.

27 Perlmutter D. *Grain Brain.* New York: Little, Brown and Co., 2013.

28 Fasano A. Zonulin, regulation of tight junctions, and autoimmune diseases. *Annals of the New York Academy of Sciences* 2012;1258:25-33.

29 wypr.publicbroadcasting.net/midday.html.

30 Biesiekierski JR, Peters SL, Newnham ED, Rosella O, Muir JG, Gibson PR. No effects of gluten in patients with self-reported non-celiac gluten sensitivity after dietary reduction of fermentable, poorly absorbed, short-chain carbohydrates. *Gastroenterology* 2013;145:320-8 e1-3.

31 Carroccio A, Brusca I, Mansueto P, et al. A comparison between two different in vitro basophil activation tests for gluten- and cow's milk protein sensitivity in irritable bowel syndrome (IBS)-like patients. *Clinical Chemistry and Laboratory Medicine* 2012:1–7.

32 Sanz Y. Effects of a gluten-free diet on gut microbiota and immune function in healthy adult humans. *Gut Microbes* 2010;1:135–37.

33 Halmos EP, Christophersen CT, Bird AR, Shepherd SJ, Gibson PR, Muir JG. Diets that differ in their FODMAP content alter the colonic luminal microenvironment. *Gut* 2014 Jul 12. [Epub ahead of print]

34 Bao Y, Han J, Hu FB, et al. Association of nut consumption with total and cause-specific mortality. *New England Journal of Medicine* 2013;369:2001-11.

35 Gulati S, Misra A, Pandey RM, Bhatt SP, Saluja S. Effects of pistachio nuts on body composition, metabolic, inflammatory and oxidative stress parameters in Asian Indians with metabolic syndrome: a 24-wk, randomized control trial. *Nutrition* 2014;30:192-97.

36 Liu Z, Lin X, Huang G, Zhang W, Rao P, Ni L. Prebiotic effects of almonds and almond skins on intestinal microbiota in healthy adult humans. *Anaerobe* 2014;26:1-6.

37 Ibid.

38 Tan SY, Dhillon J, Mattes RD. A review of the effects of nuts on appetite, food intake, metabolism, and body weight. *American Journal of Clinical Nutrition* 2014;100:412S–422S.

39 David LA, Maurice CF, Carmody RN, et al. Diet rapidly and reproducibly alters the human gut microbiome. *Nature* 2014;505:559–63.

40 Ray K. Gut microbiota: Adding weight to the microbiota's role in obesity—exposure to antibiotics early in life can lead to increased adiposity. *Nature Reviews Gastroenterology & Hepatology* 2012;9:615.

41 Tolstrup JS, Halkjaer J, Heitmann BL, et al. Alcohol drinking frequency in relation to subsequent changes in waist circumference. *American Journal of Clinical Nutrition* 2008;87:957-63.

42 Goldberg IJ, Mosca L, Piano MR, Fisher EA. AHA Science Advisory. Wine and your heart: A science advisory for healthcare professionals from the Nutrition Committee, Council on Epidemiology and Prevention, and Council on Cardiovascular Nursing of the American Heart Association. *Stroke* 2001;32:591–94.

43 Wannamethee SG, Shaper AG. Alcohol, body weight, and weight gain in middle-aged men. *American Journal of Clinical Nutrition* 2003;77:1312-17.

44 Fischer-Posovszky P, Kukulus V, Tews D, et al. Resveratrol regulates human adipocyte number and function in a Sirt1-dependent manner. *American Journal of Clinical Nutrition* 2010;92:5–15.

45 Pal S, Naissides M, Mamo J. Polyphenolics and fat absorption. *International Journal of Obesity and Related Metabolic Disorders* 2004;28:324–26.

46 Mutlu EA, Gillevet PM, Rangwala H, et al. Colonic microbiome is altered in alcoholism. *American Journal of Physiology: Gastrointestinal and Liver Physiology* 2012;302:G966–G978.

47 Mutlu E, Keshavarzian A, Engen P, Forsyth CB, Sikaroodi M, Gillevet P. Intestinal dysbiosis: a possible mechanism of alcohol-induced endotoxemia and alcoholic steatohepatitis in rats. *Alcoholism, Clinical and Experimental Research* 2009;33:1836–46.

48 Clemente-Postigo M, Queipo-Ortuno MI, Boto-Ordonez M, et al. Effect of acute and chronic red wine consumption on lipopolysaccharide concentrations. *American Journal of Clinical Nutrition* 2013;97:1053–61.

49 Riserus U, Ingelsson E. Alcohol intake, insulin resistance, and abdominal obesity in elderly men. *Obesity* 2007;15:1766–73.

50 Andreasen AS, Larsen N, Pedersen-Skovsgaard T, et al. Effects of Lactobacillus acidophilus NCFM on insulin sensitivity and the systemic inflammatory response in human subjects. *British Journal of Nutrition* 2010;104:1831–38.

51 Delzenne NM, Neyrinck AM, Backhed F, Cani PD. Targeting gut microbiota in obesity: effects of prebiotics and probiotics. *Nature Reviews Endocrinology* 2011;7:639–46.

52 Nagpal R, Kumar A, Kumar M, Behare PV, Jain S, Yadav H. Probiotics, their health benefits and applications for developing healthier foods: a review. *FEMS Microbiology Letters* 2012;334:1–15.

53 Yadav H, Lee JH, Lloyd J, Walter P, Rane SG. Beneficial metabolic effects of a probiotic via butyrate-induced GLP-1 hormone secretion. *Journal of Biological Chemistry* 2013;288:25088–97.

54 Kang JH, Yun SI, Park MH, Park JH, Jeong SY, Park HO. Anti-obesity effect of Lactobacillus gasseri BNR17 in high-sucrose diet-induced obese mice. *PLoS One* 2013;8:e54617.

55 Savignac HM, Corona G, Mills H, et al. Prebiotic feeding elevates central brain derived neurotrophic factor, N-methyl-D-aspartate receptor subunits and D-serine. *Neurochemistry International* 2013;63:756–64.

56 Chen SC, Lin YH, Huang HP, Hsu WL, Houng JY, Huang CK. Effect of conjugated linoleic acid supplementation on weight loss and body fat composition in a Chinese population. *Nutrition* 2012;28:559–65.

57 Katz SE. *The Art of Fermentation*. White River Junction, VT: Chelsea Green Publishing, 2012.

58 naturalnews.com/045791_all_natural_yogurt_aspartame_yoplait.html

59 Dhiman TR, Satter LD, Pariza MW, Galli MP, Albright K, Tolosa MX. Conjugated linoleic acid (CLA) content of milk from cows offered diets rich in linoleic and linolenic acid. *Journal of Dairy Science* 2000;83:1016–27.

60 Mullin GE, Belkoff SM. Survey of lactose maldigestion among raw milk drinkers. *Global Advances in Health and Medicine* (In press, August 2014).

61 cdc.gov/media/releases/2014/a1210-raw-milk.html

62 medpagetoday.com/MeetingCoverage/ICAAC/41531.

63 fda.gov/Food/ResourcesForYou/consumers/ucm079516.htm.

64 Moss M. *Salt Sugar Fat: How the Food Giants Hooked Us*. New York: Random House, 2013.

65 Li F, Hullar MA, Schwarz Y, Lampe JW. Human gut bacterial communities are altered by addition of cruciferous vegetables to a controlled fruit- and vegetable-free diet. *Journal of Nutrition* 2009;139:1685–91.

Chapter 7

1 fatsecret.com/calories-nutrition/usda/oat-bran?portionid=40316&portionamount=0.250.

2 Brown L, Rosner B, Willett WW, Sacks FM. Cholesterol-lowering effects of dietary fiber: a meta-analysis. *American Journal of Clinical Nutrition* 1999;69:30–42.

3 Kwiterovich PO, Jr. The role of fiber in the treatment of hypercholesterolemia in children and adolescents. *Pediatrics* 1995;96:1005–9.

4 Bazzano LA, He J, Ogden LG, et al. Dietary fiber intake and reduced risk of coronary heart disease in US men and women: the National Health and Nutrition Examination Survey I Epidemiologic Follow-up Study. *Archives of Internal Medicine* 2003;163:1897–904.

5 Anderson JW. Whole grains and coronary heart disease: the whole kernel of truth. *American Journal of Clinical Nutrition* 2004;80:1459–60.

6 van Dam RM, Hu FB, Rosenberg L, Krishnan S, Palmer JR. Dietary calcium and magnesium, major food sources, and risk of type 2 diabetes in U.S. black women. *Diabetes Care* 2006;29:2238–43.

7 Tsikitis VL, Albina JE, Reichner JS. Beta-glucan affects leukocyte navigation in a complex chemotactic gradient. *Surgery* 2004;136:384–89.

8 Suzuki R, Rylander-Rudqvist T, Ye W, Saji S, Adlercreutz H, Wolk A. Dietary fiber intake and risk of postmenopausal breast cancer defined by estrogen and progesterone receptor status–a prospective cohort study among Swedish women. *International Journal of Cancer* 2008;122:403–12.

9 Tabak C, Wijga AH, de Meer G, Janssen NA, Brunekreef B, Smit HA. Diet and asthma in Dutch school children (ISAAC-2). *Thorax* 2006;61:1048–53.

10 Al-Waili NS, Salom K, Butler G, Al Ghamdi AA. Honey and microbial infections: a review supporting the use of honey for microbial control. *Journal of Medicinal Food* 2011;14:1079–96.

11   Othmán NH. Honey and cancer: sustainable inverse relationship particularly for developing nations—a review. *Evidence-based Complementary and Alternative Medicine* 2012;2012:410406.

12   Ansorge S, Reinhold D, Lendeckel U. Propolis and some of its constituents down-regulate DNA synthesis and inflammatory cytokine production but induce TGF-beta1 production of human immune cells. *Zeitschrift fur Naturforschung Section C: Biosciences* 2003;58:580–89.

13   Al-Waili NS. Identification of nitric oxide metabolites in various honeys: effects of intravenous honey on plasma and urinary nitric oxide metabolites concentrations. *Journal of Medicinal Food* 2003;6:359–64.

14   Wong D, Alandejani T, Javer AR. Evaluation of Manuka honey in the management of allergic fungal rhinosinusitis. *Journal of Otolaryngology, Head & Neck Surgery* 2011;40:E19–E21.

15   Israili ZH. Antimicrobial properties of honey. *American Journal of Therapeutics* 2013;21:304–23.

16   Kapoor S. Systemic benefits and potential uses of tualang honey in addition to its beneficial effects on postmenopausal bone structure. *Clinics* 2012;67:1345.

17   Pecanac M, Janjic Z, Komarcevic A, Pajic M, Dobanovacki D, Miskovic SS. Burns treatment in ancient times. *Medicinski pregled* 2013;66:263–67.

18   Fashner J, Ericson K, Werner S. Treatment of the common cold in children and adults. *American Family Physician* 2012;86:153–59.

19   Erejuwa OO, Sulaiman SA, Wahab MS. Honey—a novel antidiabetic agent. *International Journal of Biological Sciences* 2012;8:913–34.

20   O'Meara S, Al-Kurdi D, Ologun Y, Ovington LG, Martyn-St James M, Richardson R. Antibiotics and antiseptics for venous leg ulcers. *Cochrane Database of Systematic Reviews* 2014;1:CD003557.

21   Burlando B, Cornara L. Honey in dermatology and skin care: a review. *Journal of Cosmetic Dermatology* 2013;12:306–13.

22   Majtan J. Honey: An immunomodulator in wound healing. *Wound Repair and Regeneration* 2014;22:187–92.

23   Sabater-Molina M, Larque E, Torrella F, Zamora S. Dietary fructooligosaccharides and potential benefits on health. *Journal of Physiology and Biochemistry* 2009;65:315–28.

24   Gautam M, Saha S, Bani S, et al. Immunomodulatory activity of Asparagus racemosus on systemic Th1/Th2 immunity: implications for immunoadjuvant potential. *Journal of Ethnopharmacology* 2009;121:241–47.

25   Shao Y, Chin CK, Ho CT, Ma W, Garrison SA, Huang MT. Anti-tumor activity of the crude saponins obtained from asparagus. *Cancer Letters* 1996;104:31–36.

26   Negi JS, Singh P, Joshi GP, Rawat MS, Bisht VK. Chemical constituents of Asparagus. *Pharmacognosy Reviews* 2010;4:215–20.

27   Kumar MC, Udupa AL, Sammodavardhana K, Rathnakar UP, Shvetha U, Kodancha GP. Acute toxicity and diuretic studies of the roots of Asparagus racemosus Willd in rats. *West Indian Medical Journal* 2010;59:3–6.

28   Sun T, Powers JR, Tang J. Enzyme-catalyzed change of antioxidants content and antioxidant activity of asparagus juice. *Journal of Agricultural and Food Chemistry* 2007;55:56–60.

29   diabetes-guide.org/american-diabetes-association-diet.htm.

30   heart.org/HEARTORG/GettingHealthy/NutritionCenter/HealthyCooking/Bean-Benefits_UCM_430105_Article.jsp.

31   centralbean.com/beans-and-your-health/beans-and-cancer/.

32   Sarmento A, Barros L, Fernandes A, Carvalho AM, Ferreira IC. Valorisation of traditional foods: nutritional and bioactive properties of Cicer arietinum L. and Lathyrus sativus L. pulses. *Journal of the Science of Food and Agriculture* 2014 Apr 18. [Epub ahead of print]

33   nutritiondata.self.com/facts/legumes-and-legume-products/4284/2.

34   Riccioni G, Sblendorio V, Gemello E, et al. Dietary fibers and cardiometabolic diseases. *International Journal of Molecular Sciences* 2012;13:1524–40.

35   Hallikainen M, Halonen J, Konttinen J, et al. Diet and cardiovascular health in asymptomatic normo- and mildly-to-moderately hypercholesterolemic participants—baseline data from the BLOOD FLOW intervention study. *Nutrition & Metabolism* 2013;10:62.

36   Paper-behind-the-green-coffee-bean-diet-craze-retracted, washingtonpost.com/news/to-your-health/wp/2014/10/22/researchers-retract-bogus-dr-oz-touted-study-on-green-coffee-bean-weight-loss-pills/

37   Espinosa-Alonso LG, Lygin A, Widholm JM, Valverde ME, Paredes-Lopez O. Polyphenols in wild and weedy Mexican common beans (Phaseolus vulgaris L.). *Journal of Agricultural and Food Chemistry* 2006;54:4436–44.

38   Zhang C, Monk JM, Lu JT, et al. Cooked navy and black bean diets improve biomarkers of colon health and reduce inflammation during colitis. *British Journal of Nutrition* 2014:1–15.

39 Preuss HG. Bean amylase inhibitor and other carbohydrate absorption blockers: effects on diabesity and general health. *Journal of the American College of Nutrition* 2009;28:266–76.

40 Tonstad S, Malik N, Haddad E. A high-fibre bean-rich diet versus a low-carbohydrate diet for obesity. *Journal of Human Nutrition and Dietetics* 2014;27 Suppl 2:109–16.

41 Hermsdorff HH, Zulet MA, Abete I, Martinez JA. A legume-based hypocaloric diet reduces proinflammatory status and improves metabolic features in overweight/obese subjects. *European Journal of Nutrition* 2011;50:61–69.

42 Queiroz Kda S, de Oliveira AC, Helbig E, Reis SM, Carraro F. Soaking the common bean in a domestic preparation reduced the contents of raffinose-type oligosaccharides but did not interfere with nutritive value. *Journal of Nutritional Science and Vitaminology* 2002;48:283–89.

43 Higdon JV, Delage B, Williams DE, Dashwood RH. Cruciferous vegetables and human cancer risk: epidemiologic evidence and mechanistic basis. *Pharmacological Research* 2007;55:224–36.

44 Kahlon TS, Chiu MC, Chapman MH. Steam cooking significantly improves in vitro bile acid binding of collard greens, kale, mustard greens, broccoli, green bell pepper, and cabbage. *Nutrition Research* 2008;28:351–57.

45 Cook NR, Appel LJ, Whelton PK. Lower levels of sodium intake and reduced cardiovascular risk. *Circulation* 2014;129:981–89.

46 Whelton PK, He J. Health effects of sodium and potassium in humans. *Current Opinion in Lipidology* 2014;25:75–79.

47 consumer.healthday.com/public-health-information-30/centers-for-disease-control-news-120/cdc-salt-guidelines-too-low-for-good-health-study-suggests-686408.html.

48 Zhu H, Pollock NK, Kotak I, et al. Dietary sodium, adiposity, and inflammation in healthy adolescents. *Pediatrics* 2014;133:e635–e642.

49 Kleinewietfeld M, Manzel A, Titze J, et al. Sodium chloride drives autoimmune disease by the induction of pathogenic TH17 cells. *Nature* 2013;496:518–22.

50 Wu C, Yosef N, Thalhamer T, et al. Induction of pathogenic TH17 cells by inducible salt-sensing kinase SGK1. *Nature* 2013;496:513–17.

51 Rodrigues Telini LS, de Carvalho Beduschi G, Caramori JC, Castro JH, Martin LC, Barretti P. Effect of dietary sodium restriction on body water, blood pressure, and inflammation in hemodialysis patients: a prospective randomized controlled study. *International Urology and Nephrology* 2014;46:91–97.

52 Kokubo Y, Iso H, Ishihara J, et al. Association of dietary intake of soy, beans, and isoflavones with risk of cerebral and myocardial infarctions in Japanese populations: the Japan Public Health Center-based (JPHC) study cohort I. *Circulation* 2007;116:2553–62.

53 Lee M, Chae S, Cha Y, Park Y. Supplementation of Korean fermented soy paste doenjang reduces visceral fat in overweight subjects with mutant uncoupling protein-1 allele. *Nutrition Research* 2012;32:8–14.

54 Tai MW, Sweet BV. Nattokinase for prevention of thrombosis. *American Journal of Health-System Pharmacy* 2006;63:1121–23.

55 Jungbauer A, Medjakovic S. Phytoestrogens and the metabolic syndrome. *Journal of Steroid Biochemistry and Molecular Biology* 2013;139:277–89.

56 Torre-Villalvazo I, Tovar AR, Ramos-Barragan VE, Cerbon-Cervantes MA, Torres N. Soy protein ameliorates metabolic abnormalities in liver and adipose tissue of rats fed a high fat diet. *Journal of Nutrition* 2008;138:462–68.

57 Lukaszuk JM, Luebbers P, Gordon BA. Preliminary study: soy milk as effective as skim milk in promoting weight loss. *Journal of the American Dietetic Association* 2007;107:1811–14.

58 Fabian E, Elmadfa I. Influence of daily consumption of probiotic and conventional yoghurt on the plasma lipid profile in young healthy women. *Annals of Nutrition & Metabolism* 2006;50:387–93.

59 Cheng S, Lyytikainen A, Kroger H, et al. Effects of calcium, dairy product, and vitamin D supplementation on bone mass accrual and body composition in 10-12-y-old girls: a 2-y randomized trial. *American Journal of Clinical Nutrition* 2005;82:1115–26; quiz 47–48.

60 Donovan SM, Shamir R. Introduction to the Yogurt in Nutrition Initiative and the First Global Summit on the Health Effects of Yogurt. *American Journal of Clinical Nutrition* 2014;99(Suppl):1209S–1211S.

61 Jones K. Probiotics: preventing antibiotic-associated diarrhea. *Journal for Specialists in Pediatric Nursing* 2010;15:160–62.

62 Guyonnet D, Woodcock A, Stefani B, Trevisan C, Hall C. Fermented milk containing Bifidobacterium lactis DN-173 010 improved self-reported digestive comfort amongst a general population of adults. A randomized, open-label, controlled, pilot study. *Journal of Digestive Diseases* 2009;10:61–70.

63 Caglar E, Kargul B, Tanboga I. Bacteriotherapy and probiotics' role on oral health. *Oral Diseases* 2005;11:131–37.

64 Pala V, Sieri S, Berrino F, et al. Yogurt consumption and risk of colorectal cancer in the Italian European prospective investigation into cancer and nutrition cohort. *International Journal of Cancer* 2011;129:2712–19.

65 biomedcentral.com/1741-7015/12/215

66 O'Connor LM, Lentjes MA, Luben RN, Khaw KT, Wareham NJ, Forouhi NG. Dietary dairy product intake and incident type 2 diabetes: a prospective study using dietary data from a 7-day food diary. *Diabetologia* 2014;57:909–17.

67 Rebello CJ, Liu AG, Greenway FL, Dhurandhar NV. Dietary strategies to increase satiety. *Advances in Food and Nutrition Research* 2013;69:105–82.

68 Chung KH, Shin KO, Yoon JA, Choi KS. Study on the obesity and nutrition status of housewives in Seoul and Kyunggi area. *Nutrition Research and Practice* 2011;5:140–49.

69 Chang BJ, Park SU, Jang YS, et al. Effect of functional yogurt NY-YP901 in improving the trait of metabolic syndrome. *European Journal of Clinical Nutrition* 2011;65:1250–55.

70 Diepvens K, Soenen S, Steijns J, Arnold M, Westerterp-Plantenga M. Long-term effects of consumption of a novel fat emulsion in relation to body-weight management. *International Journal of Obesity* 2007;31:942–49.

71 Zemel MB, Richards J, Mathis S, Milstead A, Gebhardt L, Silva E. Dairy augmentation of total and central fat loss in obese subjects. *International Journal of Obesity* 2005;29:391–97.

72 Martinez-Gonzalez MA, Sayon-Orea C, Ruiz-Canela M, de la Fuente C, Gea A, Bes-Rastrollo M. Yogurt consumption, weight change and risk of overweight/obesity: the SUN cohort study. *Nutrition, Metabolism, and Cardiovascular Diseases*: NMCD November 2014, vol. 24, issue 11:1189–96.

73 Carlsson M, Gustafson Y, Haglin L, Eriksson S. The feasibility of serving liquid yoghurt supplemented with probiotic bacteria, Lactobacillus rhamnosus LB 21, and Lactococcus lactis L1A–a pilot study among old people with dementia in a residential care facility. *Journal of Nutrition, Health & Aging* 2009;13:813–19.

74 Mason C, Xiao L, Imayama I, et al. Vitamin D$_3$ supplementation during weight loss: a double-blind randomized controlled trial. *American Journal of Clinical Nutrition* 2014;99:1015–25.

75 Anderson GH, Luhovyy B, Akhavan T, Panahi S. Milk proteins in the regulation of body weight, satiety, food intake and glycemia. *Nestlé Nutrition Workshop Series Paediatric Programme* 2011;67:147–59.

76 Ludwig DS, Willett WC. Three daily servings of reduced-fat milk: an evidence-based recommendation? *JAMA Pediatrics* 2013;167:788–89.

77 Martinez-Gonzalez MA et al. Yogurt consumption, weight change and risk of overweight/obesity; Louie JC, Flood VM, Hector DJ, Rangan AM, Gill TP. Dairy consumption and overweight and obesity: a systematic review of prospective cohort studies. *Obesity Reviews*: an official journal of the International Association for the Study of Obesity 2011;12:e582–592.

78 aboutyogurt.com/Live-Culture.

79 Patterson E, Larsson SC, Wolk A, Akesson A. Association between dairy food consumption and risk of myocardial infarction in women differs by type of dairy food. *Journal of Nutrition* 2013;143:74–79.

80 Soedamah-Muthu SS, Ding EL, Al-Delaimy WK, et al. Milk and dairy consumption and incidence of cardiovascular diseases and all-cause mortality: dose-response meta-analysis of prospective cohort studies. *American Journal of Clinical Nutrition* 2011;93:158–71.

81 Dalmeijer GW, Struijk EA, van der Schouw YT, et al. Dairy intake and coronary heart disease or stroke–a population-based cohort study. *International Journal of Cardiology* 2013;167:925–29.

82 aboutyogurt.com/Live-Culture.

83 Lopitz-Otsoa F, Rementeria A, Elguezabal N, Garaizar J. Kefir: a symbiotic yeasts-bacteria community with alleged healthy capabilities. *Revista iberoamericana de micologia* 2006;23:67–74.

84 Margulis L, Sagan D, Thomas L. *Microcosmos: Four Billion Years of Microbial Evolution.* Berkeley: University of California Press, 1997.

85 de Oliveira Leite AM, Miguel MA, Peixoto RS, Rosado AS, Silva JT, Paschoalin VM. Microbiological, technological and therapeutic properties of kefir: a natural probiotic beverage. *Brazilian Journal of Microbiology* 2013;44:341–49.

86 Kabeerdoss J, Devi RS, Mary RR, et al. Effect of yoghurt containing Bifidobacterium lactis Bb12(R) on faecal excretion of secretory immunoglobulin A and human beta-defensin 2 in healthy adult volunteers. *Nutrition Journal* 2011;10:138.

87 Grishina A, Kulikova I, Alieva L, Dodson A, Rowland I, Jin J. Antigenotoxic effect of kefir and ayran supernatants on fecal water-induced DNA damage in human colon cells. *Nutrition and Cancer* 2011; 63:73–79.

88 Chen YP, Lee TY, Hong WS, Hsieh HH, Chen MJ. Effects of Lactobacillus kefiranofaciens M1 isolated from kefir grains on enterohemorrhagic Escherichia coli infection using mouse and intestinal cell models. *Journal of Dairy Science* 2013;96:7467–77.

89 Hertzler SR, Clancy SM. Kefir improves lactose digestion and tolerance in adults with lactose maldigestion. *Journal of the American Dietetic Association* 2003;103:582–87.

90 Furuno T, Nakanishi M. Kefiran suppresses antigen-induced mast cell activation. *Biological & Pharmaceutical Bulletin* 2012;35:178–83.

91 Liu JR, Wang SY, Lin YY, Lin CW. Antitumor activity of milk kefir and soy milk kefir in tumor-bearing mice. *Nutrition and Cancer* 2002;44:183–87.

92 Ishida Y, Nakamura F, Kanzato H, et al. Effect of milk fermented with Lactobacillus acidophilus strain L-92 on symptoms of Japanese cedar pollen allergy: a randomized placebo-controlled trial. *Bioscience, Biotechnology, and Biochemistry* 2005;69:1652–60.

93 Anderson JW, Gilliland SE. Effect of fermented milk (yogurt) containing Lactobacillus acidophilus L1 on serum cholesterol in hypercholesterolemic humans. *Journal of the American College of Nutrition* 1999;18:43–50.

94 Guzel-Seydim ZB, Kok-Tas T, Greene AK, Seydim AC. Review: functional properties of kefir. *Critical Reviews in Food Science and Nutrition* 2011;51:261–68.

95 Ho JN, Choi JW, Lim WC, Kim MK, Lee IY, Cho HY. Kefir inhibits 3T3-L1 adipocyte differentiation through down-regulation of adipogenic transcription factor expression. *Journal of the Science of Food and Agriculture* 2012;93:485–90.

96 Park KY, Jeong JK, Lee YE, Daily JW, 3rd. Health benefits of kimchi (Korean fermented vegetables) as a probiotic food. *Journal of Medicinal Food* 2014;17:6–20.

97 Yoon JY, Kim SH, Jung KO, Park KY. Antiobesity effect of baek-kimchi (whitish baechu kimchi) in rats fed high fat diet. *Journal of Food Science and Nutrition* 2004;9:259–64.

98 Choi SH, Suh BS, Kozukue E, Kozukue N, Levin CE, Friedman M. Analysis of the contents of pungent compounds in fresh Korean red peppers and in pepper-containing foods. *Journal of Agricultural and Food Chemistry* 2006;54:9024–31.

99 Ahn SJ. The effect of kimchi powder supplement on the body weight reduction of obese adult women [MS thesis]. Busan, Korea: Pusan National University, 2007.

100 Kim EK, An SY, Lee MS, et al. Fermented kimchi reduces body weight and improves metabolic parameters in overweight and obese patients. *Nutrition Research* 2011;31:436–43.

101 Kwon M J C, Song YS, Song YO. Daily kimchi consumption and its hypolipidemic effect in middle-aged men. *Journal of the Korean Society of Food Science and Nutrition* 1998;28:1144–50.

102 Park K. The nutritional evaluation, and antimutagenic and anticancer effects of kimchi. *Journal of the Korean Society of Food Science and Nutrition* 1995;24:169–82.

103 Kim KH, Park KY. Effects of kimchi extracts on production of nitric oxide by activated macrophages, transforming growth factor β1 of tumor cells and interleukin-6 in splenocytes. *Journal of Food Science and Nutrition* 2001;6:126–32.

104 Ngo ST, Li MS. Curcumin binds to Abeta1-40 peptides and fibrils stronger than ibuprofen and naproxen. *Journal of Physical Chemistry B* 2012;116:10165–75.

105 Asher GN, Spelman K. Clinical utility of curcumin extract. *Alternative Therapies in Health and Medicine* 2013;19:20–22.

106 Ginter E, Simko V. Plant polyphenols in prevention of heart disease. *Bratislavske lekarske listy* 2012;113:476–80.

107 Bereswill S, Munoz M, Fischer A, et al. Anti-inflammatory effects of resveratrol, curcumin and simvastatin in acute small intestinal inflammation. *PLoS One* 2010;5:e15099.

108 Ejaz A, Wu D, Kwan P, Meydani M. Curcumin inhibits adipogenesis in 3T3-L1 adipocytes and angiogenesis and obesity in $C5_{7/8}L$ mice. *Journal of Nutrition* 2009;139:919–25.

109 Yu Y, Hu SK, Yan H. [The study of insulin resistance and leptin resistance on the model of simplicity obesity rats by curcumin]. *Zhonghua yu fang yi xue za zhi* [Chinese Journal of Preventive Medicine] 2008;42:818–22.

110 Weisberg SP, Leibel R, Tortoriello DV. Dietary curcumin significantly improves obesity-associated inflammation and diabetes in mouse models of diabesity. *Endocrinology* 2008;149:3549–58.

111 Cao H. Adipocytokines in obesity and metabolic disease. *Journal of Endocrinology* 2014;220:T47–T59.

112 Ouchi N, Parker JL, Lugus JJ, Walsh K. Adipokines in inflammation and metabolic disease. *Nature Reviews Immunology* 2011;11:8597.

113 Kim CY, Kim KH. Curcumin prevents leptin-induced tight junction dysfunction in intestinal Caco-2 BBe cells. *Journal of Nutritional Biochemistry* 2014;25:26–35.

114 Mangge H, Summers K, Almer G, et al. Antioxidant food supplements and obesity-related inflammation. *Current Medicinal Chemistry* 2013;20:2330–37.

115 Jang EM, Choi MS, Jung UJ, et al. Beneficial effects of curcumin on hyperlipidemia and insulin resistance in high-fat-fed hamsters. *Metabolism: Clinical and Experimental* 2008;57:1576–83.

116 Tang Y, Chen A. Curcumin eliminates the effect of advanced glycation end-products (AGEs) on the divergent regulation of gene expression of receptors of AGEs by interrupting leptin signaling. *Laboratory Investigation* 2014;94:503–16.

117 Lee YK, Lee WS, Hwang JT, Kwon DY, Surh YJ, Park OJ. Curcumin exerts antidifferentiation effect through AMPKalpha-PPAR-gamma in 3T3-L1 adipocytes and antiproliferatory effect through AMPKalpha-COX-2 in cancer cells. *Journal of Agricultural and Food Chemistry* 2009;57:305–10.

118 Dagon Y, Avraham Y, Berry EM. AMPK activation regulates apoptosis, adipogenesis, and lipolysis by eIF2alpha in adipocytes. *Biochemical and Biophysical Research Communications* 2006;340:43–47.

119 Al-Suhaimi EA, Al-Riziza NA, Al-Essa RA. Physiological and therapeutical roles of ginger and turmeric on endocrine functions. *American Journal of Chinese Medicine* 2011;39:215–31.

120 Jang EM, Choi MS, Jung UJ, et al. Beneficial effects of curcumin on hyperlipidemia and insulin resistance in high-fat-fed hamsters. *Metabolism: Clinical and Experimental* 2008;57:1576–83.

121 Shin SK, Ha TY, McGregor RA, Choi MS. Long-term curcumin administration protects against atherosclerosis via hepatic regulation of lipoprotein cholesterol metabolism. *Molecular Nutrition & Food Research* 2011;55:1829–40.

122 Soni KB, Kuttan R. Effect of oral curcumin administration on serum peroxides and cholesterol levels in human volunteers. *Indian Journal of Physiology and Pharmacology* 1992;36:273–75.

123 Ibid.

124 Jaruszewski KM, Curran GL, Swaminathan SK, et al. Multimodal nanoprobes to target cerebrovascular amyloid in Alzheimer's disease brain. *Biomaterials* 2014;35:1967–76.

125 vinegarworkswonders.com/history.asp.

126 Johnston CS, Gaas CA. Vinegar: medicinal uses and antiglycemic effect. *Medscape General Medicine* 2006;8:61.

127 Johnston CS, Kim CM, Buller AJ. Vinegar improves insulin sensitivity to a high-carbohydrate meal in subjects with insulin resistance or type 2 diabetes. *Diabetes Care* 2004;27:281–82.

128 Gambon DL, Brand HS, Veerman EC. [Unhealthy weight loss. Erosion by apple cider vinegar]. *Nederlands tijdschrift voor tandheelkunde* 2012;119:589–91.

129 Tong LT, Katakura Y, Kawamura S, et al. Effects of Kurozu concentrated liquid on adipocyte size in rats. *Lipids in Health and Disease* 2010;9:134.

130 Kondo T, Kishi M, Fushimi T, Ugajin S, Kaga T. Vinegar intake reduces body weight, body fat mass, and serum triglyceride levels in obese Japanese subjects. *Bioscience, Biotechnology, and Biochemistry* 2009;73:1837–43.

131 Mushref MA, Srinivasan S. Effect of high fat-diet and obesity on gastrointestinal motility. *Annals of Translational Medicine* 2013;1:14.

132 Lee JH, Cho HD, Jeong JH, et al. New vinegar produced by tomato suppresses adipocyte differentiation and fat accumulation in 3T3-L1 cells and obese rat model. *Food Chemistry* 2013;141:3241–49.

133 Kondo T, Kishi M, Fushimi T, Kaga T. Acetic acid upregulates the expression of genes for fatty acid oxidation enzymes in liver to suppress body fat accumulation. *Journal of Agricultural and Food Chemistry* 2009;57:5982–86.

Chapter 8

1 webmd.com/diet/grapefruit-diet.

2 Ayyad C, Andersen T. Long-term efficacy of dietary treatment of obesity: a systematic review of studies published between 1931 and 1999. *Obesity Reviews* 2000;1:113–19.

3 Anderson JW, Konz EC, Frederich RC, Wood CL. Long-term weight-loss maintenance: a meta-analysis of US studies. *American Journal of Clinical Nutrition* 2001;74:579–84.

4 Lagerros YT, Rossner S. Obesity management: what brings success? *Therapeutic Advances in Gastroenterology* 2013;6:77–88.

5 Wing RR, Lang W, Wadden TA, et al. Benefits of modest weight loss in improving cardiovascular risk factors in overweight and obese individuals with type 2 diabetes. *Diabetes Care* 2011;34:1481–86.

6   Willett WC, Sacks F, Trichopoulou A, et al. Mediterranean diet pyramid: a cultural model for healthy eating. *American Journal of Clinical Nutrition* 1995;61:1402S–1406S.

7   Estruch R, Ros E, Martinez-Gonzalez MA. Mediterranean diet for primary prevention of cardiovascular disease. *New England Journal of Medicine* 2013;369:676–77.

8   Estruch R, Ros E, Salas-Salvado J, et al. Primary prevention of cardiovascular disease with a Mediterranean diet. *New England Journal of Medicine* 2013;368:1279–90.

9   Estruch R, Martinez-Gonzalez MA, Corella D, et al. Effects of a Mediterranean-style diet on cardiovascular risk factors: a randomized trial. *Annals of Internal Medicine* 2006;145:1–11.

10 Estruch R, Ros E, Martinez-Gonzalez MA. Mediterranean diet for primary prevention of cardiovascular disease. *New England Journal of Medicine* 2013;369:676–77.

11 Rees K, Hartley L, Flowers N, et al. 'Mediterranean' dietary pattern for the primary prevention of cardiovascular disease. *Cochrane Database of Systematic Reviews* 2013;8:CD009825.

12 Perona JS, Cabello-Moruno R, Ruiz-Gutierrez V. The role of virgin olive oil components in the modulation of endothelial function. *Journal of Nutritional Biochemistry* 2006;17:429–45.

13 Salas-Salvado J, Bullo M, Estruch R, et al. Prevention of diabetes with Mediterranean diets: a subgroup analysis of a randomized trial. *Annals of Internal Medicine* 2014;160:1–10.

14 Andersen CJ, Fernandez ML. Dietary strategies to reduce metabolic syndrome. *Reviews in Endocrine & Metabolic Disorders* 2013;14:241–54.

15 Richard C, Royer MM, Couture P, et al. Effect of the Mediterranean diet on plasma adipokine concentrations in men with metabolic syndrome. *Metabolism: Clinical and Experimental* 2013;62:1803–10.

16 Richard C, Couture P, Desroches S, Lamarche B. Effect of the Mediterranean diet with and without weight loss on markers of inflammation in men with metabolic syndrome. *Obesity* 2013;21:51–57.

17 Gotsis E, Anagnostis P, Mariolis A, Vlachou A, Katsiki N, Karagiannis A. Health benefits of the Mediterranean diet: an update of research over the last 5 years. *Angiology* 2014 Apr 27. [Epub ahead of print]

18 Funtikova AN, Benitez-Arciniega AA, Gomez SF, Fito M, Elosua R, Schroder H. Mediterranean diet impact on changes in abdominal fat and 10-year incidence of abdominal obesity in a Spanish population. *British Journal of Nutrition* 2014;111:1481–87.

19 Steinle N CS, Ryan K, Fraser C, Shuldiner A, Mongodin E. Increased gut microbiome diversity following a high fiber Mediterranean style diet. *FASEB Journal* 2013;27:1056.3.

20 Gotsis E, Anagnostis P, Mariolis A, Vlachou A, Katsiki N, Karagiannis A. Health benefits of the Mediterranean diet: an update of research over the last 5 years. *Angiology* 2014 Apr 27. [Epub ahead of print]

21 Bourlioux P. [Current view on gut microbiota]. *Annales pharmaceutiques françaises* 2014;72:15–21.

22 Olveira C, Olveira G, Espildora F, et al. Mediterranean diet is associated on symptoms of depression and anxiety in patients with bronchiectasis. *General Hospital Psychiatry* 2014;36:277–83.

23 Sanchez-Villegas A, Martinez-Gonzalez MA, Estruch R, et al. Mediterranean dietary pattern and depression: the PREDIMED randomized trial. *BMC Medicine* 2013;11:208.

24 Caracciolo B, Xu W, Collins S, Fratiglioni L. Cognitive decline, dietary factors and gut-brain interactions. *Mechanisms of Ageing and Development* 2014;136–137:59–69.

25 Otaegui-Arrazola A, Amiano P, Elbusto A, Urdaneta E, Martinez-Lage P. Diet, cognition, and Alzheimer's disease: food for thought. *European Journal of Nutrition* 2014;53:1–23.

26 Goulet J, Lamarche B, Nadeau G, Lemieux S. Effect of a nutritional intervention promoting the Mediterranean food pattern on plasma lipids, lipoproteins and body weight in healthy French-Canadian women. *Atherosclerosis* 2003;170:115–24.

27 Perez-Guisado J, Munoz-Serrano A, Alonso-Moraga A. Spanish ketogenic Mediterranean diet: a healthy cardiovascular diet for weight loss. *Nutrition Journal* 2008;7:30.

28 Paoli A, Bianco A, Grimaldi KA, Lodi A, Bosco G. Long term successful weight loss with a combination biphasic ketogenic Mediterranean diet and Mediterranean diet maintenance protocol. *Nutrients* 2013;5:5205–17.

29 Kanerva N, Loo BM, Eriksson JG, et al. Associations of the Baltic Sea diet with obesity-related markers of inflammation. *Annals of Medicine* 2014;46:90–96.

30 Nova E, Baccan GC, Veses A, Zapatera B, Marcos A. Potential health benefits of moderate alcohol consumption: current perspectives in research. *Proceedings of the Nutrition Society* 2012;71:307–15.

31 Kanerva N, Kaartinen NE, Schwab U, Lahti-Koski M, Mannisto S. Adherence to the Baltic Sea diet consumed in the Nordic countries is associated with lower abdominal obesity. *British Journal of Nutrition* 2013;109:520–28.

32 Ibid.

33 Ibid.

34 Rehm J, Shield K. Alcohol consumption. In: Stewart BW, Wild CB, eds. World Cancer Report 2014. Lyon, France: International Agency for Research on Cancer; 2014. worldcat.org/oclc/636655624/editions ?editionsView=true&referer=di

35 ncbi.nlm.nih.gov/pubmed/25505228

36 Kanerva N, Kaartinen NE, Schwab U, Lahti-Koski M, Mannisto S. The Baltic Sea Diet Score: a tool for assessing healthy eating in Nordic countries. *Public Health Nutrition* 2013:1-9.

37 Ali RE, Rattan SI. Curcumin's biphasic hormetic response on proteasome activity and heat-shock protein synthesis in human keratinocytes. *Annals of the New York Academy of Sciences* 2006;1067:394-99.

38 Prickett CD, Lister E, Collins M, et al. Alcohol: friend or foe? Alcoholic beverage hormesis for cataract and atherosclerosis is related to plasma antioxidant activity. *Nonlinearity in Biology, Toxicology, Medicine* 2004;2:353-70.

39 Mullin GE. Search for the optimal diet. *Nutrition in Clinical Practice* 2010;25:581-84.

40 Mozaffarian D, Hao T, Rimm EB, Willett WC, Hu FB. Changes in diet and lifestyle and long-term weight gain in women and men. *New England Journal of Medicine* 2011;364:2392-404.

41 Ibid.

42 oldwayspt.org/about-us/our-mission, #78494.

43 Oyebode O, Gordon-Dseagu V, Walker A, Mindell JS. Fruit and vegetable consumption and all-cause, cancer and CVD mortality: analysis of Health Survey for England data. *Journal of Epidemiology and Community Health* 2014;68:856-62.

44 Wise J. The health benefits of vegetables and fruit rise with consumption, finds study. *BMJ* 2014;348:g2434.

45 Holt SH, Miller JC, Petocz P, Farmakalidis E. A satiety index of common foods. *European Journal of Clinical Nutrition* 1995;49:675-90.

46 Langholf V. *Medical Theories in Hippocrates: Early Texts and the "Epidemics."* Berlin; New York: W. de Gruyter, 1990.

47 Sinclair TR SC. *Bread, Beer and the Seeds of Change: Agriculture's Imprint on World History* Wallingford, UK: CABI; 2010.

48 Larsson SC, Giovannucci E, Wolk A. Folate and risk of breast cancer: a meta-analysis. *Journal of the National Cancer Institute* 2007;99:64-76.

49 Zhang SM, Hankinson SE, Hunter DJ, Giovannucci EL, Colditz GA, Willett WC. Folate intake and risk of breast cancer characterized by hormone receptor status. *Cancer Epidemiology, Biomarkers & Prevention* 2005;14:2004-8.

50 Hamajima N, Hirose K, Tajima K, et al. Alcohol, tobacco and breast cancer–collaborative reanalysis of individual data from 53 epidemiological studies, including 58,515 women with breast cancer and 95,067 women without the disease. *British Journal of Cancer* 2002;87:1234-45.

51 Kuijer RG, Boyce JA. Chocolate cake. Guilt or celebration? Associations with healthy eating attitudes, perceived behavioural control, intentions and weight-loss. *Appetite* 2014;74:48-54.

52 Mullin GE, Swift KM. *The Inside Tract.* New York: Rodale, 2011.

Chapter 9

1 umm.edu/health/medical/altmed/supplement/omega6-fatty-acids

2 Matsumoto R, Tu NP, Haruta S, Kawano M, Takeuchi I. Polychlorinated biphenyl (PCB) concentrations and congener composition in masu salmon from Japan: a study of all 209 PCB congeners by high-resolution gas chromatography/high-resolution mass spectrometry (HRGC/HRMS). *Marine Pollution Bulletin* 2014;85:549-57.

3 Zacs D, Rjabova J, Bartkevics V. Occurrence of brominated persistent organic pollutants (PBDD/DFs, PXDD/DFs, and PBDEs) in Baltic wild salmon (Salmo salar) and correlation with PCDD/DFs and PCBs. *Environmental Science & Technology* 2013;47:9478-86.

4 Perlmutter D. *Grain Brain.* New York: Little, Brown and Co., 2013.

5 Fan YY, Ran Q, Toyokuni S, et al. Dietary fish oil promotes colonic apoptosis and mitochondrial proton leak in oxidatively stressed mice. *Cancer Prevention Research* 2011;4:1267-74.

6 Ramel A, Parra D, Martinez JA, Kiely M, Thorsdottir I. Effects of seafood consumption and weight loss on fasting leptin and ghrelin concentrations in overweight and obese European young adults. *European Journal of Nutrition* 2009;48:107-14.

7   Ramel A, Martinez JA, Kiely M, Bandarra NM, Thorsdottir I. Effects of weight loss and seafood consumption on inflammation parameters in young, overweight and obese European men and women during 8 weeks of energy restriction. *European Journal of Clinical Nutrition* 2010;64:987–93.

8   Thorsdottir I, Birgisdottir B, Kiely M, Martinez J, Bandarra N. Fish consumption among young overweight European adults and compliance to varying seafood content in four weight loss intervention diets. *Public Health Nutrition* 2009;12:592–98.

9   Poulsen SK, Due A, Jordy AB, et al. Health effect of the New Nordic Diet in adults with increased waist circumference: a 6-month randomized controlled trial. *American Journal of Clinical Nutrition* 2014;99:35–45.

10   Ramel A, Jonsdottir MT, Thorsdottir I. Consumption of cod and weight loss in young overweight and obese adults on an energy reduced diet for 8 weeks. *Nutrition, Metabolism, and Cardiovascular Diseases* 2009;19:690–96.

11   Ibid.

12   nrdc.org/health/effects/mercury/guide.asp.

13   Ibid.

14   seafoodwatch.org/cr/cr_seafoodwatch/content/media/MBA_SeafoodWatch_NationalGuide.pdf; wholefoodsmarket.com/blog/what%E2%80%99s-so-great-about-our-tilapia-we%E2%80%99ll-tell-you.

15   Benjamin RM. Dietary guidelines for Americans, 2010: the cornerstone of nutrition policy. *Public Health Reports* 2011;126:310–11.

16   Walker KZ, O'Dea K. Is a low fat diet the optimal way to cut energy intake over the long term in overweight people? *Nutrition, Metabolism, and Cardiovascular Diseases* 2001;11:244–48.

17   Lasa A, Miranda J, Bullo M, et al. Comparative effect of two Mediterranean diets versus a low-fat diet on glycaemic control in individuals with type 2 diabetes. *European Journal of Clinical Nutrition* 2014;68:767–72.

18   Frank S, Linder K, Fritsche L, et al. Olive oil aroma extract modulates cerebral blood flow in gustatory brain areas in humans. *American Journal of Clinical Nutrition* 2013;98:1360–66.

19   Alfenas RC, Mattes RD. Effect of fat sources on satiety. *Obesity Research* 2003;11:183–87.

20   Kozimor A, Chang H, Cooper JA. Effects of dietary fatty acid composition from a high fat meal on satiety. *Appetite* 2013;69:39–45.

21   Virruso C, Accardi G, Colonna Romano G, Candore G, Vasto S, Caruso C. Nutraceutical properties of extra virgin olive oil: a natural remedy for age-related disease? *Rejuvenation Research* 2013;17:217–20.

22   Martin-Pelaez S, Covas MI, Fito M, Kusar A, Pravst I. Health effects of olive oil polyphenols: recent advances and possibilities for the use of health claims. *Molecular Nutrition & Food Research* 2013;57:760–71.

23   Reaven P, Parthasarathy S, Grasse BJ, et al. Feasibility of using an oleate-rich diet to reduce the susceptibility of low-density lipoprotein to oxidative modification in humans. *American Journal of Clinical Nutrition* 1991;54:701–6.

24   Mensink RP, Katan MB. Effect of monounsaturated fatty acids versus complex carbohydrates on high-density lipoproteins in healthy men and women. *Lancet* 1987;1:122–25.

25   Ibid.

26   Ulbricht TL, Southgate DA. Coronary heart disease: seven dietary factors. *Lancet* 1991;338:985–92.

27   Willett WC, Sacks F, Trichopoulou A, et al. Mediterranean diet pyramid: a cultural model for healthy eating. *American Journal of Clinical Nutrition* 1995;61:1402S–1406S.

28   Bertoli S, Spadafranca A, Bes-Rastrollo M, et al. Adherence to the Mediterranean diet is inversely related to binge eating disorder in patients seeking a weight loss program. *Clinical Nutrition* 2014 Feb 14. [Epub ahead of print]

29   Ibid.

30   Flynn MM, Reinert SE. Comparing an olive oil-enriched diet to a standard lower-fat diet for weight loss in breast cancer survivors: a pilot study. *Journal of Women's Health* 2010;19:1155–61.

31   Puel C, Quintin A, Agalias A, et al. Olive oil and its main phenolic micronutrient (oleuropein) prevent inflammation-induced bone loss in the ovariectomised rat. *British Journal of Nutrition* 2004;92:119–27.

32   Condezo-Hoyos L, Mohanty IP, Noratto GD. Assessing non-digestible compounds in apple cultivars and their potential as modulators of obese faecal microbiota in vitro. *Food Chemistry* 2014;161;208–15.

33   Sesso HD, Gaziano JM, Liu S, Buring JE. Flavonoid intake and the risk of cardiovascular disease in women. *American Journal of Clinical Nutrition* 2003;77:1400–1408.

34   Knekt P, Jarvinen R, Reunanen A, Maatela J. Flavonoid intake and coronary mortality in Finland: a cohort study. *BMJ* 1996;312:478–81.

35   Knekt P, Isotupa S, Rissanen H, et al. Quercetin intake and the incidence of cerebrovascular disease. *European Journal of Clinical Nutrition* 2000;54:415–17.

36 Arts IC, Jacobs DR, Jr., Harnack LJ, Gross M, Folsom AR. Dietary catechins in relation to coronary heart disease death among postmenopausal women. *Epidemiology* 2001;12:668–75.

37 Hertog MG, Feskens EJ, Hollman PC, Katan MB, Kromhout D. Dietary antioxidant flavonoids and risk of coronary heart disease: the Zutphen Elderly Study. *Lancet* 1993;342:1007–11.

38 Aprikian O, Duclos V, Guyot S, et al. Apple pectin and a polyphenol-rich apple concentrate are more effective together than separately on cecal fermentations and plasma lipids in rats. *Journal of Nutrition* 2003;133:1860–65.

39 Feskanich D, Ziegler RG, Michaud DS, et al. Prospective study of fruit and vegetable consumption and risk of lung cancer among men and women. *Journal of the National Cancer Institute* 2000;92:1812–23.

40 Le Marchand L, Murphy SP, Hankin JH, Wilkens LR, Kolonel LN. Intake of flavonoids and lung cancer. *Journal of the National Cancer Institute* 2000;92:154–60.

41 Woods RK, Walters EH, Raven JM, et al. Food and nutrient intakes and asthma risk in young adults. *American Journal of Clinical Nutrition* 2003;78:414–21.

42 Butland BK, Fehily AM, Elwood PC. Diet, lung function, and lung function decline in a cohort of 2512 middle aged men. *Thorax* 2000;55:102–8.

43 Knekt P, Kumpulainen J, Jarvinen R, Rissanen H, Heliovaura M, Reunanen A, Hakulinen T, Aromaa A. Flavenoid intake and risk of chronic diseases. *American Journal of Clinical Nutrition* 2002;76:560–68.

44 Conceicao de Oliveira M, Sichieri R, Sanchez Moura A. Weight loss associated with a daily intake of three apples or three pears among overweight women. *Nutrition* 2003;19:253–56.

45 Cho KD, Han CK, Lee BH. Loss of body weight and fat and improved lipid profiles in obese rats fed apple pomace or apple juice concentrate. *Journal of Medicinal Food* 2013;16:823–30.

46 Ravn-Haren G, Dragsted LO, Buch-Andersen T, et al. Intake of whole apples or clear apple juice has contrasting effects on plasma lipids in healthy volunteers. *European Journal of Nutrition* 2013;52:1875–89.

47 Licht TR, Hansen M, Bergstrom A, et al. Effects of apples and specific apple components on the cecal environment of conventional rats: role of apple pectin. *BMC Microbiology* 2010;10:13.

48 Crozier SJ, Preston AG, Hurst JW, et al. Cacao seeds are a "super fruit": a comparative analysis of various fruit powders and products. *Chemistry Central Journal* 2011;5:5.

49 Franco OH, Bonneux L, de Laet C, Peeters A, Steyerberg EW, Mackenbach JP. The Polymeal: a more natural, safer, and probably tastier (than the Polypill) strategy to reduce cardiovascular disease by more than 75%. *BMJ* 2004;329:1447–50.

50 Zeng H, Locatelli M, Bardelli C, et al. Anti-inflammatory properties of clovamide and Theobroma cacao phenolic extracts in human monocytes: evaluation of respiratory burst, cytokine release, NF-kappaB activation, and PPARgamma modulation. *Journal of Agricultural and Food Chemistry* 2011;59:5342–50.

51 Wan Y, Vinson JA, Etherton TD, Proch J, Lazarus SA, Kris-Etherton PM. Effects of cocoa powder and dark chocolate on LDL oxidative susceptibility and prostaglandin concentrations in humans. *American Journal of Clinical Nutrition* 2001;74:596–602.

52 Faridi Z, Njike VY, Dutta S, Ali A, Katz DL. Acute dark chocolate and cocoa ingestion and endothelial function: a randomized controlled crossover trial. *American Journal of Clinical Nutrition* 2008;88:58–63.

53 Grassi D, Necozione S, Lippi C, et al. Cocoa reduces blood pressure and insulin resistance and improves endothelium-dependent vasodilation in hypertensives. *Hypertension* 2005;46:398–405.

54 Ibid.

55 Jacques PF, Cassidy A, Rogers G, Peterson JJ, Meigs JB, Dwyer JT. Higher dietary flavonol intake is associated with lower incidence of type 2 diabetes. *Journal of Nutrition* 2013;143:1474–80.

56 Wedick NM, Pan A, Cassidy A, et al. Dietary flavonoid intakes and risk of type 2 diabetes in US men and women. *American Journal of Clinical Nutrition* 2012;95:925–33.

57 Tzounis X, Rodriguez-Mateos A, Vulevic J, Gibson GR, Kwik-Uribe C, Spencer JP. Prebiotic evaluation of cocoa-derived flavanols in healthy humans by using a randomized, controlled, double-blind, crossover intervention study. *American Journal of Clinical Nutrition* 2011;93:62–72.

58 latimes.com/science/sciencenow/la-sci-sn-secret-to-dark-chocolates-health-benefits-20140318-story.html.

59 Cuenca-Garcia M, Ruiz JR, Ortega FB, Castillo MJ, group Hs. Association between chocolate consumption and fatness in European adolescents. *Nutrition* 2014;30:236–69.

60 Dorenkott MR, Griffin LE, Goodrich KM, et al. Oligomeric cocoa procyanidins possess enhanced bioactivity compared to monomeric and polymeric cocoa procyanidins for preventing the development of obesity, insulin resistance, and impaired glucose tolerance during high-fat feeding. *Journal of Agricultural and Food Chemistry* 2014;62:2216–27.

61   Asai A, Terasaki M, Nagao A. An epoxide-furanoid rearrangement of spinach neoxanthin occurs in the gastrointestinal tract of mice and in vitro: formation and cytostatic activity of neochrome stereoisomers. *Journal of Nutrition* 2004;134:2237–43.

62   Ibid.

63   Gates MA, Tworoger SS, Hecht JL, De Vivo I, Rosner B, Hankinson SE. A prospective study of dietary flavonoid intake and incidence of epithelial ovarian cancer. *International Journal of Cancer Journal* 2007;121:2225–32.

64   Edenharder R, Keller G, Platt KL, Unger KK. Isolation and characterization of structurally novel antimutagenic flavonoids from spinach (Spinacia oleracea). *Journal of Agricultural and Food Chemistry* 2001;49:2767–73.

65   Kirsh VA, Peters U, Mayne ST, et al. Prospective study of fruit and vegetable intake and risk of prostate cancer. *Journal of the National Cancer Institute* 2007;99:1200–1209.

66   Yang Y, Marczak ED, Yokoo M, Usui H, Yoshikawa M. Isolation and antihypertensive effect of angiotensin I-converting enzyme (ACE) inhibitory peptides from spinach Rubisco. *Journal of Agricultural and Food Chemistry* 2003;51:4897–902.

67   Lucarini M, Lanzi S, D'Evoli L, Aguzzi A, Lombardi-Boccia G. Intake of vitamin A and carotenoids from the Italian population–results of an Italian total diet study. *International Journal for Vitamin and Nutrition Research* 2006;76:103–9.

68   Ozsoy-Sacan O, Karabulut-Bulan O, Bolkent S, Yanardag R, Ozgey Y. Effects of chard (Beta vulgaris L. var cicla) on the liver of the diabetic rats: a morphological and biochemical study. *Bioscience, Biotechnology, and Biochemistry* 2004;68:1640–48.

69   Wu QJ, Yang Y, Wang J, Han LH, Xiang YB. Cruciferous vegetable consumption and gastric cancer risk: a meta-analysis of epidemiological studies. *Cancer Science* 2013;104:1067–73.

70   Liu X, Lv K. Cruciferous vegetables intake is inversely associated with risk of breast cancer: a meta-analysis. *Breast* 2013;22:309–13.

71   Wang LI, Giovannucci EL, Hunter D, Neuberg D, Su L, Christiani DC. Dietary intake of Cruciferous vegetables, Glutathione S-transferase (GST) polymorphisms and lung cancer risk in a Caucasian population. *Cancer Causes & Control* 2004;15:977–85.

72   Higdon JV, Delage B, Williams DE, Dashwood RH. Cruciferous vegetables and human cancer risk: epidemiologic evidence and mechanistic basis. *Pharmacological Research* 2007;55:224–36.

73   Tang L, Zirpoli GR, Guru K, et al. Consumption of raw cruciferous vegetables is inversely associated with bladder cancer risk. *Cancer Epidemiology, Biomarkers & Prevention* 2008;17:938–44.

74   Higdon JV, Delage B, Williams DE, Dashwood RH. Cruciferous vegetables and human cancer risk: epidemiologic evidence and mechanistic basis. *Pharmacological Research* 2007;55:224–36.

75   Kim MK, Park JH. Conference on "Multidisciplinary approaches to nutritional problems." Symposium on "Nutrition and health." Cruciferous vegetable intake and the risk of human cancer: epidemiological evidence. *Proceedings of the Nutrition Society* 2009;68:103–10.

76   Higdon JV, Delage B, Williams DE, Dashwood RH. Cruciferous vegetables and human cancer risk: epidemiologic evidence and mechanistic basis. *Pharmacological Research* 2007;55:224–36.

77   Clarke JD, Dashwood RH, Ho E. Multi-targeted prevention of cancer by sulforaphane. *Cancer Letters* 2008;269:291–304.

78   Kahlon TS, Chiu MC, Chapman MH. Steam cooking significantly improves in vitro bile acid binding of collard greens, kale, mustard greens, broccoli, green bell pepper, and cabbage. *Nutrition Research* 2008;28:351–57.

79   Angeloni C, Leoncini E, Malaguti M, Angelini S, Hrelia P, Hrelia S. Modulation of phase II enzymes by sulforaphane: implications for its cardioprotective potential. *Journal of Agricultural and Food Chemistry* 2009;57:5615–22.

80   Cornelis MC, El-Sohemy A, Campos H. GSTT1 genotype modifies the association between cruciferous vegetable intake and the risk of myocardial infarction. *American Journal of Clinical Nutrition* 2007;86:752–58.

81   Liu S, Serdula M, Janket SJ, et al. A prospective study of fruit and vegetable intake and the risk of type 2 diabetes in women. *Diabetes Care* 2004;27:2993–96.

82   Mulabagal V, Ngouajio M, Nair A, Zhang Y, Gottumukkala AL, Nair MG. In vitro evaluation of red and green lettuce (Lactuca sativa) for functional food properties. *Food Chemistry* 2010;118:300–306.

83   Becker C, Klaering HP, Schreiner M, Kroh LW, Krumbein A. Unlike quercetin glycosides, cyanidin glycoside in red leaf lettuce responds more sensitively to increasing low radiation intensity before than after head formation has started. *Journal of Agricultural and Food Chemistry* 2014;62:6911–17.

84 Mulabagal V, Ngouajio M, Nair A, Zhang Y, Gottumukkala AL, Nair MG. In vitro evaluation of red and green lettuce (Lactuca sativa) for functional food properties. *Food Chemistry* 2010;118:300–306.

85 Azadbakht L, Haghighatdoost F, Karimi G, Esmaillzadeh A. Effect of consuming salad and yogurt as preload on body weight management and cardiovascular risk factors: a randomized clinical trial. *International Journal of Food Sciences and Nutrition* 2013;64:392–99.

86 Rolls BJ. Dietary strategies for weight management. *Nestlé Nutrition Institute Workshop Series* 2012;73:37–48.

87 Flood JE, Rolls BJ. Soup preloads in a variety of forms reduce meal energy intake. *Appetite* 2007;49:626–34.

88 Ma J, Stevens JE, Cukier K, et al. Effects of a protein preload on gastric emptying, glycemia, and gut hormones after a carbohydrate meal in diet-controlled type 2 diabetes. *Diabetes Care* 2009;32:1600–1602.

89 Marciani L, Hall N, Pritchard SE, et al. Preventing gastric sieving by blending a solid/water meal enhances satiation in healthy humans. *Journal of Nutrition* 2012;142:1253–58.

90 Rolls BJ, Roe LS, Beach AM, Kris-Etherton PM. Provision of foods differing in energy density affects long-term weight loss. *Obesity Research* 2005;13:1052–60.

91 Zhu Y, Hollis JH. Soup consumption is associated with a lower dietary energy density and a better diet quality in US adults. *British Journal of Nutrition* 2014;111:1474–80.

92 Rolls BJ, Roe LS, Beach AM, Kris-Etherton PM. Provision of foods differing in energy density affects long-term weight loss. *Obesity Research* 2005;13:1052–60.

93 Zhu Y, Hollis JH. Soup consumption is associated with a reduced risk of overweight and obesity but not metabolic syndrome in US adults: NHANES 2003-2006. *PLoS One* 2013;8:e75630.

94 ——. Soup consumption is associated with a lower dietary energy density and a better diet quality in US adults. *British Journal of Nutrition* 2014;111:1474–80.

95 Kuroda M, Ohta M, Okufuji T, et al. Frequency of soup intake is inversely associated with body mass index, waist circumference, and waist-to-hip ratio, but not with other metabolic risk factors in Japanese men. *Journal of the American Dietetic Association* 2011;111:137–42.

96 ——. Frequency of soup intake and amount of dietary fiber intake are inversely associated with plasma leptin concentrations in Japanese adults. *Appetite* 2010;54:538–43.

97 Perez-Jimenez J, Neveu V, Vos F, Scalbert A. Identification of the 100 richest dietary sources of polyphenols: an application of the Phenol-Explorer database. *European Journal of Clinical Nutrition* 2010;64(Suppl 3):S112–S20.

98 Woting A, Clavel T, Loh G, Blaut M. Bacterial transformation of dietary lignans in gnotobiotic rats. *FEMS Microbiology Ecology* 2010;72:507–14.

99 Ibrugger S, Kristensen M, Mikkelsen MS, Astrup A. Flaxseed dietary fiber supplements for suppression of appetite and food intake. *Appetite* 2012;58:490–95.

100 Khan MI, Anjum FM, Sohaib M, Sameen A. Tackling metabolic syndrome by functional foods. *Reviews in Endocrine & Metabolic Disorders* 2013;14:287–97.

101 Adlercreutz H. Lignans and human health. *Critical Reviews in Clinical Laboratory Sciences* 2007;44:483–525.

102 Sturgeon SR, Heersink JL, Volpe SL, et al. Effect of dietary flaxseed on serum levels of estrogens and androgens in postmenopausal women. *Nutrition and Cancer* 2008;60:612–18.

103 Rhee Y, Brunt A. Flaxseed supplementation improved insulin resistance in obese glucose intolerant people: a randomized crossover design. *Nutrition Journal* 2011;10:44.

104 Dodin S, Lemay A, Jacques H, Legare F, Forest JC, Masse B. The effects of flaxseed dietary supplement on lipid profile, bone mineral density, and symptoms in menopausal women: a randomized, double-blind, wheat germ placebo-controlled clinical trial. *Journal of Clinical Endocrinology and Metabolism* 2005;90:1390–97.

105 Kristensen M, Jensen MG, Aarestrup J, et al. Flaxseed dietary fibers lower cholesterol and increase fecal fat excretion, but magnitude of effect depend on food type. *Nutrition & Metabolism* 2012;9:8.

106 Fukumitsu S, Aida K, Shimizu H, Toyoda K. Flaxseed lignan lowers blood cholesterol and decreases liver disease risk factors in moderately hypercholesterolemic men. *Nutrition Research* 2010;30:441–46.

107 Baranowski M, Enns J, Blewett H, Yakandawala U, Zahradka P, Taylor CG. Dietary flaxseed oil reduces adipocyte size, adipose monocyte chemoattractant protein-1 levels and T-cell infiltration in obese, insulin-resistant rats. *Cytokine* 2012;59:382–91.

108 Fukumitsu S, Aida K, Ueno N, Ozawa S, Takahashi Y, Kobori M. Flaxseed lignan attenuates high-fat diet-induced fat accumulation and induces adiponectin expression in mice. *British Journal of Nutrition* 2008;100:669–76.

109 Cintra DE, Ropelle ER, Moraes JC, et al. Unsaturated fatty acids revert diet-induced hypothalamic inflammation in obesity. *PLoS One* 2012;7:e30571.

110 Morisset AS, Lemieux S, Veilleux A, Bergeron J, John Weisnagel S, Tchernof A. Impact of a lignan-rich diet on adiposity and insulin sensitivity in post-menopausal women. *British Journal of Nutrition* 2009;102:195–200.

111 Bao Y, Han J, Hu FB, et al. Association of nut consumption with total and cause-specific mortality. *New England Journal of Medicine* 2013;369:2001–11.

112 Bao Y, Rosner BA, Fuchs CS. Nut consumption and mortality. *New England Journal of Medicine* 2014;370:882.

113 Fraser GE, Sabate J, Beeson WL, Strahan TM. A possible protective effect of nut consumption on risk of coronary heart disease. The Adventist Health Study. *Archives of Internal Medicine* 1992;152:1416–24.

114 Sabate J, Fraser GE, Burke K, Knutsen SF, Bennett H, Lindsted KD. Effects of walnuts on serum lipid levels and blood pressure in normal men. *New England Journal of Medicine* 1993;328:603–7.

115 Kelly JH, Jr., Sabate J. Nuts and coronary heart disease: an epidemiological perspective. *British Journal of Nutrition* 2006;96(Suppl 2):S61–S67.

116 Albert CM, Gaziano JM, Willett WC, Manson JE. Nut consumption and decreased risk of sudden cardiac death in the Physicians' Health Study. *Archives of Internal Medicine* 2002;162:1382–87.

117 Sabate J, Oda K, Ros E. Nut consumption and blood lipid levels: a pooled analysis of 25 intervention trials. *Archives of Internal Medicine* 2010;170:821–27.

118 Banel DK, Hu FB. Effects of walnut consumption on blood lipids and other cardiovascular risk factors: a meta-analysis and systematic review. *American Journal of Clinical Nutrition* 2009;90:56–63.

119 Jiang R, Jacobs DR, Jr., Mayer-Davis E, et al. Nut and seed consumption and inflammatory markers in the multi-ethnic study of atherosclerosis. *American Journal of Epidemiology* 2006;163:222–31.

120 Mantzoros CS, Williams CJ, Manson JE, Meigs JB, Hu FB. Adherence to the Mediterranean dietary pattern is positively associated with plasma adiponectin concentrations in diabetic women. *American Journal of Clinical Nutrition* 2006;84:328–35.

121 Salas-Salvado J, Garcia-Arellano A, Estruch R, et al. Components of the Mediterranean-type food pattern and serum inflammatory markers among patients at high risk for cardiovascular disease. *European Journal of Clinical Nutrition* 2008;62:651–59.

122 Lopez-Uriarte P, Bullo M, Casas-Agustench P, Babio N, Salas-Salvado J. Nuts and oxidation: a systematic review. *Nutrition Reviews* 2009;67:497–508.

123 Jaceldo-Siegl K, Haddad E, Oda K, Fraser GE, Sabate J. Tree nuts are inversely associated with metabolic syndrome and obesity: the Adventist health study-2. *PLoS One* 2014;9:e85133.

124 Rebello CJ, Liu AG, Greenway FL, Dhurandhar NV. Dietary strategies to increase satiety. *Advances in Food and Nutrition Research* 2013;69:105–82.

125 Tan SY, Mattes RD. Appetitive, dietary and health effects of almonds consumed with meals or as snacks: a randomized, controlled trial. *European Journal of Clinical Nutrition* 2013;67:1205–14.

126 Cassady BA, Hollis JH, Fulford AD, Considine RV, Mattes RD. Mastication of almond: effects of lipid bioaccessibility, appetite, and hormone response. *American Journal of Clinical Nutrition* 2009;89:794–800.

127 Pasman WJ, Heimerikx J, Rubingh CM, et al. The effect of Korean pine nut oil on in vitro CCK release, on appetite sensations and on gut hormones in post-menopausal overweight women. *Lipids in Health and Disease* 2008;7:10.

128 Mattes RD. The energetics of nut consumption. *Asia Pacific Journal of Clinical Nutrition* 2008;17(Suppl 1): 337–79.

129 Mattes RD, Dreher ML. Nuts and healthy body weight maintenance mechanisms. *Asia Pacific Journal of Clinical Nutrition* 2010;19:137–41.

130 Mattes RD, Kris-Etherton PM, Foster GD. Impact of peanuts and tree nuts on body weight and healthy weight loss in adults. *Journal of Nutrition* 2008;138:1741S–45S.

131 Casas-Agustench P, Lopez-Uriarte P, Bullo M, Ros E, Cabre-Vila JJ, Salas-Salvado J. Effects of one serving of mixed nuts on serum lipids, insulin resistance and inflammatory markers in patients with the metabolic syndrome. *Nutrition, Metabolism, and Cardiovascular Diseases* 2011;21:126–35.

132 Mozaffarian D, Hao T, Rimm EB, Willett WC, Hu FB. Changes in diet and lifestyle and long-term weight gain in women and men. *New England Journal of Medicine* 2011;364:2392–404.

133 Bes-Rastrollo M, Sabate J, Gomez-Gracia E, Alonso A, Martinez JA, Martinez-Gonzalez MA. Nut consumption and weight gain in a Mediterranean cohort: the SUN study. *Obesity* 2007;15:107–16.

134 Bes-Rastrollo M, Wedick NM, Martinez-Gonzalez MA, Li TY, Sampson L, Hu FB. Prospective study of nut consumption, long-term weight change, and obesity risk in women. *American Journal of Clinical Nutrition* 2009;89:1913–19.

135 Mozaffarian D, Hao T, Rimm EB, Willett WC, Hu FB. Changes in diet and lifestyle and long-term weight gain in women and men. *New England Journal of Medicine* 2011;364:2392–404.

136 Dreher ML. Pistachio nuts: composition and potential health benefits. *Nutrition Reviews* 2012;70:234–40.

137 Ibid.

138 Kennedy-Hagan K, Painter JE, Honselman C, Halvorson A, Rhodes K, Skwir K. The effect of pistachio shells as a visual cue in reducing caloric consumption. *Appetite* 2011;57:418–20.

139 Honselman CS, Painter JE, Kennedy-Hagan KJ, et al. In-shell pistachio nuts reduce caloric intake compared to shelled nuts. *Appetite* 2011;57:414–17.

140 Li Z, Song R, Nguyen C, et al. Pistachio nuts reduce triglycerides and body weight by comparison to refined carbohydrate snack in obese subjects on a 12-week weight loss program. *Journal of the American College of Nutrition* 2010;29:198–203.

141 Tan SY, Dhillon J, Mattes RD. A review of the effects of nuts on appetite, food intake, metabolism, and body weight. *American Journal of Clinical Nutrition* 2014;100:412S–22S.

142 berkeleywellness.com/healthy-eating/food/article/decaf-healthy-choice.

143 health.harvard.edu/fhg/updates/update0406c.shtml.

144 Steffen M, Kuhle C, Hensrud D, Erwin PJ, Murad MH. The effect of coffee consumption on blood pressure and the development of hypertension: a systematic review and meta-analysis. *Journal of Hypertension* 2012;30:2245–54.

145 Freedman ND, Park Y, Abnet CC, Hollenbeck AR, Sinha R. Association of coffee drinking with total and cause-specific mortality. *New England Journal of Medicine* 2012;366:1891–904.

146 Keijzers GB, De Galan BE, Tack CJ, Smits P. Caffeine can decrease insulin sensitivity in humans. *Diabetes Care* 2002;25:364–69.

147 Johnston KL, Clifford MN, Morgan LM. Coffee acutely modifies gastrointestinal hormone secretion and glucose tolerance in humans: glycemic effects of chlorogenic acid and caffeine. *American Journal of Clinical Nutrition* 2003;78:728–33.

148 Greenberg JA, Boozer CN, Geliebter A. Coffee, diabetes, and weight control. *American Journal of Clinical Nutrition* 2006;84:682–93.

149 Rodriguez-Moran M, Guerrero-Romero F. Oral magnesium supplementation improves the metabolic profile of metabolically obese, normal-weight individuals: a randomized double-blind placebo-controlled trial. *Archives of Medical Research* 2014;45:388–93.

150 Rodriguez-Moran M, Guerrero-Romero F. Oral magnesium supplementation improves insulin sensitivity and metabolic control in type 2 diabetic subjects: a randomized double-blind controlled trial. *Diabetes Care* 2003;26:1147–52.

151 Kovacs EM, Lejeune MP, Nijs I, Westerterp-Plantenga MS. Effects of green tea on weight maintenance after body-weight loss. *British Journal of Nutrition* 2004;91:431–37.

152 Lopez-Garcia E, van Dam RM, Rajpathak S, Willett WC, Manson JE, Hu FB. Changes in caffeine intake and long-term weight change in men and women. *American Journal of Clinical Nutrition* 2006;83:674–80.

153 St-Onge MP, Salinardi T, Herron-Rubin K, Black RM. A weight-loss diet including coffee-derived mannooligosaccharides enhances adipose tissue loss in overweight men but not women. *Obesity* 2012;20:343–48.

154 Lucas M, Mirzaei F, Pan A, et al. Coffee, caffeine, and risk of depression among women. *Archives of Internal Medicine* 2011;171:1571–78.

155 Kokubo Y, Iso H, Saito I, et al. The impact of green tea and coffee consumption on the reduced risk of stroke incidence in Japanese population: the Japan public health center-based study cohort. *Stroke* 2013;44:1369–74.

156 Sinha R, Cross AJ, Daniel CR, et al. Caffeinated and decaffeinated coffee and tea intakes and risk of colorectal cancer in a large prospective study. *American Journal of Clinical Nutrition* 2012;96:374–81.

157 de la Figuera von Wichmann M. [Coffee consumption and hepatobilliary system]. *Medicina clinica* 2008;131:594–97.

158 Derkinderen P, Shannon KM, Brundin P. Gut feelings about smoking and coffee in Parkinson's disease. *Movement Disorders* 2014;29:976–79.

159 Freedman ND, Everhart JE, Lindsay KL, et al. Coffee intake is associated with lower rates of liver disease progression in chronic hepatitis C. *Hepatology* 2009;50:1360–69.

160 Molloy JW, Calcagno CJ, Williams CD, Jones FJ, Torres DM, Harrison SA. Association of coffee and caffeine consumption with fatty liver disease, nonalcoholic steatohepatitis, and degree of hepatic fibrosis. *Hepatology* 2012;55:429–36.

161 Saab S, Mallam D, Cox GA, 2nd, Tong MJ. Impact of coffee on liver diseases: a systematic review. *Liver International* 2014;34:495–504.

162 Ambrosone CB, Tang L. Cruciferous vegetable intake and cancer prevention: role of nutrigenetics. *Cancer Prevention Research* 2009;2:298–300.

163 Kirsh VA, Peters U, Mayne ST et al. Prospective study of fruit and vegetable intake and risk of prostate cancer. *Journal of the National Cancer Institute* 2007;99:1200–1209.

164 Traka M, Gasper AV, Melchini A, et al. Broccoli consumption interacts with GSTM1 to perturb oncogenic signalling pathways in the prostate. *PLoS One* 2008;3:e2568.

165 Steinbrecher A, Linseisen J. Dietary intake of individual glucosinolates in participants of the EPIC-Heidelberg cohort study. *Annals of Nutrition & Metabolism* 2009;54:87–96.

166 Bahadoran Z, Mirmiran P, Azizi F. Potential efficacy of broccoli sprouts as a unique supplement for management of type 2 diabetes and its complications. *Journal of Medicinal Food* 2013;16:375–82.

167 Choi Y, Um SJ, Park T. Indole-3-carbinol directly targets SIRT1 to inhibit adipocyte differentiation. *International Journal of Obesity* 2013;37:881–84.

168 Bahadoran Z, Mirmiran P, Hosseinpanah F, Hedayati M, Hosseinpour-Niazi S, Azizi F. Broccoli sprouts reduce oxidative stress in type 2 diabetes: a randomized double-blind clinical trial. *European Journal of Clinical Nutrition* 2011;65:972–77.

169 Bahadoran Z, Tohidi M, Nazeri P, Mehran M, Azizi F, Mirmiran P. Effect of broccoli sprouts on insulin resistance in type 2 diabetic patients: a randomized double-blind clinical trial. *International Journal of Food Sciences and Nutrition* 2012;63:767–71.

170 pages.jh.edu/~jhumag/0408web/talalay.html.

171 Lopez-Molina D, Navarro-Martinez MD, Rojas Melgarejo F, Hiner AN, Chazarra S, Rodriguez-Lopez JN. Molecular properties and prebiotic effect of inulin obtained from artichoke (Cynara scolymus L.). *Phytochemistry* 2005;66:1476–84.

172 Costabile A, Kolida S, Klinder A, et al. A double-blind, placebo-controlled, cross-over study to establish the bifidogenic effect of a very-long-chain inulin extracted from globe artichoke (Cynara scolymus) in healthy human subjects. *British Journal of Nutrition* 2010;104:1007–17.

173 Ibid.

174 Rondanelli M, Giacosa A, Opizzi A, et al. Beneficial effects of artichoke leaf extract supplementation on increasing HDL-cholesterol in subjects with primary mild hypercholesterolaemia: a double-blind, randomized, placebo-controlled trial. *International Journal of Food Sciences and Nutrition* 2013;64:7–15.

175 Barrat E, Zair Y, Ogier N, et al. A combined natural supplement lowers LDL cholesterol in subjects with moderate untreated hypercholesterolemia: a randomized placebo-controlled trial. *International Journal of Food Sciences and Nutrition* 2013;64:882–89.

176 Rondanelli M, Opizzi A, Faliva M, et al. Metabolic management in overweight subjects with naive impaired fasting glycaemia by means of a highly standardized extract from Cynara scolymus: a double-blind, placebo-controlled, randomized clinical trial. *Phytotherapy Research* 2014;28:33–41.

177 Kovacs EM, Lejeune MP, Nijs I, Westerterp-Plantenga MS. Effects of green tea on weight maintenance after body-weight loss. *British Journal of Nutrition* 2004;91:431–37.

Chapter 10

1 cbsnews.com/news/cdc-80-percent-of-american-adults-dont-get-recommended-exercise/.

2 americashealthrankings.org/all/sedentary.

3 sciencedaily.com/releases/2009/08/090810024825.htm.

4 Mons U, Hahmann H, Brenner H. A reverse J-shaped association of leisure time physical activity with prognosis in patients with stable coronary heart disease: evidence from a large cohort with repeated measurements. *Heart* 2014;100:1043–49.

5 apa.org/news/press/releases/stress/2011/final-2011.pdf.

6 Kessler RC, Chiu WT, Demler O, Merikangas KR, Walters EE. Prevalence, severity, and comorbidity of 12-month DSM-IV disorders in the National Comorbidity Survey Replication. *Archives of General Psychiatry* 2005;62:617–27.

7 Kessler RC, Demler O, Frank RG, et al. Prevalence and treatment of mental disorders, 1990 to 2003. *New England Journal of Medicine* 2005;352:2515–23.

8 apa.org/news/press/releases/stress/2012/generations.aspx.

9 apa.org/news/press/releases/stress/2011/final-2011.pdf.

10 Morton NM, Seckl JR. 11beta-hydroxysteroid dehydrogenase type 1 and obesity. *Frontiers of Hormone Research* 2008;36:146–64.

11 Black PH. The inflammatory consequences of psychologic stress: relationship to insulin resistance, obesity, atherosclerosis and diabetes mellitus, type II. *Medical Hypotheses* 2006;67:879–91.

12 Peeke PM, Chrousos GP. Hypercortisolism and obesity. *Annals of the New York Academy of Sciences* 1995;771:665–76.

13 Huang CJ, Webb HE, Zourdos MC, Acevedo EO. Cardiovascular reactivity, stress, and physical activity. *Frontiers in Physiology* 2013;4:314.

14 Redmond N, Richman J, Gamboa CM, et al. Perceived stress is associated with incident coronary heart disease and all-cause mortality in low- but not high-income participants in the Reasons for Geographic and Racial Differences in Stroke study. *Journal of the American Heart Association* 2013;2:e000447.

15 Bacon SL, Campbell TS, Arsenault A, Lavoie KL. The impact of mood and anxiety disorders on incident hypertension at one year. *International Journal of Hypertension* 2014;2014:953094.

16 Whitworth JA, Williamson PM, Mangos G, Kelly JJ. Cardiovascular consequences of cortisol excess. *Vascular Health and Risk Management* 2005;1:291–99.

17 Ventura T, Santander J, Torres R, Contreras AM. Neurobiologic basis of craving for carbohydrates. *Nutrition* 2014;30:252–56.

18 Bailey MT, Dowd SE, Galley JD, Hufnagle AR, Allen RG, Lyte M. Exposure to a social stressor alters the structure of the intestinal microbiota: implications for stressor-induced immunomodulation. *Brain, Behavior, and Immunity* 2011;25:397–407.

19 Cryan JF, Dinan TG. Mind-altering microorganisms: the impact of the gut microbiota on brain and behaviour. *Nature Reviews Neuroscience* 2012;13:701–12.

20 Sapolsky RM. *Why Zebras Don't Get Ulcers*, 3rd ed. New York: Holt Paperbacks; 2004.

21 news.ca.uky.edu/article/uk-researcher-finds-stress-management-may-contribute-weight-loss.

22 Mathieu J. What should you know about mindful and intuitive eating? *Journal of the American Dietetic Association* 2009;109:1982–87.

23 Schaefer JT, Magnuson AB. A review of interventions that promote eating by internal cues. *Journal of the Academy of Nutrition and Dietetics* 2014;114:734–60.

24 Kidd LI, Graor CH, Murrock CJ. A mindful eating group intervention for obese women: a mixed methods feasibility study. *Archives of Psychiatric Nursing* 2013;27:211–18.

25 Godsey J. The role of mindfulness based interventions in the treatment of obesity and eating disorders: an integrative review. *Complementary Therapies in Medicine* 2013;21:430–39.

26 May M. *Eat What You Love, Love What You Eat: How to Break Your Eat-Repent-Repeat Cycle: Am I Hungry?* Austin, TX: Greenleaf, 2011.

27 Breslau N. The epidemiology of trauma, PTSD, and other posttrauma disorders. *Trauma, Violence & Abuse* 2009;10:198–210.

28 Lopez-Diazguerrero NE, Gonzalez Puertos VY, Hernandez-Bautista RJ, Alarcon-Aguilar A, Luna-Lopez A, Konigsberg Fainstein M. [Hormesis: What doesn't kill you makes you stronger]. *Gaceta medica de Mexico* 2013;149:438–47.

29 Nunn AV, Guy GW, Brodie JS, Bell JD. Inflammatory modulation of exercise salience: using hormesis to return to a healthy lifestyle. *Nutrition & Metabolism* 2010;7:87.

30 apa.org/helpcenter/road-resilience.aspx#.

31 Southwick SM. *Resilience: The Science of Mastering Life's Greatest Challenges*. New York: Cambridge University Press; 2012.

32 Hughes V. Stress: the roots of resilience. *Nature* 2012;490:165–67.

33 Hingle MD, Wertheim BC, Tindle HA, et al. Optimism and diet quality in the Women's Health Initiative. *Journal of the Academy of Nutrition and Dietetics* 2014;114:1036–45.

34 Sarkar M, Fletcher D. Psychological resilience in sport performers: a review of stressors and protective factors. *Journal of Sports Sciences* 2014;32:1419–34.

35 Martin AS, Distelberg B, Palmer BW, Jeste DV. Development of a new multidimensional individual and interpersonal resilience measure for older adults. *Aging & Mental Health* 2014:1–14.

36 cptryon.org/prayer/special/serenity.html.

37 Gard T, Taquet M, Dixit R, et al. Fluid intelligence and brain functional organization in aging yoga and meditation practitioners. *Frontiers in Aging Neuroscience* 2014;6:76.

38 Childs E, de Wit H. Regular exercise is associated with emotional resilience to acute stress in healthy adults. *Frontiers in Physiology* 2014;5:161.

39 imdb.com/title/tt0479143/.

40 samplage.com/movie-quotes/it-aint-about-how-hard-you-hit/.

41 Dawson MA, Hamson-Utley JJ, Hansen R, Olpin M. Examining the effectiveness of psychological strategies on physiologic markers: evidence-based suggestions for holistic care of the athlete. *Journal of Athletic Training* 2014;49:331–37.

42 Prinsloo GE, Derman WE, Lambert MI, Laurie Rauch HG. The effect of a single session of short duration biofeedback-induced deep breathing on measures of heart rate variability during laboratory-induced cognitive stress: a pilot study. *Applied Psychophysiology and Biofeedback* 2013;38:81–90.

43 Shah M, Copeland J, Dart L, Adams-Huet B, James A, Rhea D. Slower eating speed lowers energy intake in normal-weight but not overweight/obese subjects. *Journal of the Academy of Nutrition and Dietetics* 2014;114:393–402.

44 okinawa-diet.com/okinawa_diet/hara_hachi_bu.html.

45 nhlbi.nih.gov/guidelines/obesity/prctgd_c.pdf.

46 Johnson PM, Kenny PJ. Dopamine D2 receptors in addiction-like reward dysfunction and compulsive eating in obese rats. *Nature Neuroscience* 2010;13:635–41.

47 Mantzios M, Giannou K. Group vs. single mindfulness meditation: exploring avoidance, impulsivity, and weight management in two separate mindfulness meditation settings. *Applied Psychology Health and Well-being* 2014;6:173–91.

48 clinicaltrials.gov/ct2/show/NCT01619384?term=bowel&recr=Open&cntry1=NA%3AUS&rank=69.

49 Goyal M, Singh S, Sibinga EM, et al. Meditation programs for psychological stress and well-being: a systematic review and meta-analysis. *JAMA Internal Medicine* 2014;174:357–68.

50 Daubenmier J, Kristeller J, Hecht FM, et al. Mindfulness intervention for stress eating to reduce cortisol and abdominal fat among overweight and obese women: an exploratory randomized controlled study. *Journal of Obesity* 2011;2011:651936.

51 Kristal AR, Littman AJ, Benitez D, White E. Yoga practice is associated with attenuated weight gain in healthy, middle-aged men and women. *Alternative Therapies in Health and Medicine* 2005;11:28–33.

52 Bernstein A BJ, Ehrman JP, Goulbic M,Roizen MF. Yoga in the management of overweight and obesity. *American Journal of Lifestyle Medicine* 2014;8:33-41.

53 Gurgevich S. *The Self-Hypnosis Diet Book*. Boulder, CO: Sounds True, 2009.

54 sleepandhypnosis.org/pdf/15_1_1.pdf.

55 Yeo S, Kim KS, Lim S. Randomised clinical trial of five ear acupuncture points for the treatment of overweight people. *Acupuncture in Medicine* 2014;32:132–38.

56 Sui Y, Zhao HL, Wong VC, et al. A systematic review on use of Chinese medicine and acupuncture for treatment of obesity. *Obesity Reviews* 2012;13:409–30.

57 Bernstein A BJ, Ehrman JP, Goulbic M, Roizen MF. Yoga in the management of overweight and obesity. *American Journal of Lifestyle Medicine* 2014;8(1):33–41.

58 Rioux J, Thomson C, Howerter A. A pilot feasibility study of whole-systems Ayurvedic medicine and yoga therapy for weight loss. *Global Advances in Health and Medicine* 2014;3(1):28–35.

59 Bernstein A BJ, Ehrman JP, Goulbic M, Roizen MF. Yoga in the management of overweight and obesity. *American Journal of Lifestyle Medicine* 2014;8(1):33–41.

60 Sarvottam K, Yadav TK. Obesity-related inflammation and cardiovascular disease: efficacy of a yoga-based lifestyle intervention. *Indian Journal of Medical Research* 2014;139(6):822–34.

61 Ibid.

62 Sui Y, Zhao HL, Wong VC, et al. A systematic review on use of Chinese medicine and acupuncture for treatment of obesity. *Obesity Reviews* 2012;13:409–30.

63 Cabyoglu MT, Ergene N, Tan U. The treatment of obesity by acupuncture. *The International Journal of Neuroscience* 2006;116:165-75.

64 jstor.org/stable/30038995.

65 Cho JH, Jae SY, Choo IL, Choo J. Health-promoting behaviour among women with abdominal obesity: a conceptual link to social support and perceived stress. *Journal of Advanced Nursing* 2014;70:1381–90.

66 Robertson C, Archibald D, Avenell A, et al. Systematic reviews of and integrated report on the quantitative, qualitative and economic evidence base for the management of obesity in men. *Health Technology Assessment* 2014;18:1–424.

67 Cacioppo JT, Cacioppo S. Social relationships and health: the toxic effects of perceived social isolation. *Social and Personality Psychology Compass* 2014;8:58–72.

68 Konturek PC, Brzozowski T, Konturek SJ. Gut clock: implication of circadian rhythms in the gastrointestinal tract. *Journal of Physiology and Pharmacology* 2011;62:139–50.

69 Fu XY, Li Z, Zhang N, Yu HT, Wang SR, Liu JR. Effects of gastrointestinal motility on obesity. *Nutrition & Metabolism* 2014;11:3.

70 sleepfoundation.org.

71 Schmid SM, Hallschmid M, Schultes B. The metabolic burden of sleep loss. *Lancet Diabetes & Endocrinology* 2014 Mar 25. [Epub ahead of print]

72 Schmid SM, Hallschmid M, Jauch-Chara K, Born J, Schultes B. A single night of sleep deprivation increases ghrelin levels and feelings of hunger in normal-weight healthy men. *Journal of Sleep Research* 2008;17:331–34.

73 Copinschi G. Metabolic and endocrine effects of sleep deprivation. *Essential Psychopharmacology* 2005;6:341–47.

74 Depner CM, Stothard ER, Wright KP, Jr. Metabolic consequences of sleep and circadian disorders. *Current Diabetes Reports* 2014;14:507.

75 Ferrie JE, Shipley MJ, Cappuccio FP, et al. A prospective study of change in sleep duration: associations with mortality in the Whitehall II cohort. *Sleep* 2007;30:1659–66.

76 Gilbert-Diamond D, Li Z, Adachi-Mejia AM, McClure AC, Sargent JD. Association of a television in the bedroom with increased adiposity gain in a nationally representative sample of children and adolescents. *JAMA Pediatrics* 2014;168:427–34.

77 Taveras EM, Gillman MW, Pena MM, Redline S, Rifas-Shiman SL. Chronic sleep curtailment and adiposity. *Pediatrics* 2014;133:1013–22.

78 Fisher A, McDonald L, van Jaarsveld CH, et al. Sleep and energy intake in early childhood. *International Journal of Obesity* 2014;38:926–29.

79 Hart CN, Carskadon MA, Considine RV, et al. Changes in children's sleep duration on food intake, weight, and leptin. *Pediatrics* 2013;132:e1473–80.

80 Nedeltcheva AV, Kilkus JM, Imperial J, Schoeller DA, Penev PD. Insufficient sleep undermines dietary efforts to reduce adiposity. *Annals of Internal Medicine* 2010;153:435–41.

81 Khosro S, Alireza S, Omid A, Forough S. Night work and inflammatory markers. *Indian Journal of Occupational and Environmental Medicine* 2011;15:38–41.

82 Malmberg B, Kecklund G, Karlson B, Persson R, Flisberg P, Orbaek P. Sleep and recovery in physicians on night call: a longitudinal field study. *BMC Health Services Research* 2010;10:239.

83 Ibid.

84 Palma JA, Urrestarazu E, Iriarte J. Sleep loss as risk factor for neurologic disorders: a review. *Sleep Medicine* 2013;14:229–36.

85 Ruggiero JS, Redeker NS. Effects of napping on sleepiness and sleep-related performance deficits in night-shift workers: a systematic review. *Biological Research for Nursing* 2014;16:134–42.

86 Ali T, Choe J, Awab A, Wagener TL, Orr WC. Sleep, immunity and inflammation in gastrointestinal disorders. *World Journal of Gastroenterology* 2013;19:9231–39.

87 Noguti J, Andersen ML, Cirelli C, Ribeiro DA. Oxidative stress, cancer, and sleep deprivation: is there a logical link in this association? *Sleep & Breathing* 2013;17:905–10.

88 Palma JA, Urrestarazu E, Iriarte J. Sleep loss as risk factor for neurologic disorders: a review. *Sleep Medicine* 2013;14:229–36.

89 Ruggiero JS, Redeker NS. Effects of napping on sleepiness and sleep-related performance deficits in night-shift workers: a systematic review. *Biological Research for Nursing* 2014;16:134–42.

90 Ali T, Choe J, Awab A, Wagener TL, Orr WC. Sleep, immunity and inflammation in gastrointestinal disorders. *World Journal of Gastroenterology* 2013;19:9231–39.

91 Noguti J, Andersen ML, Cirelli C, Ribeiro DA. Oxidative stress, cancer, and sleep deprivation: is there a logical link in this association? *Sleep & Breathing* 2013;17:905–10.

92 Palagini L, Bruno RM, Gemignani A, Baglioni C, Ghiadoni L, Riemann D. Sleep loss and hypertension: a systematic review. *Current Pharmaceutical Design* 2013;19:2409–19.

93 Wiebe ST, Cassoff J, Gruber R. Sleep patterns and the risk for unipolar depression: a review. *Nature and Science of Sleep* 2012;4:63–71.

94 Cassoff J, Wiebe ST, Gruber R. Sleep patterns and the risk for ADHD: a review. *Nature and Science of Sleep* 2012;4:73–80.

95 Wolk R, Somers VK. Sleep and the metabolic syndrome. *Experimental Physiology* 2007;92:67–78.

96 Pigeon WR, Carr M, Gorman C, Perlis ML. Effects of a tart cherry juice beverage on the sleep of older adults with insomnia: a pilot study. *Journal of Medicinal Food* 2010;13:579–83.

97 Choi JJ, Eum SY, Rampersaud E, Daunert S, Abreu MT, Toborek M. Exercise attenuates PCB-induced changes in the mouse gut microbiome. *Environmental Health Perspectives* 2013;121:725–30.

98 nytimes.com/health/guides/specialtopic/physical-activity/print.html.

99 van der Ploeg HP, Chey T, Korda RJ, Banks E, Bauman A. Sitting time and all-cause mortality risk in 222 497 Australian adults. *Archives of Internal Medicine* 2012;172:494–500.

100 Jeon CY, Lokken RP, Hu FB, van Dam RM. Physical activity of moderate intensity and risk of type 2 diabetes: a systematic review. *Diabetes Care* 2007;30:744–52.

101 Oguma Y, Shinoda-Tagawa T. Physical activity decreases cardiovascular disease risk in women: review and meta-analysis. *American Journal of Preventive Medicine* 2004;26:407–18.

102 Gregg EW, Gerzoff RB, Caspersen CJ, Williamson DF, Narayan KM. Relationship of walking to mortality among US adults with diabetes. *Archives of Internal Medicine* 2003;163:1440–47.

103 Trapp EG, Chisholm DJ, Freund J, Boutcher SH. The effects of high-intensity intermittent exercise training on fat loss and fasting insulin levels of young women. *International Journal of Obesity* 2008;32:684–91.

104 Teixeira-Lemos E, Nunes S, Teixeira F, Reis F. Regular physical exercise training assists in preventing type 2 diabetes development: focus on its antioxidant and anti-inflammatory properties. *Cardiovascular Diabetology* 2011;10:12.

105 DiPietro L, Dziura J, Yeckel CW, Neufer PD. Exercise and improved insulin sensitivity in older women: evidence of the enduring benefits of higher intensity training. *Journal of Applied Physiology* 2006;100:142–49.

Chapter 11

1 Hamrick K, et al. How much time do Americans spend on food? Economic Information Bulletin No. 86 (EIB-86), November 2011.

2 Cutler D, Glaeser E, Shapiro J. Why have Americans become obese? *Journal of Economic Perspectives* 2003;17:93–118.

INDEX

Bold page references indicate pictures. <u>Underscored</u> page references indicate boxed text and tables.